Catheter Ablation of Atrial Fibrillation

Catheter Ablation of Atrial Fibrillation

EDITED BY

Etienne Aliot
Michel Haïssaguerre
Warren M. Jackman

Blackwell Futura

Blackwell Futura is an imprint of Blackwell Publishing

Blackwell Publishing, Inc., 350 Main Street, Malden, Massachusetts 02148-5020, USA
Blackwell Publishing Ltd, 9600 Garsington Road, Oxford OX4 2DQ, UK
Blackwell Publishing Asia Pty Ltd, 550 Swanston Street, Carlton, Victoria 3053, Australia

First published 2008
1 2008

ISBN: 978-1-4051-6349-1

Library of Congress Cataloging-in-Publication Data

Catheter ablation of atrial fibrillation / edited by Etienne Aliot, Michel Haissguerre, Warren M. Jackman.
p. ; cm.
Includes bibliographical references.
ISBN 978-1-4051-6349-1 (Hbk trade version)
978-1-4051-8665-0 (Customised version, not for trade sale)
1. Catheter ablation. 2. Atrial fibrillation – Surgery. I. Aliot, Etienne. II. Ha?ssaguerre, Michel. III. Jackman, Warren M.
[DNLM: 1. Atrial Fibrillation – surgery. 2. Atrial Fibrillation – therapy. 3. Catheter Ablation – methods. WG 330 C3628 2008]

RD598.35.C39C383 2008
616.1′28–dc22 2007049865

A catalogue record for this title is available from the British Library

Commissioning Editor: Gina Almond
Development Editor: Beckie Brand
Editorial Assistant: Jamie Hartmann-Boyce
Production Controller: Debbie Wyer

Set in 9.5/12 pt Minion by Graphicraft Limited, Hong Kong
Printed and bound in Singapore by Fabulous Printers Pte Ltd

For further information on Blackwell Publishing, visit our website:
www.blackwellcardiology.com

The publisher's policy is to use permanent paper from mills that operate a sustainable forestry policy, and which has been manufactured from pulp processed using acid-free and elementary chlorine-free practices. Furthermore, the publisher ensures that the text paper and cover board used have met acceptable environmental accreditation standards.

Contents

Part 3 Special challenges in atrial fibrillation

Contributors

Joseph Akar, MD, PHD
Center for Heart and Cardiovascular Medicine,
Loyola University Health System,
Maywood, Illinois, USA

Etienne Aliot, MD
Department of Cardiology,
University of Nancy,
Vandoeuvre les Nancy,
France

Maurits Allessie, MD, PhD
Department of Physiology,
Cardiovascular Research Institute Maastricht (CARIM),
Maastricht University, Maastricht,
The Netherlands

Matthias Antz, MD
Oberärztin Magn. Navigation,
Hanseatic Heart Center St. Georg,
Hamburg, Germany

Leonardo Arantès, MD
Hôpital Cardiologique du Haut-Lévêque and the
Université Victor Segalen Bordeaux II,
Bordeaux, France

Dietmar Bänsch, MD
Oberärztin Magn. Navigation,
Hanseatic Heart Center St. Georg,
Hamburg, Germany

Omer Berenfeld, PhD
Department of Pharmacology and the Institute for
Cardiovascular Research,
SUNY Upstate Medical University,
Syracuse, New York, USA

Pierre Bordachar, MD
Hôpital Cardiologique du Haut-Lévêque and the
Université Victor Segalen Bordeaux II,
Bordeaux, France

Neil Brysiewicz, BSE
Center for Heart and Cardiovascular Medicine,
Loyola University Health System,
Maywood, Illinois, USA

José Angel Cabrera, MD, PhD
Arrhythmia Unit, Hospital Quiron-Madrid,
Universidad Europea de Madrid,
Madrid, Spain

Domenico Caponi, MD
Cardinal Massaia Hospital,
Asti, AT Italy

Shih-Ann Chen, MD
Division of Cardiology and Cardiovascular Research
Center, National Yang-Ming University, School of
Medicine and Taipei Veterans General Hospital,
Taiwan

Julian K.R. Chun, MD
Oberärztin Magn. Navigation,
Hanseatic Heart Center St. Georg,
Hamburg, Germany

Jacques Clémenty, MD
Hôpital Cardiologique du Haut-Lévêque and the
Université Victor Segalen Bordeaux II,
Bordeaux, France

Lam Dang, PhD
Swiss Federal Institute of Technology,
Lausanne, Switzerland

D. Wyn Davies, MD, FRCP
St. Mary's Hospital,
Waller Department of Cardiology,
London, UK

Christian de Chillou, MD, PHD
Department of Cardiology,
Nancy University Hospital,
Nancy, France

Natasja de Groot, MD, PHD
Department of Physiology,
Cardiovascular Research Institute Maastricht (CARIM),
Maastricht University, Maastricht,
The Netherlands

Isabel Deisenhofer, MD
Deutsches Herzzentrum München,
Klinik an der Technischen,
Universität München,
München, Germany

Antoine Deplagne, MD
Hôpital Cardiologique du Haut-Lévêque and the Université
Victor Segalen Bordeaux II,
Bordeaux, France

Nicolas Derval, MD
Hôpital Cardiologique du Haut-Lévêque and the
Université Victor Segalen Bordeaux II,
Bordeaux, France

Sabine Ernst, MD, PHD
Imperial College,
National Heart and Lung Institute,
Royal Brompton and Harefield Hospital,
London, UK

Thomas H. Everett, IV, PhD
Division of Cardiology and the Cardiovascular
Research Institute, University of California
San Francisco, San Francisco,
California, USA

Jerónimo Farré, MD, PhD, FESC
Department of Cardiology,
Fundación Jiménez Díaz-Capio,
Universidad Autónoma de Madrid,
Madrid, Spain

Fiorenzo Gaita, MD
Department of Cardiology,
Cardinal Massaia Hospital, Asti,
AT, Italy

Michel Haïssaguerre, MD
Hôpital Cardiologique du Haut-Lévêque and the
Université Victor Segalen Bordeaux II,
Bordeaux, France

Siew Yen Ho, PhD, FRCPath
National Heart and Lung Institute,
Imperial College and the Royal Brompton and
Harefield NHS Trust,
London, UK

Mélèze Hocini, MD
Hôpital Cardiologique du Haut-Lévêque and the
Université Victor Segalen Bordeaux II,
Bordeaux, France

Li-Fern Hsu, MB, BS
Hôpital Cardiologique du Haut-Lévêque and the
Université Victor Segalen Bordeaux II,
Bordeaux, France

Pierre Jaïs, MD
Hôpital Cardiologique du Haut-Lévêque and the
Université Victor Segalen Bordeaux II,
Bordeaux, France

José Jalife, MD
Department of Pharmacology and Institute for
Cardiovascular Research,
SUNY Upstate Medical University,
Syracuse, New York, USA

Bobby John, MD
Cardiovascular Research Centre,
Department of Cardiology,
Royal Adelaide Hospital and the Disciplines of
Medicine and Physiology, University of Adelaide,
Adelaide, Australia

Anders Jönsson, MD
Hôpital Cardiologique du Haut-Lévêque and the
Université Victor Segalen Bordeaux II,
Bordeaux, France

Jérôme Kalifa, MD, PhD
Department of Pharmacology and Institute for
Cardiovascular Research,
SUNY Upstate Medical University,
Syracuse, New York, USA

Lukas Kappenberger, MD
CardioMet, Centre Hospitalier Universitaire Vaudois,
Lausanne, Switzerland

Mohammed Nasir Khan, MD
Cardiovascular Associates,
Elk Grove Village,
Illinois, USA

George J. Klein, MD
University of Western Ontario, University Hospital,
London, Ontario, Canada

Sébastien Knecht, MD
Hôpital Cardiologique du Haut-Lévêque and the
Université Victor Segalen Bordeaux II,
Bordeaux, France

Sathish Kodali, MD
Hôpital Cardiologique du Haut-Lévêque and the
Université Victor Segalen Bordeaux II,
Bordeaux, France

Karl-Heinz Kück, MD
Oberärztin Magn. Navigation,
Hanseatic Heart Center St. Georg,
Hamburg, Germany

Pawel Kuklik, BSC
Cardiovascular Research Centre, Department of Cardiology, Royal Adelaide Hospital and the Disciplines of Medicine and Physiology, University of Adelaide, Adelaide, Australia

Dennis H. Lau, MB, BS
Cardiovascular Research Centre, Department of Cardiology, Royal Adelaide Hospital and the Disciplines of Medicine and Physiology, University of Adelaide, Adelaide, Australia

Kang Teng Lim, MB, BS
Hôpital Cardiologique du Haut-Lévêque and the Université Victor Segalen Bordeaux II, Bordeaux, France

Lorraine Mackenzie, PHD
Cardiovascular Research Centre, Department of Cardiology, Royal Adelaide Hospital and the Disciplines of Medicine and Physiology, University of Adelaide, Adelaide, Australia

Seiichiro Matsuo, MD
Hôpital Cardiologique du Haut-Lévêque and the Université Victor Segalen Bordeaux II, Bordeaux, France

Antonio Montefusco, MD
Cardinal Massaia Hospital, Asti, AT, Italy

Andrea Natale, MD
Adjunct Professor, Stanford University, Palo Alto, California, USA

Stanley Nattel, MD
Department of Medicine and Research Center, Montreal Heart Institute and Université de Montréal and Department of Pharmacology and Therapeutics, McGill University, Montreal, Quebec, Canada

Jeffrey E. Olgin, MD
Division of Cardiology and the Cardiovascular Research Institute, University of California San Francisco, San Francisco, California, USA

Mark D. O'Neill, MB, BCH, DPHIL
Hôpital Cardiologique du Haut-Lévêque and the Université Victor Segalen Bordeaux II, Bordeaux, France

Feifan Ouyang, MD
Oberärztin Magn. Navigation, Hanseatic Heart Center St. Georg, Hamburg, Germany

Carlo Pappone, MD, PHD
Department of Cardiology, Electrophysiology and Cardiac Pacing Unit, San Raffaele Scientific Institute, Milan, Italy

Ibrahim Abu Romeh, MD
Heart Failure and Transplant Fellow, University of Utah, Utah, USA

Thomas Rostock, MD
Hôpital Cardiologique du Haut-Lévêque and the Université Victor Segalen Bordeaux II, Bordeaux, France

Martin Rotter, MD
Hôpital Cardiologique du Haut-Lévêque and the Université Victor Segalen Bordeaux II, Bordeaux, France

Patrick Ruchat, MD
Service de Chirurgie Cardio-Vasculaire, Centre Hospitalier Universitaire Vaudois, Lausanne, Switzerland

Frédéric Sacher, MD
Hôpital Cardiologique du Haut-Lévêque and the Université Victor Segalen Bordeaux II, Bordeaux, France

Damián Sánchez-Quintana, MD, PhD
Department of Human Anatomy and Cell Biology, Faculty of Medicine, University of Extremadura, Badajoz, Spain

Prashanthan Sanders, MB, BS, PHD
Hôpital Cardiologique du Haut-Lévêque and the Université Victor Segalen Bordeaux II, Bordeaux, France and Cardiovascular Research Centre, Department of Cardiology, Royal Adelaide Hospital and the Disciplines of Medicine and Physiology, University of Adelaide, Adelaide, Australia

Vincenzo Santinelli, MD
Department of Cardiology, Electrophysiology and Cardiac Pacing Unit, San Raffaele Scientific Institute, Milan, Italy

Peter Santucci, MD
Center for Heart and Cardiovascular Medicine,
Loyola University Health System,
Maywood, Illinois, USA

Juerg Schlaepfer, MD
Service de Cardiologie,
Centre Hospitalier Universitaire Vaudois,
Lausanne, Switzerland

Claus Schmitt, MD
Medizinischen Klinik,
Klinikum Karlsruhe,
Karlsruhe, Germany

Martin K. Stiles, MB, CHB
Cardiovascular Research Centre,
Department of Cardiology,
Royal Adelaide Hospital and the Disciplines of
Medicine and Physiology, University of Adelaide,
Adelaide, Australia

Rajesh Subbiah, BSC(MED), MB, BS, PHD
Hôpital Cardiologique du Haut-Lévêque and the
Université Victor Segalen Bordeaux II,
Bordeaux, France

Yoshihide Takahashi, MD
Hôpital Cardiologique du Haut-Lévêque and the
Université Victor Segalen Bordeaux II,
Bordeaux, France

Hsuan-Ming Tsao, MD
Department of Internal Medicine, National Yang-Ming
University Hospital, Taiwan

Els Tuyls, MSc
Department of Physiology,
Cardiovascular Research Institute Maastricht (CARIM),
Maastricht University,
Maastricht, The Netherlands

Sander Verheule, PhD
Department of Physiology, Cardiovascular Research
Institute Maastricht (CARIM),
Maastricht University, Maastricht,
The Netherlands

Nathalie Virag, PhD
Medtronic Europe,
Tolochenaz, Switzerland

David J. Wilber, MD
Center for Heart and Cardiovascular Medicine,
Loyola University Health System,
Maywood, Illinois, USA

Scott Willoughby, PHD
Cardiovascular Research Centre, Department of
Cardiology, Royal Adelaide Hospital
and the Disciplines of Medicine and Physiology,
University of Adelaide,
Adelaide, Australia

Matthew Wright, MBBS, PHD
St. Mary's Hospital,
Waller Department of Cardiology,
London, UK

Mei-Han Wu, MD
Division of Radiology, National Yang-Ming University,
School of Medicine and Taipei Veterans General Hospital,
Taiwan

Glenn D. Young, MB, BS
Cardiovascular Research Centre,
Department of Cardiology,
Royal Adelaide Hospital and the Disciplines of
Medicine and Physiology,
University of Adelaide,
Adelaide, Australia

Introduction

Atrial fibrillation (AF) has long been a field for experimental, pharmacological, and clinical investigations. After initial surgical attempts to cure AF using multiple incisions, the observation that the pulmonary veins were mainly involved in the genesis of AF has promoted the use of catheter techniques for curative approaches.

This book provides a collective text that integrates advances in basic and clinical electrophysiology that have emerged in the last 10 years. Our goal is to produce a treatise that electrophysiologists, allied healthcare professionals, and industry personnel will use as a guide to assist in patient care, to stimulate research projects, and to continue the remarkable advances in the treatment of AF.

A major message appears to be the complexity of underlying factors initiating and perpetuating AF, and the need for combined approaches to involve these different mechanisms. Another message is to acknowledge the limitations of present technologies which, despite achieving dramatic termination of most AF, require additional interventions for tissue recovery or new substrate.

The book is divided into several parts. The first part (Chapters 1–7) is devoted to the fundamental concepts of AF, origin of signals, computer simulation, and updated reviews of ablation tools. The anatomy chapter is richly illustrated by numerous high quality images. This information is necessary for appropriate clinical practice. The second part (Chapters 8–12) provides the present practical approaches to the ablation of specific targets in the fibrillating atria including pulmonary veins, fragmented electrograms, and linear lesions and details the strategies in paroxysmal or chronic AF or facing left atrial tachycardias. The final part (Chapters 13–18) addresses the special challenge of heart failure patients, the impact of ablation on mortality, atrial mechanical function, and lessons from surgical AF ablation.

Each chapter is written by experienced and internationally recognized authors, most being the leading experts in this field.

We hope that this book may become a reference text for many and will be followed by future editions to provide up to date information in this rapidly developing area.

Etienne Aliot
Michel Haïssaguerre
Warren M. Jackman

PART 1

Fundamental concepts of atrial fibrillation

CHAPTER 1

Anatomy of the left atrium relevant to atrial fibrillation ablation

José Angel Cabrera, Jerónimo Farré, Siew Yen Ho, & Damián Sánchez-Quintana

Introduction

Atrial fibrillation (AF) is an arrhythmia most likely due to multiple etiopathogenic mechanisms. In spite of a still incomplete understanding of the anatomo-functional basis for the initiation and maintenance of AF, various radiofrequency catheter ablation (RFCA) techniques have been shown to modify the substrate of the arrhythmia and/or its neurovegetative modulators, achieving in a high proportion of cases a sustained restoration of a stable sinus rhythm [1–26]. Catheter ablation techniques in patients with AF have evolved from an initial approach focused on the pulmonary veins (PVs) and their junctions with the left atrium (LA), to a more extensive intervention mainly, but not exclusively, on the left atrial myocardium and its neurovegetative innervation [27–32]. We firmly believe that progress is still required to refine the currently accepted catheter ablation approaches to AF. Because the LA is the main target of catheter ablation in patients with AF, in this chapter we review the gross morphological and architectural features of this chamber and its relations with extracardiac structures. The latter have also become relevant because of some extracardiac complications of AF ablation, such as injuries of the phrenic and vagal plexus nerves, or the devastating left atrioesophageal fistula formation [33–40].

Catheter Ablation of Atrial Fibrillation Edited by Etienne Aliot, Michel Haïssaguerre and Warren M. Jackman

Components of the left atrium

From a gross anatomical viewpoint the LA has four components: (1) a venous part that receives the PVs; (2) a vestibule that conducts to the mitral valve; (3) the left atrial appendage (LAA); and (4) the so-called interatrial septum. We want to emphasize that the true interatrial septum is the oval fossa, a depression in the right atrial aspect of the area traditionally considered to be the interatrial septum [41–46] (Figures 1.1–1.4). At the left atrial level, a membranous valve covers this region and conceptually represents the only true interatrial septum in the sense that it can be crossed without exiting the heart. The rest of the "muscular interatrial septum" is formed by the apposition of the right and left atrial myocardia that are separated by vascularized fibro-fatty tissues extending from the extracardiac fat. This is why we prefer to use the term *interatrial groove* rather than muscular interatrial septum, a concept that is not only of academic interest because trans-septal punctures to access the LA should be performed through the oval fossa (Figure 1.2). Thus, a puncture throughout the interatrial groove (the muscular interatrial septum)

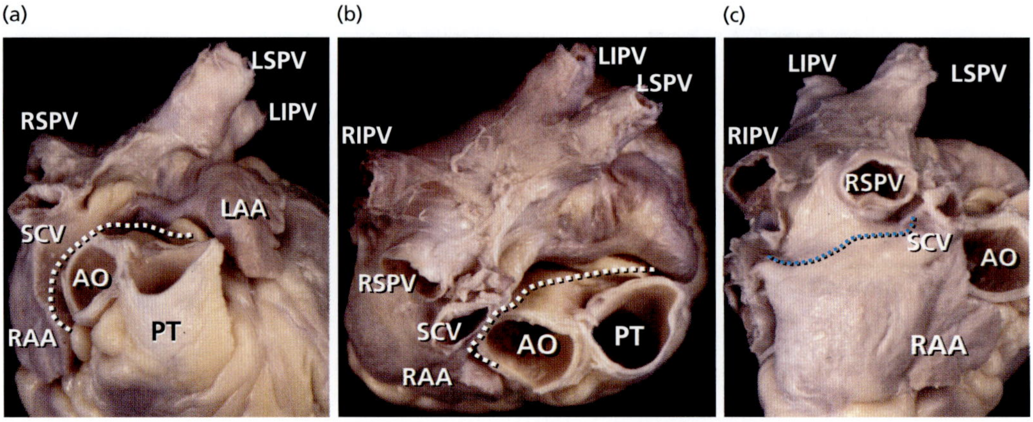

Figure 1.1 External appearances of the right and left atriums viewed from anterior (a), superior (b), and right lateral (c) views. Note the location of the transverse sinus (white dotted lines) and its relationship to the aorta and atrial walls (a, b). The superior and posterior walls of the LA were anchored by the entrance of one PV at each of the four corners. (c) Site of the interatrial groove (Waterston's groove, blue dotted line). AO, aorta; LAA, left atrial appendage; LIPV, left inferior pulmonary vein; LSPV, left superior PV; PT, pulmonary trunk; RAA, right atrial appendage; RIPV, right inferior pulmonary vein; RSPV, right superior pulmonary vein; SCV, superior caval vein.

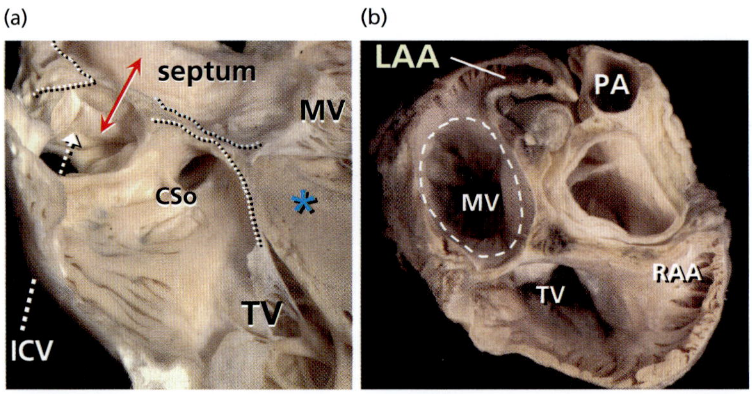

Figure 1.2 (a) Four-chamber section through the heart showing the offset arrangement of the mitral valve (MV) and tricuspid valve (TV) which produces the so-called muscular atrioventricular septum (*) and the deep infolding of the atrial wall superior to the floor of the oval fossa (dotted lines). The true septal area is considerably smaller. (b) The cardiac base (short axis) is dissected by removing most of the atrium's aspects. The right pectinate muscles skirt around the vestibule of the right atrium and reach the orifice of the coronary sinus. Note that the pectinate muscles in the LA are limited mostly within the appendage and the dotted line marking the vestibule of the mitral annulus. CSo, coronary sinus orifice; ICV, inferior caval vein; LAA, left atrial appendage; PA, pulmonary artery; RAA, right atrial appendage.

may result in hemopericardium in a highly anticoagulated patient because blood will dissect the vascularized fibro-fatty tissue that is sandwiched between the right and left atrial myocardium at this level [47–49].

The major part of the endocardial LA including the septal and interatrial groove component is relatively smooth walled. The left aspect of the interatrial groove, apart from a small crescent-like edge, is almost indistinguishable from the parietal atrial wall. The smoothest parts are the superior and posterior walls, which make up the pulmonary venous component, and the vestibule surrounding the mitral orifice. Behind the posterior portion of

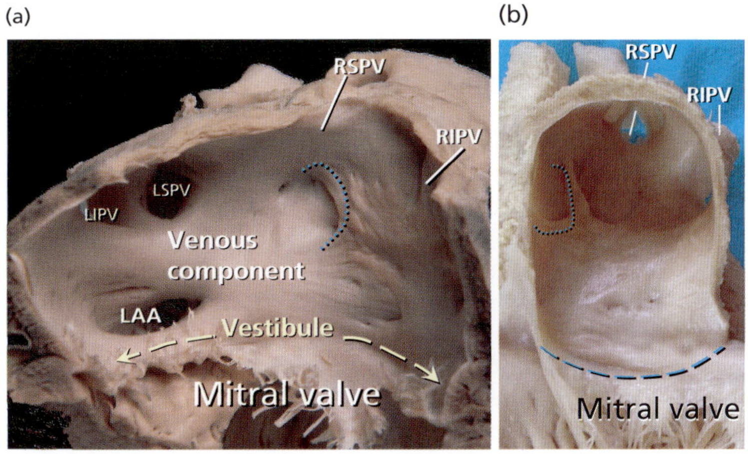

Figure 1.3 (a) Dissection of the posterior wall of the LA close to Waterston's groove. The smooth-walled venous component of the LA is the most extensive. The septal aspect of the LA shows the crescentic line of the free edge (dotted line) of the flap valve against the rim of the oval fossa. (b) The orifices of the right superior and inferior pulmonary veins (RSPV and RIPV) are adjacent to the plane of the septal aspect of the LA (dotted line). The dashed blue line marks the hinge of the mitral valve. LAA, left atrial appendage; LIPV, left inferior pulmonary vein; LSPV, left superior pulmonary vein.

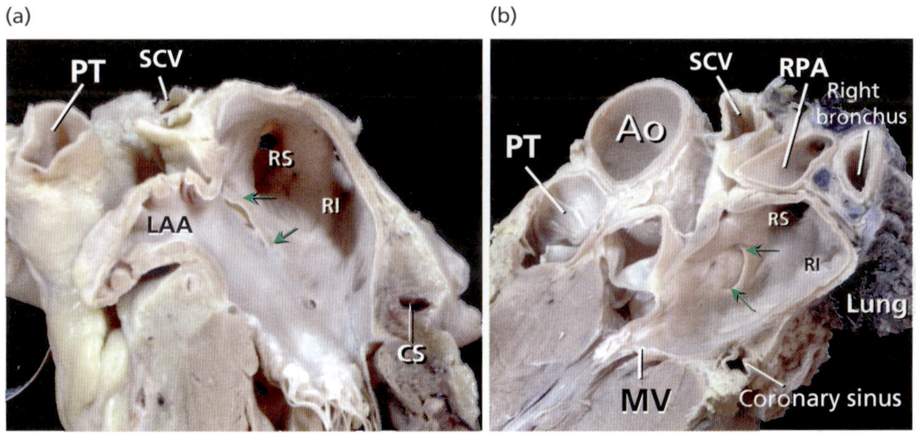

Figure 1.4 Longitudinal sections through the left atrial appendage (LAA) showing the orifices of the right PV; the flap valve of the oval fossa overlaps (arrows) the rim to form the septal aspect of the LA. Note the relation of the superior caval vein (SCV) to the right superior pulmonary vein (RS). (b) Longitudinal section to show the relationship of the roof of the left atrium with the right pulmonary artery (RPA) and right bronchus. Ao, aorta; CS, coronary sinus; MV, mitral valve; PT, pulmonary trunk, RI, right inferior pulmonary vein; RS, right superior pulmonary vein.

the vestibular component of the LA is the anterior wall of the coronary sinus [41] (Figures 1.3 and 1.4).

The walls of the left atrium and the septum

The left atrial wall and its thickness

The walls of LA, excluding the LAA, can be described as anterior, superior, left lateral, septal, and posterior. The anterior wall is located behind the ascending aorta and the transverse pericardial sinus. From epicardium to endocardium its width is 3.3 ± 1.2 mm (range 1.5–4.8 mm) in unselected necropsic heart specimens, but this wall can become very thin at the area near the vestibule of the mitral annulus where it measures an average of 2 mm in thickness in our autopsy studies. The roof or superior wall of the LA is in close proximity to the right pulmonary artery and its width ranges from 3.5 to 6.5 mm (mean 4.5 ± 0.6 mm). The thickness of the lateral wall ranges between 2.5 and 4.9 mm (mean 3.9 ± 0.7 mm) [41].

As already stated, an anatomic septum is like a wall that separates adjacent chambers so that perforation of a septal wall would enable us to enter from a chamber to the opposite one without exiting the heart. Thus, the true atrial septal wall is confined to the flap valve of the oval fossa. The flap valve is hinged from the muscular rim that, deriving from the septum secundum, is seen from the right atrial aspect of the interatrial wall. At its anteroinferior portion the rim separates the foramen ovale from the coronary sinus and the vestibule of the tricuspid valve [48] (Figure 1.2). On the left atrial aspect there is no visible rim and the flap valve overlaps the oval rim quite considerably and two horns mark the usual site of fusion with the rim (Figure 1.3 and 1.4). The measurement of the mean thickness of the atrial septum in normal hearts at the level of the anteroinferior portion of the muscular rim is 5.5 ± 2.3 mm, and the mean thickness of the flap valve is 1.5 ± 0.6 mm [41]. These results agree with previously published echocardiographic studies [50]. The major portion of the rim around the fossa is an infolding of the muscular atrial wall that is filled with epicardial fat. Superiorly and posteriorly there is an interatrial groove, also known as Waterston's groove, whose dissection permits the separation of the right and left atrial myocardial walls and to enter the LA without transgressing into the right atrium. Anteriorly and inferiorly, the rim and its continuation into the atrial vestibules overlies the myocardial masses of the ventricles from which they are separated by the fat-filled inferior pyramidal space [48,51] (Figures 1.2–1.4).

The posterior wall of the LA is a target of currently used ablation procedures in patients with AF. Early surgical interventions aimed at reducing the critical mass of atrial tissues created long transmural linear lesions incorporating the posterior LA wall. The posterior wall of the LA is related to the esophagus and its nerves (vagal nerves) and the thoracic aorta, and its inferior portion is related to the coronary sinus. In a previous study in 26 unselected human heart specimens the overall thickness of the posterior LA wall was 4.1 ± 0.7 mm (range 2.5–5.3 mm) [41]. In a subsequent study we measured the thickness of the posterior wall from the epicardium to endocardium, obtaining sagittal and transverse sections through the LA at three levels (superior, middle, and inferior close to the coronary sinus) in three different LA regions (right venoatrial junction, mid-posterior atrial wall, and left venoatrial junction) [52]. We also analyzed the myocardial content of the LA wall at all these predefined sites. The region with the thickest myocardial content was the mid-posterior LA wall (2.9 ± 0.5 mm, range 0.6–4.2 mm). The inferior level, immediately superior to the coronary sinus and between 6 and 15 mm from the mitral annulus, had the thickest posterior LA wall (6.5 ± 2.5 mm, range 2.8–12 mm). The latter thickness was due to a rather bulky myocardial layer (4.3 ± 0.8 mm) and the presence of a profuse amount of fibro-fatty tissue, both components being less developed at more superior levels of the posterior LA wall. The wall at the plane of the right or left venoatrial junction had the thinnest musculature (2.2 ± 0.3 mm, range 1.2–4.5 mm) and a very scanty content of fibro-fatty tissue [52]. In some samples of histological sections obtained at the PV and posterior atrial wall, the myocardial layer had small areas of discontinuities that were filled with fibrous tissue [42,53].

The myoarchitecture of the left atrial wall

Detailed dissections of the subendocardial and subepicardial myofibers along the entire thickness of the LA walls have shown a complex architecture of overlapping bands of aligned myocardial bundles [41,51] (Figures 1.5 and 1.6). The term "fibers" describes the macroscopic appearance of strands of cardiomyocytes. These fibers are circumferential when they run parallel to the mitral annulus and longitudinal when they are approximately perpendicular to the mitral orifice. Although there are some individual variations, our epicardial dissections of the LA have shown a predominant pattern of arrangement of the myocardial fibers [41]. On the subepicardial aspect of the LA, the fibers in the anterior wall consisted of a main bundle that was parallel to the atrioventricular groove. This was the continuation of the interatrial bundle (Bachmann's bundle) [54], which could be traced rightward to the junction between the right atrium and the superior caval vein. In the LA, the interatrial bundle

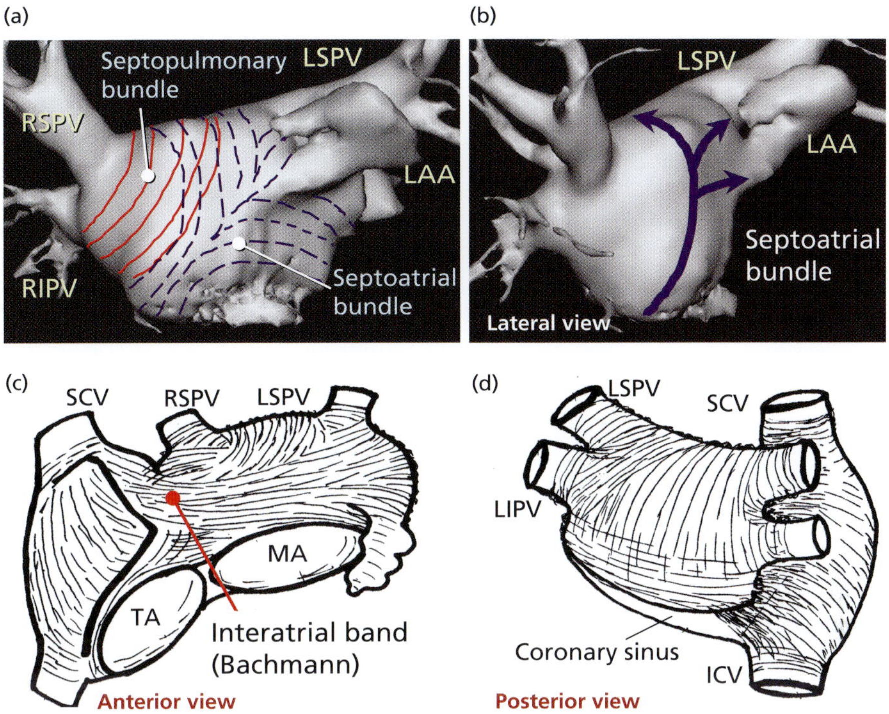

Figure 1.5 Schematic representation of the general arrangement of the subepicardial and subendocardial fibers of the LA, viewed from the anterior (a, c) and posterior (b, d) aspect. (b) Note the three major subendocardial fascicles of the septoatrial bundle. ICV, inferior caval vein; LAA, left atrial appendage; LIPV, left inferior pulmonary vein; LSPV, left superior pulmonary vein; MA, mitral valve; RIPV, right inferior pulmonary vein; RSPV, right superior pulmonary vein; SCV, superior caval vein; TA, tricuspid valve.

was joined inferiorly at the septal raphe (the portion that is buried in the atrial septum) by fibers arising from the anterior rim of the oval foramen. Superiorly, it blended with a broad band of circumferential fibers that arose from the anterosuperior part of the septal raphe to sweep leftward into the lateral wall. Reinforced superficially by the interatrial bundle, these circumferential fibers passed to either side of the neck of the atrial appendage to encircle the appendage, and reunited as a broad circumferential band around the inferior part of the posterior wall to enter the posterior septal raphe (Figures 1.5 and 1.6). The epicardial fibers of the superior wall are composed of longitudinal or oblique fibers, (named by Papez as the "septopulmonary bundle" in 1920) [55] that arise from the anterosuperior septal raphe, beneath the circumferential fibers of the Bachmann's bundle. As they ascend the roof, they fan out to pass in front, between, and behind the insertions of the pulmonary veins and the myocardial sleeves that surround the venous orifices. On the posterior wall, the septopulmonary bundle often bifurcates to become two oblique branches. The leftward branch fused with, and was indistinguishable from, the circumferential fibers of the anterior and lateral walls, whereas the rightward branch turned into the posterior septal raphe. Often, extensions from the rightward branch passed over the septal raphe to blend with right atrial fibers and others toward the septal mitral valve annulus, forming a line that marked an abrupt change in subendocardial fiber orientation.

On the subendocardial aspect of the LA, most specimens showed a common pattern of general architecture. The dominant fibers in the anterior wall were those orginating from a bundle described by Papez as the septoatrial bundle [55]. The fibers of this bundle ascended obliquely from the anterior interatrial raphe and combined with longitudinal fibers arising from the vestibule. They passed the posterior aspect of the LA between the left and right pulmonary veins, blending with longitudinal

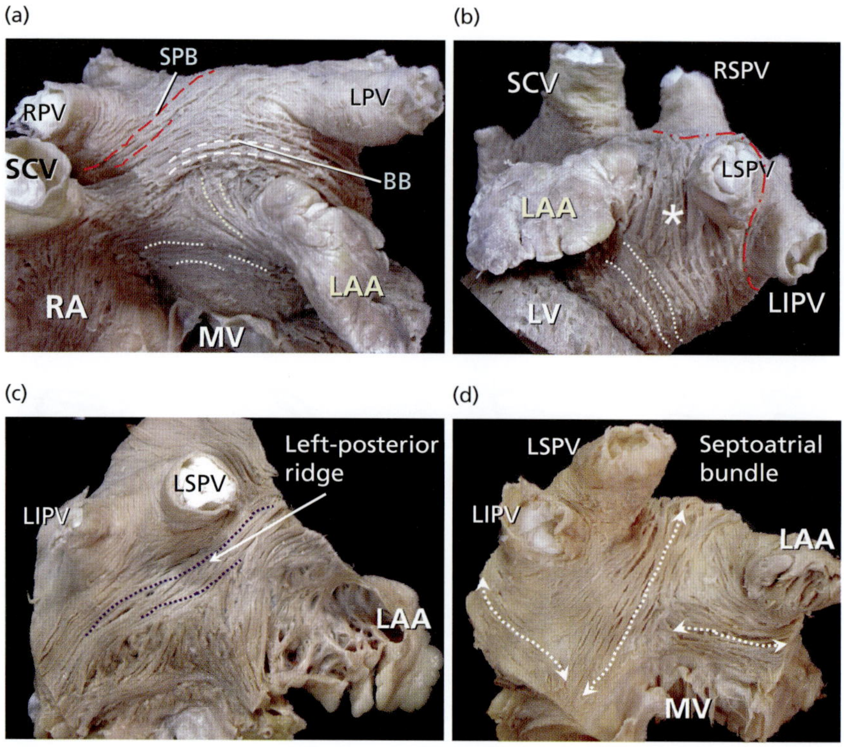

Figure 1.6 (a, b) Dissections of the subepicardial fibers viewed from the anterior and left lateral aspects. The interatrial (Bachmann) bundle (BB, white dashed lines) crosses the septal raphe and blends into the circumferential fibers of the anterior wall (dotted lines), passes to either side of the neck of the atrial appendage and runs parallel to the posterolateral aspect (*) of the LA. Oblique fibers of the septopulmonary bundle (SPB) become longitudinal as they cross the roof between the left and right PVs (red dashed lines). (c, d) The left atrium everted to show the subendocardial fibers and the fiber arrangement of the septoatrial bundle and its three major fascicles (double-headed arrows). Note that endocardially the myocardial content of the left posterior ridge is the prolongation of leftward fibers from the septoatrial bundle that run toward the orifices of the left-sided PVs and the mouth of the left atrial appendage (LAA, blue dotted lines). LIPV, left inferior pulmonary vein; LPV, left pulmonary vein; LSPV, left superior pulmonary vein; LV, left ventricle; MV, mitral valve; RA, right atrium; RPV, right pulmonary vein; RSPV, right superior pulmonary vein; SCV, superior caval vein.

or oblique fibers of the septopulmonary bundle from the subepicardial layer. The septoatrial bundle also passed leftward, superior and inferior to the mouth of the atrial appendage to reach the lateral and posterior walls. Some of these fibers encircled the mouth of the LA appendage and continued into the pectinate muscles within the appendage (Figures 1.5 and 1.6). The subendocardial fibers at the orifices of the PVs were usually loop-like extensions from the longitudinal fibers. These fibers became circular at varying distances into the venous walls and were continuous with the subepicardial fibers. In some specimens, however, the subendocardial fibers were longitudinal or oblique, whereas the subepicardial fibers were circular, or vice versa. The distal margins of the muscular sleeves were highly irregular in the majority of veins.

Pulmonary veins and their ending into the left atrium

Clinical imaging studies using magnetic resonance imaging (MRI) and multislice computed tomography (CT) demonstrated the complex anatomy of the PVs with significant variability in dimensions, shape, and branching patterns [56–63]. When assessed in a correct attitudinal orientation, the left PVs are located more superiorly than the right-sided veins [64] (Figure 1.7). The superior PVs run cranially and more anteriorly, whereas the

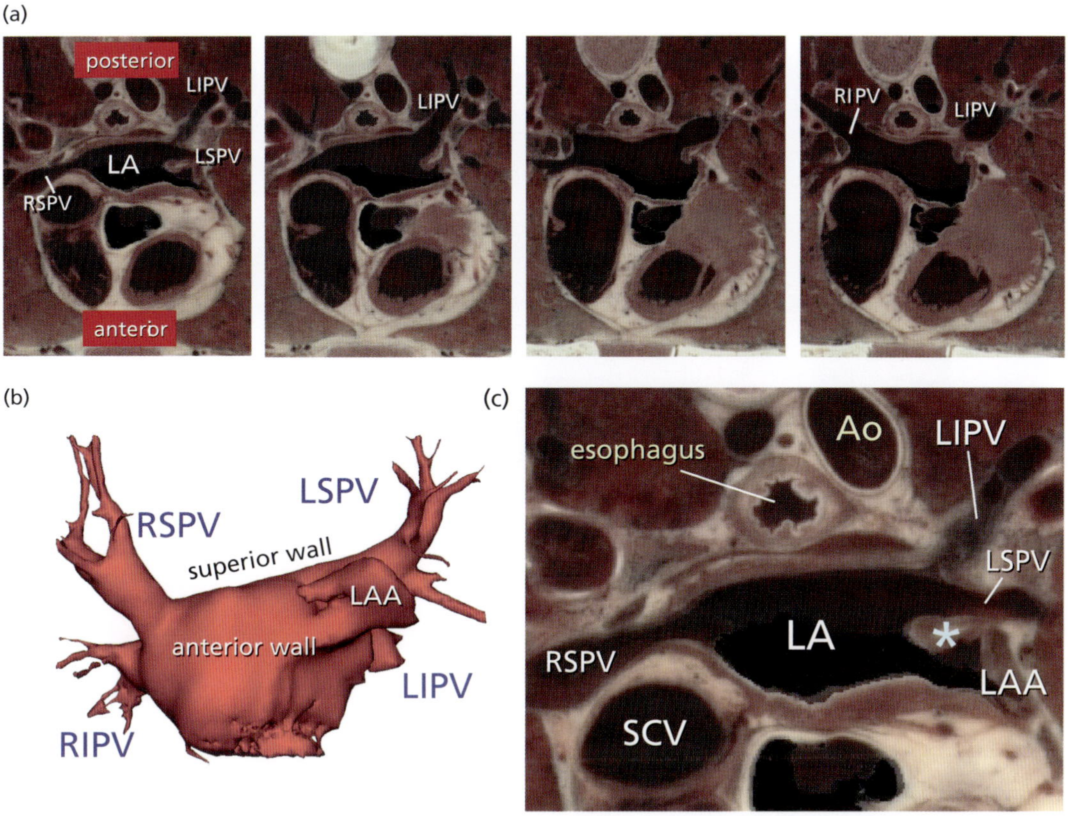

Figure 1.7 Left atrial anatomy as depicted on axial slices obtained with the "Visible Human Slice and Surface Server" [46] and three-dimensional reconstruction of the left atrium (LA) and pulmonary veins (PV) using the NavX® system from data obtained with a 32-slice multidetector CT scanner. (a) Four successive slides obtained from a cranial to caudal direction. Note that the left PVs are located more superiorly than the right-sided veins. The superior PVs run cranially and more anteriorly and the inferior veins have a more posterior and lateral course. (b) The NavX system allows better geometric visualization of the LA, left atrial appendage (LAA), and PVs in a correct attitudinal orientation. The LAA is anterior to the left superior PV (LSPV). (c) The right superior PV (RSPV) is seen behind the superior caval vein (SCV). Note the posterior wall of the LA related to the esophagus and aorta and the infold (*) of the posterolateral atrial wall protuding into the endocardial LA surface as a prominent ridge. Ao, aorta; LIPV, left inferior pulmonary vein; RIPV, right inferior pulmonary vein.

inferior veins have a more posterior and lateral course. The right superior PV runs near the posterior aspect of the right atrium immediately behind the superior caval vein. The right PVs are also related to the right pulmonary artery, which passes close to the roof of the LA [46] (Figure 1.8).

The orifices of the right PVs are directly adjacent to the plane of the atrial septum (see Figures 1.3 and 1.4). The left superior PV lies superiorly and posteriorly to the mouth of the LAA, separated endocardially by a posterolateral ridge which, epicardially, is a fold that frequently extends to the origin of the left inferior PV [41,46,61–63]. Although textbooks typically depict four venous orifices, anatomic observations confirmed by MRI and CT studies in structurally normal hearts, have demonstrated the variability of the ending of the PVs into the LA. In our series of 35 postmortem human hearts, we found 26 specimens (74%) with two PVs on each side [44]. Of these 26 hearts, 15 (69%) had four separate openings of the PVs into the LA and the remaining 11 specimens (31%) had a "vestibule-like" portion for both PVs before opening via a common orifice into the atrium (Figures 1.9 and 1.10). The venous vestibule is more frequently found on the left than on the right side and its length ranged from 3 to 15 mm (7 ± 3 mm). A single common PV, defined as a vein branching at the

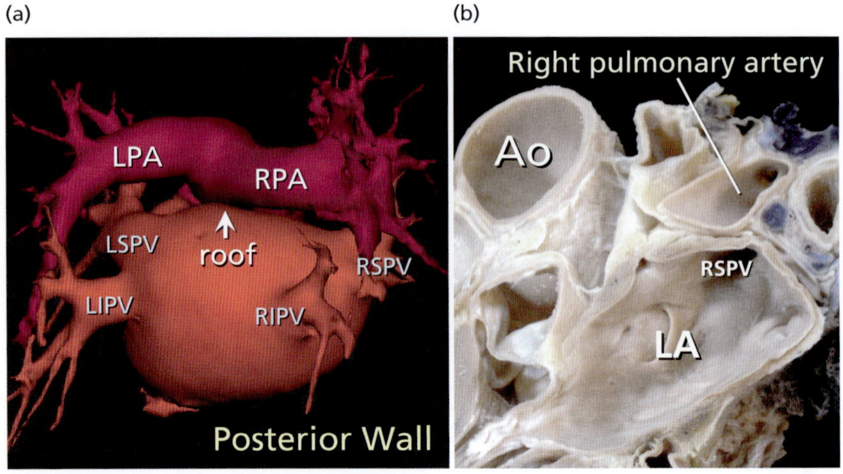

Figure 1.8 (a, b) The right superior pulmonary vein (RSPV) is related to the right pulmonary artery (RPA) that passes close to the roof of the left atrium (LA). Ao, aorta; LIPV, left inferior pulmonary vein; LPA, left pulmonary artery; LSPV, left superior pulmonary vein; RIPV, right inferior pulmonary vein.

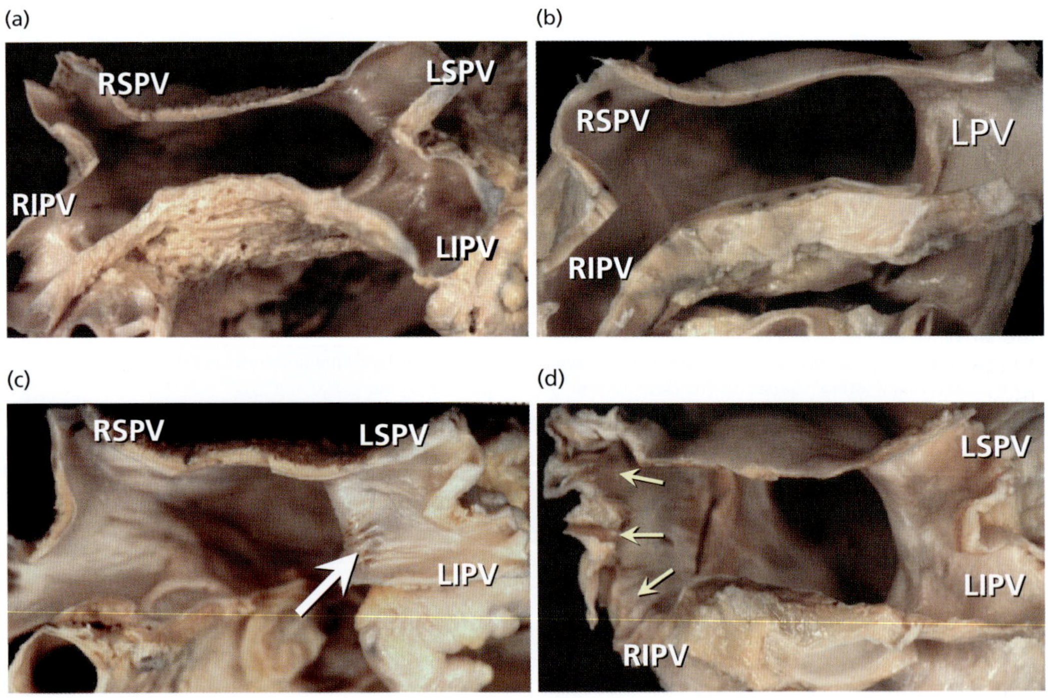

Figure 1.9 Four heart specimens sectioned tranversally with the roof of the LA removed and viewed from above to shows the entrance of the pulmonary veins (PVs). (a) The arrangement of four individualized ending of the PVs into the LA. (b) A single left PV (LPV). (c) Four PVs; the left PV has a "vestibule-like" portion (white arrow) for both the left superior PV (LSPV) and left inferior PV (LIPV) before opening via a common orifice into the left atrium. (c) This heart displayed more than four PVs: three orifices on the right (yellow arrows) and two on the left. RIPV, right inferior pulmonary vein; RSPV, right superior pulmonary vein.

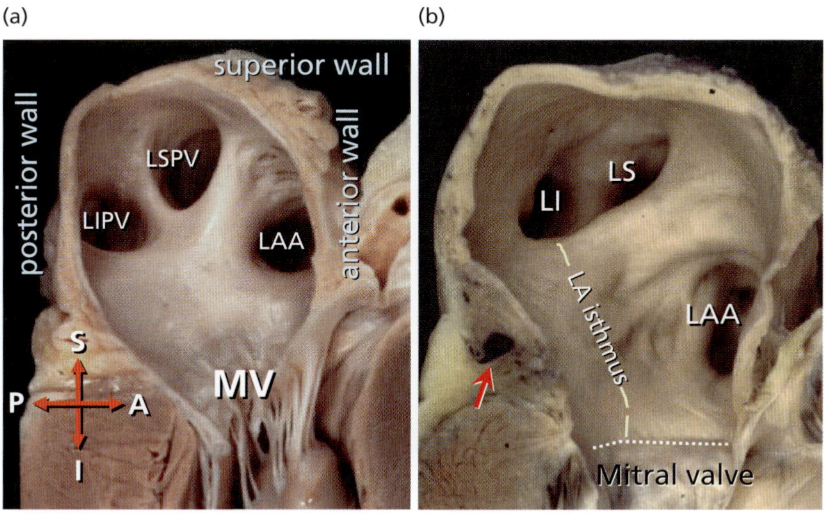

Figure 1.10 Longitudinal sections of two hearts illustrating endings of the pulmonary veins (PVs) into the LA. (a) An individualized ending of the left superior PV (LSPV) and the left inferior PV (LIPV) into the LA. The left PVs lie superior and posterior to the mouth of the left atrial appendage (LAA), both separated by a muscular fold. (b) Heart showing a common vestibule for both left PVs. Note the larger anteroposterior diameter than the superoinferior one and the line connecting the inferior margin of the ostium of the left inferior PV to the mitral annulus called the left atrial isthmus. The red arrow marks the coronary sinus. LI, left inferior PV; LS, left superior PV; MV, mitral valve.

level of the hilum of the lung, was found in three hearts (9%), two on the left side and one on the right. Six hearts (17%) displayed more than four pulmonary veins (three orifices on the right and two on the left). Clinical examination demonstrated four venous orifices in 81% of patients, while 3% had three orifices and 16% had five orifices [59]. The most common variation is a separate origin of the vein coming from the right middle lobe of the lung (Figure 1.9). The distance between the orifices of the right PVs ranged from 3 to 14 mm (mean 7.3 ± 2.7 mm), and in the left PVs from 2 to 16 mm (mean 7.5 ± 2.8 mm). A thin inter-orifice left atrial rim between the superior and inferior PVs (measuring from 1 to 3 mm) was found in 50% of the hearts. Endocardial examination of the LA using three-dimensional MRI has shown that the shortest distance between the right and left PVs, the so-called roof line, was 29.9 ± 5.9 mm, ranging between 18.9 and 39.2 mm [62].

Anatomic studies and clinical imaging investigations have shown that the PV ending in the LA is not perfectly cylindrical but has a funnel-shaped morphology, making it difficult to identify a sharp landmark for the anatomic limits of the PV ostium [41,56,57]. Discounting the common vestibule, the diameter of the venous orifices at the venoatrial junction ranged in our anatomic specimens from 8 to 21 mm (12.5 ± 3 mm). The transversal diameter of the common vestibule is longer than its superoinferior diameter (19.5 ± 3 mm vs.13.5 ± 1 mm) [41]. Early studies demonstrated a strong correlation between the degree of left atrial dilation and both occurrence and duration of AF [65]. Imaging studies of the PVs demonstrated that the ostial diameters of the superior PV were greater in patients with AF than in controls [60,66].

Gross anatomy of the left posterolateral ridge

The posterolateral ridge between the orifices of the left PVs and the mouth of the LAA is the most relevant structural prominence of the endocardial LA (Figure 1.11). Although already described in 1907 by Arthur Keith [67] as the "left tænia terminalis" (terminal band or strip) and 13 years later by James Papez [55] as the "left posterior crest", the LA posterolateral ridge actually is a fold of the posterolateral left atrial wall protruding into the endocardial LA surface as a prominent crest or ridge (Figure 1.11). Epicardially, this broad bundle is in continuity with the uppermost and distal part of the interatrial band (Bachmann's bundle).

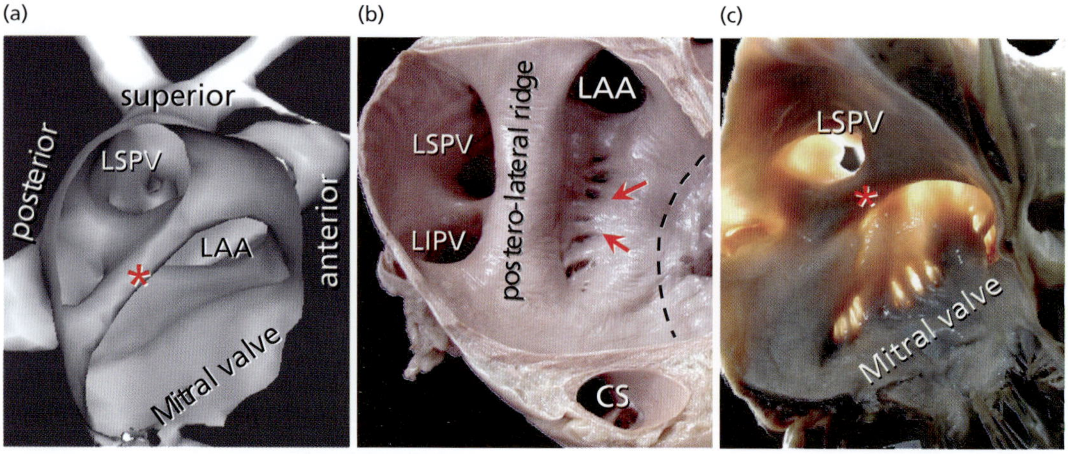

Figure 1.11 Endocardial visualization of the left posterolateral wall. (a) Three-dimensional reconstruction of the endocardial left atrium using the NavX system from data obtained with a 32-slice multidetector CT scanner. Note the prominent posterolateral ridge (*) between the left atrial appendage (LAA) and the left superior pulmonary vein (LSPV) along the lateral wall from its anterosuperior to posteroinferior region. (b, c) Two postmortem heart specimens showing prominent endocardial posterolateral ridges, extending in (b) to the inferior margin of the left inferior pulmonary vein (LIPV). Observe the muscular trabeculations extending inferiorly from the left appendage to the vestibule of the mitral valve (red arrows). (c) Transillumination of the left lateral wall to illustrate the extra-appendicular posterior pectinate muscle and the thinnest muscular wall in between the muscular trabeculae. CS, coronary sinus.

Endocardially, the myocardial content is the prolongation of leftward fibers from the septoatrial bundle that run toward the orifices of the left-sided PVs and the mouth of the LAA (see Figure 1.6). The shape and size of this posterolateral LA ridge is of relevance during catheter ablation of AF when encircling the orificies of the left PVs or during ablation of extrapulmonary vein triggers arising around or inside the LAA. Anatomic information of this structure may be useful in order to perform ablation techniques more efficiently and safely, and it can be obtained with current multislice CT and MRI reconstructions of the endocardial aspect of the LA [61–63]. The ridge extends along the lateral wall of the LA from the anterosuperior to posteroinferior region. A recent three-dimensional MRI study showed that the ridge was narrowest between the left superior PV and the LAA in 84% of patients. In this study, the mean distance between the left superior PV and the LAA, and between the left inferior PV and the LAA, were found to be 3.8 ± 1.1 mm and 5.8 ± 2.0 mm, respectively. The ridge was narrower than 5 mm in the majority of patients, thus determining the possibility of obtaining stable catheter position in this region [61]. Our recent anatomic study of 32 structurally normal human heart necropsic specimens also revealed a thicker myocardial wall of the ridge at its inferior level adjacent to the inferior PV, with a range between 1.5 and 4.2 mm (mean 2.8 ± 1.1 mm). The mean length of the ridge was 24.2 ± 5.3 mm (range 14.2–32.5 mm) with a constant superior insertion at the lateral roof of the LA extending inferiorly to reach the posteroinferior margin of the inferior PV in 88% of hearts (unpublished observations). A CT scan study showed a prominent ridge in all subjects extending from the superior part of the left superior PV to the inferior PV in 70–72% of patients [63]. These investigators also found no significant differences in the length and width of the ridge between patients with AF and controls [63].

Gross anatomy of the left atrial appendage

The LAA is characteristically a small finger-like extension of the LA with a multilobulated appearance in 80% of hearts [68,69] (Figure 1.12). A quantitative study of the normal LAA in 500 autopsy hearts showed that the mean length, width, and size of the appendage increased with age up 20 years [69]. In adult postmortem hearts the mean orifice

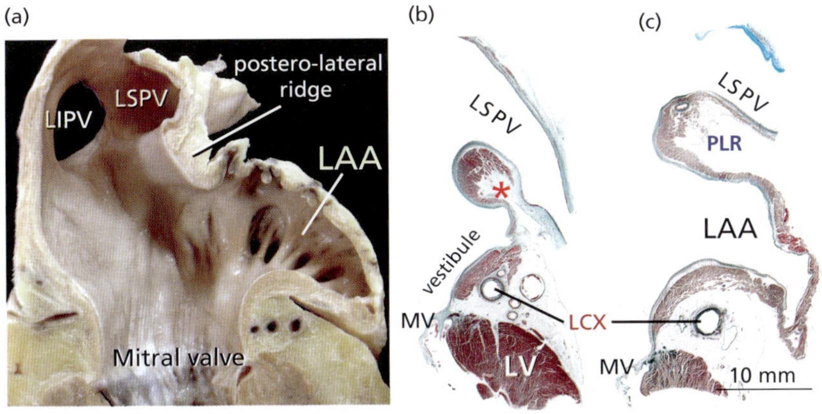

Figure 1.12 (a) Longitudinal section through left atrial appendage (LAA) showing the orifices of the left pulmonary veins, and the left posterolateral ridge. (b, c) Longitudinal sections through the left superior pulmonary vein (LSPV) and left atrial appendage (LAA) and left superior pulmonary vein (LSPV) stained with Masson's trichrome. Note the myocardium and fat tissue (*) of the posterolateral ridge and the left circumflex artery (LCX) closer to the vestibule of the left atrium in (b). LIPV, left inferior pulmonary vein; LV, left ventricle; MV, mitral valve; PLR, posterolateral ridge.

diameter of the LAA was 1.07 cm in women and 1.16 cm in men, in contrast with morphological examinations of LAA orifices using CT scans that showed a mean longitudinal and transverse diameter of 3.2 ± 0.6 mm and 1.9 ± 0.5 mm, respectively [63,69]. The greater diameters in the in vivo human studies as compared to necropsic measurements most likely is due to tissue retraction produced by the fixation of the specimens in the latter studies. The LAA orifice and volume of patients with AF is greater than that observed in controls.

Reinforced superficially by the interatrial bundle, circumferential fibers that arise from the anterosuperior part of the septal raphe pass to either side of the neck of the left appendage to form broad bundles of muscular connections between the appendage and the body of the LA. A recent study has shown that to electrically disconnect the LAA it is necessary to apply long-lasting radiofrequency pulses that gradually change the activation sequence, thus suggesting a dense circumferential connection of the appendage to the LA [32]. A narrow, oval-shaped mouth marks the junction between the LAA and the venous component of the LA. The myocardial ridge and an inflection of the endocardial surface bounded the ostial borders of the appendage in most hearts. In the LA, the pectinate muscles are mostly confined within the left appendage. They form a complicated network of muscular strips lining the endocardial surface. In some 28% of our human heart specimens the anterior ostial margin of the appendage does not present as a clear-cut border and muscular trabeculations can be found extending inferiorly from the appendage to the vestibule of the mitral valve (see Figure 1.11). These extra-appendicular myocardial bands correspond to the small posterior set of pectinate muscles originating from the septoatrial bundle to embrace the left appendage. In those hearts with extra-appendicular posterior pectinate muscles, the areas in between the muscular trabeculae had the thinnest muscular walls (0.5 ± 0.2 mm) (see Figures 1.6 and 1.11). In other specimens (15%), remnants of pectinate muscles between the ostium of the left inferior PV and vestibule of the mitral annulus can be found. A previous histological study of the mitral isthmus described "small isthmus crevices" present in almost all patients that may entrap the tip of the ablation catheter, which may lead to excessive tissue heating and tamponade.

The left circumflex coronary artery runs epicardially in the fat-filled atrioventricular groove, related to the smooth anterior vestibule and in close proximity to the inferior border of the orifice of the LAA (Figure 1.12). The shortest distance from the left appendage orifice and the circumflex artery was < 3–5 mm in 80% of our unselected human heart necropsic specimens. In CT in vivo studies the left circumflex coronary artery ran < 2 mm from the LAA orifice in 74% of cases, an anatomic detail to be considered when ablating inside or around the orifice of the LAA.

Architecture of the left posterolateral ridge: the Marshall structures

The posterolateral ridge is more than a simple endocardial fold of the lateral LA wall that influences the stability of the contact of the tip of the catheter with the endocardium during an ablation procedure. Electrophysiological and surgical investigations demonstrated extra-PV atrial foci after PV isolation originating from the LAA [22,32]. In addition, the junctional area between the LAA and the LA body has a relevant impact on the fibrillatory process, acting as a source of activity spreading to the rest of the atrium and contributing to the maintenance of atrial fibrillation [19,21–23, 70–72]. Because of the potential relevance for current and future endocardial catheter ablation techniques we will describe the architectural arrangement of myocardial bundles forming the posterolateral LA ridge and its vascular and autonomic nervous system content, as well as the anatomic relations with the Marshall structures (the oblique vein and ligament).

The so-called oblique vein of Marshall is part of the ligament of Marshall (LOM), formed by the venous element and fibro-fatty tissue, muscular bundle and autonomic nerves, all forming a vestigial fold of the pericardium described by John Marshall in 1850 [73] (Figure 1.13). The LOM courses obliquely above the LAA and can be traced laterally to the left superior PV bundle in the epicardial aspect of the left atrial fold that forms the left posterior "crest". Sherlag et al. [74] first demonstrated the existence of muscular left atrial "tracts" within this vestigial fold and found electrical activity arising from the LOM. In their study, Sherlag et al. recorded double potentials from the ligament, advancing the hypothesis that this structure could play a role in arrhythmogenesis [74]. More recently, the so-called Marshall bundles have been thought to be the origin of certain forms of focal AF and that a considerable percentage of non-pulmonary vein foci may arise from the LOM [30,31,75–79]. Electroanatomic mapping showed a common pattern of electrical connection between the LOM and coronary sinus muscular sleeves, resulting in early activation of the low posterolateral wall of the LA. In addition, some patients had distal electrical connections at the floor of the left inferior PV or anterolateral wall of the left superior PV [75,76].

In an elegant histological examination, Kim et al. [80] demonstrated multiple myocardial "tracts" present within the LOM that directly insert into the coronary sinus musculature near the origin of the vein of Marshall or distally into the posterior free wall of the LA. They found in 57% of specimens both superficial and deep muscular "tracts" in

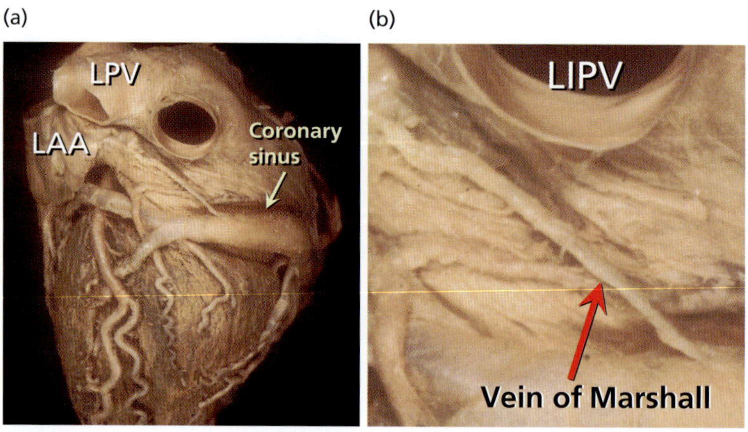

Figure 1.13 (a) Heart specimen showing the spatial relationship of the coronary sinus and the vein/ligament of Marshall. The coronary sinus runs along the epicardial portion of the vestibular component of the LA surrounding circumferentially the orifice of the mitral valve. (b) Note in the enlarged figure, the left atrial oblique vein of Marshall formed by the venous element with fibro-fatty tissue and small muscular bundles. LAA, left atrial appendage; LIPV, left inferior pulmonary vein; LPV, left pulmonary vein.

relation to the oblique vein of Marshall with an overall mean length and diameter of 7.8 ± 3.9 mm and 0.7 ± 0.2 mm, respectively. Electrical activity originating from the LOM can be recorded from the endocardial aspect of the LA in or around the orifices of the left PV. A recent anatomic study showed that Marshall bundles gradually diminished in density towards the distal venous branch and reached the left inferior PV–LA junction and left superior PV–LA junction in 76% and 24% of cases, respectively [81]. In patients with AF undergoing ablation of the LOM, it has been shown that most arrhythmic episodes arise from the distal segment of the ligament close to the left superior PVs [75,77,79]. An angiographic study also revealed that the distal end of the vein of Marshall and its branches are likely to be distributed around the left superior PV or the left inferior PV ostia, especially in patients with arrhythmogenic foci [79]. Studies of endocardial ablation to eliminate activation from Marshall bundles recognize that the most frequently successful ablation site is at the inferior border of the ostium of the left inferior PV. We have studied the Marshall structures, demonstrating that they course along the left posterior ridge and that they are in close proximity to the endocardial aspect of the left atrium (Figure 1.14). In 73% of specimens the oblique vein of Marshall or its ligament runs at a distance less than 3 mm from the superior level of the endocardial ridge. Throughout the trajectory of the vein in relation to the left posterior ridge, we observed in all specimens small muscular bundles that crossed the oblique vein to connect with the left atrial free wall.

The Marshall ligament is richly innervated by sympathetic nerve fibers [80,81]. Adrenergic

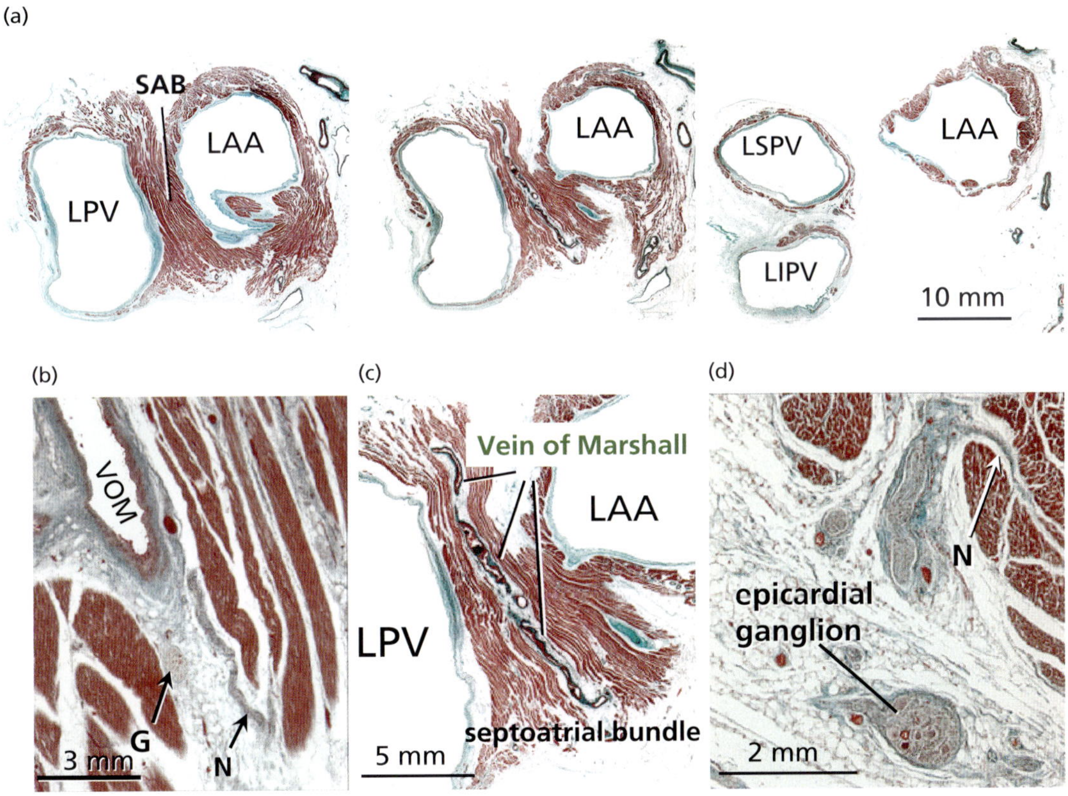

Figure 1.14 (a) Transverse sections at different levels of the myocardial sleeve of the left pulmonary vein (LPV), septoatrial bundle (SAB), and left atrial appendage (LAA) from a 56-year-old man. (b) Transverse section showing the oblique vein of Marshall (VOM). The arrows (G) and (N) indicate the ganglion and nerve bundles in the vicinity of the vein, respectively. (c) An enlargement of the septoatrial bundle shown in (a). Note that the VOM was found in direct contact with the myocardium of the septoatrial bundle. (d) Transverse section showing the epicardial ganglion and nerve bundles (N) in the vicinity of the myocardium of the septoatrial bundle. (Trichrome stain.) LIPV, left inferior pulmonary vein; LSPV, left superior pulmonary vein.

sensitivity of the myocardial tissues within the LOM may be responsible for atrial tachyarrhythmias arising from the LA [78]. Both focal sources arising from Marshall structures and muscular connections with the epicardial interatrial Bachmann's bundle and the inner septoatrial bundle may have implications in the fibrillatory process and spread of AF activity between both atria (Figure 1.14). Recent reports have shown that left-to-right interatrial conduction occurs predominantly through the Bachmann bundle and that sinus impulses propagated through this interatrial bundle could excite the Marshall musculature and the nearby left atrium simultaneously [82,83].

The left atrial isthmus

Linear ablation connecting the inferior margin of the ostium of the left inferior PV to the mitral annulus appears to increase the success rate of catheter ablation in patients with AF [13,84]. Although this posteroinferior wall of the LA between the orifice of the left inferior PV and the mitral annulus cannot be considered an anatomic entity, it is being named by electrophysiologist as the left atrial isthmus or mitral isthmus (Figure 1.15). In a recent anatomic study of 20 hearts, Anton Becker [85] showed marked variability in the dimensions of the mitral isthmus with considerable differences in thickness of the left atrial myocardium at various levels and among different hearts. This study also showed the close anatomic relation between the isthmus area with the great cardiac vein and the left circumflex artery. The mean distance between the left inferior PV and the mitral annulus ranged between 17 and 51 mm (mean 34.6 mm). In some hearts the left atrial myocardium extended into the atrial aspect of the mitral valve leaflets. Gaps in the lesion line may result in conduction delay and facilitate left atrial flutter. Therefore, the variable thickness of the left atrial myocardial tissue is highly relevant to achieving an adequate transmural linear lesion across the

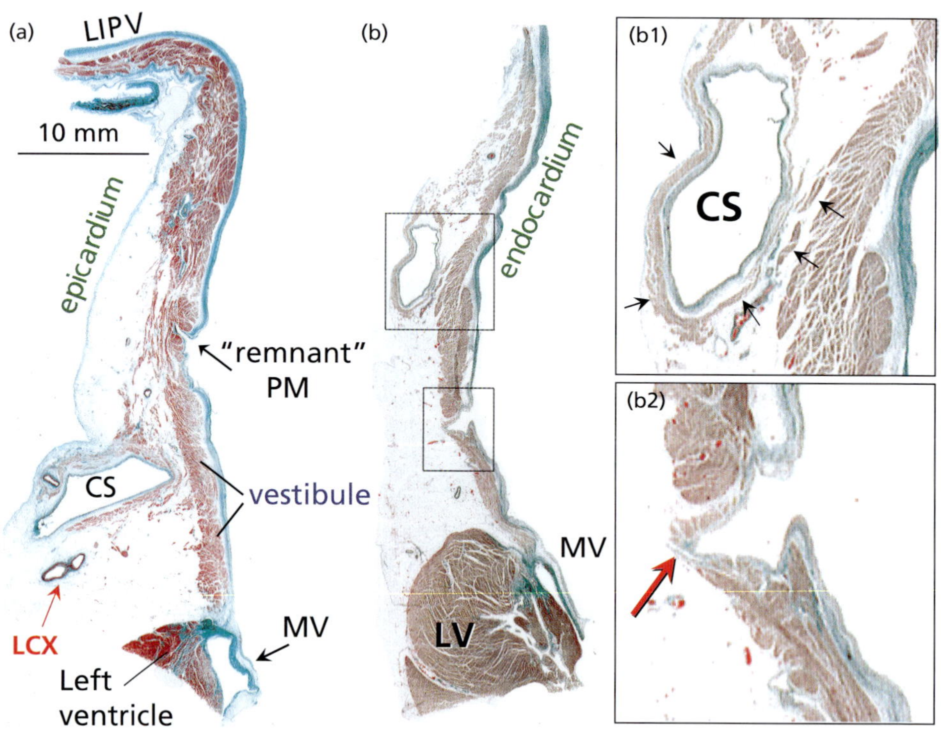

Figure 1.15 (a, b) Longitudinal sections at the mitral isthmus to illustrate its anatomic relations with the coronary sinus (CS) and circumflex artery (LCX). (b) The coronary sinus is surrounded by a sleeve of muscle from the left atrial wall (arrows in b1). Note in (b2) the space between the pectinate muscles where the left posterior atrial wall becomes thinner (red arrow). Note also the distance of the coronary sinus to the hingeline of the mitral valve. (Trichrome stain.) LIPV, left inferior pulmonary vein; LV, left ventricle; MV, mitral valve.

isthmus. The study by Becker showed that the mean myocardial thickness of the mitral isthmus at the level of the PV orifice was 3.0 mm (range 1.4–7.7 mm). The thickness midway in between the PV and the mitral annulus was 2.8 mm (range 1.2–4.4 mm) and that at the mitral valve annulus was 1.2 mm (range 0–3.2 mm) [85]. By contrast, a recent histological examination revealed that the thickest atrial wall was midway between the mitral annulus and the left inferior PV with tapering at either end of the isthmus [86]. Wittkampf et al. have suggested that the muscle sleeve around the coronary sinus and the close anatomic proximity of the circumflex artery are the two major anatomic determinants for the creation of mitral isthmus conduction block [86]. Atrial arteries fully embedded in atrial myocardium closer than 5 mm from the endocardium are likely to be damaged by transmural lesions. In addition, local cooling mediated by atrial arteries and veins may protect the surrounding left atrial myocardium, preventing the formation of transmural lesions by radiofrequency current applications, thus making it difficult or impossible for the creation of conduction block through the mitral isthmus. Also relevant is the presence of small crevices close to the base of the LAA that may entrap the tip of the ablation catheter, increasing the risk of isthmus perforation [86] (Figure 1.15).

During the ablation procedure, the position of the catheter introduced in the coronary sinus is used as an anatomic marker of the mitral annulus. However, previous anatomic studies showed that the great cardiac vein is not a good landmark to spot the mitral annulus [85,86]. This venous structure runs on the atrial side of the left atrioventricular groove at a considerable distance from the mitral annulus (6 mm in the most distal sector of the great cardiac vein, and up to 11 mm in the most proximal portion close to the ostium of the coronary sinus).

Architecture of the PV–atrial junction and left posterior atrial wall: relevance to atrial fibrillation ablation

Muscular myoarchitecture of the venoatrial junction and pulmonary veins

The presence of atrial myocardial tissue extending over the wall of the PVs has been confirmed both macroscopically and histologically by many investigators (Figure 1.16). The studies of Burch and Romey [87] and Nathan and Eliakim (88) in the mid 20th century drew attention to the potential function of these muscular sleeves. At that time, the role of myocardial sleeves in the pulmonary veins was thought to be that of a sphincter capable of acting like a "throttle valve" and causing pulmonary edema. It is also recognized that the PVs are capable of generating electrical impulses independently [89–91]. The venous wall in humans shows an innermost layer wall formed by a thin endothelium overlying an irregular media of connective tissue and smooth muscle cells, and a thick outer layer of fibrous adventitia. At the PV–atrial junction, the endocardium of the LA is in continuity with the

(a)

(b)

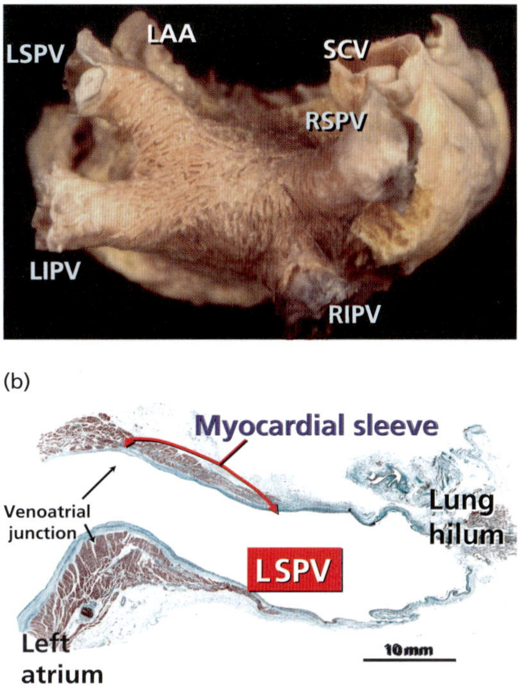

Figure 1.16 (a) Arrangement of the subepicardial myofibers around the pulmonary venous orifices. The myocardial tissue encircles the venoatrial junction forming the myocardial sleeve. The right superior pulmonary vein (RSPV) lies immediately behind the superior caval vein (SCV). (b) Histological longitudinal sections through a left superior pulmonary vein (LSPV). The myocardial sleeve extends over the wall of the PV from the LA. The sleeve are thicker at the venoatrial junction and thinner towards the lung hilum. LAA, left atrial appendage; LIPV, left inferior pulmonary vein; RIPV, right inferior pulmonary vein.

endothelial lining of the vein. The transition from the venous media to the left atrial subendocardial region is represented by a gradual decline in the number of smooth muscle cells. In most PVs (96%) the smooth muscle of the venous wall overlaps with a layer of myocardial bundles extending over the inner layer but is separated from it by a thin plane of fibro-fatty tissue. This intermediate myocardial layer, between the adventitia and the venous media, is the myocardial continuity from the left atrial wall (so-called myocardial sleeves) in a fine matrix composed of collagen, elastic fibers, and blood vessels [41,42]. Therefore, as seen in longitudinal sections, the extension of the left atrial musculature lies external to the venous wall and within the epicardium/adventitia.

In our histological study on 65 veins [42], the thickness of the smooth muscle ranged from 0.05 to 1 mm at the venoatrial junction, diminishing to 0.03–0.5 mm at a distance of 10 mm from the junction. The lengths of the sleeves varied from vein to vein, and the distal margins were irregular in most of the specimens, especially those of the inferior veins which tended to have less myocardial coverage than the superior veins. In keeping with previous anatomic studies, the sleeves in the superior right and left PVs were longer than those observed in the inferior veins. The sleeves were thickest at the venoatrial junction (1.88 ± 0.45 mm, range 1.2–2.8 mm) and then tapered toward the lung hilums, but the decrease in thickness was not uniform circumferentially. The atrial myocardial sleeves in the superior veins were thickest inferiorly (at 6 o'clock), and thinnest superiorly (at 12 o'clock), whereas an opposite pattern was found in the inferior veins. When superior and inferior veins were compared, the sleeves were thickest in the left superior veins. The mean thickness of adventitia and endocardium/venous wall also decreased from the venoatrial junction toward the lungs. Electrophysiological studies using a circular multielectrode catheter to obtain a circumferential mapping of the PVs demonstrated a non-homogeneous pattern of PV activation and revealed the presence of critical sites of atriovenous connection that enable us to achieve the electrical isolation of the PV without a circumferential ablation. Ablation confirms that these critical sites of myocardial venoatrial connection are most often located at the bottom of the superior PVs (85% of the cases) and at the top of inferior PVs (75% of the cases) [92].

The anatomic orientation of the myocardial fibers making up the sleeves is highly variable. Although the sleeves are mainly composed of circularly orientated bundles, oblique and longitudinally oriented fibers are also common [41,93]. These architectural observations are consistent with mapping studies of the PVs in the living human heart, demonstrating conduction patterns in a longitudinal and transverse direction [94]. A longitudinal pattern of activation is a strong predictor of ostial sites that require the application of ablative energy to electrically isolate the PV, whereas those with a transverse activation pattern are much less likely to require ablation. Recent electrophysiological studies in humans have demonstrated the presence of electrical conduction between the upper and lower left PVs, which may imply isolation of contiguous vessels from a single or circumscribed region to achieve complete PV electrical disconnection [95,96]. At the level of the venoatrial junction, we found in our specimens myocardial fibers crossing the isthmus between the superior and inferior venous orifices in both right and left PVs (Figure 1.17). These crossing fibers were found in 41% of the hearts at the level of the left PVs, and in the right PVs in 25% of hearts. Histological examinations showed that the myocardial fibers connecting the two contiguous PVs run along the posterior wall of the superior PVs and cross through the interpulmonary isthmus to the anterior margin of the inferior PV in 63% of hearts, whereas a reverse orientation (from anterior to posterior PV wall) was observed in another 37% of the connecting veins. The histological thickness of the crossing fibers showed variations in the maximal thickness at the venoatrial junctions ranging from 0.2 to 2.5 mm. The prevalence of muscular connections between the veins at the level of the venoatrial junction was independent of the distance between the orifices of the right and left PVs.

At the venoatrial junction, gaps of myocardial tissue of irregular morphology and small areas of myocardial degeneration with fibrous replacement can be found in 34% of the veins across the age range of the people from whom the specimens

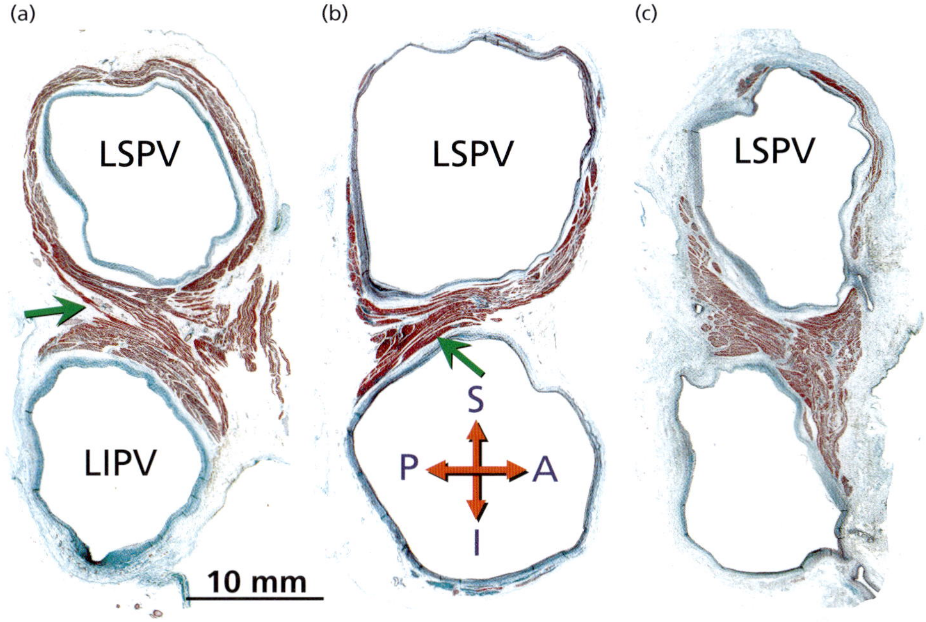

Figure 1.17 Histological cross-sections through three sets of left pulmonary veins (PVs) showing the variation in circumferential arrangement and thickness of the myocardial sleeves (a, b, c). The myocardial thickness varied from vein to vein and the sleeves are thicker in the area close to adjacent veins. The inferior veins have less myocardial coverage than the superior veins. (a, b) Myocardial fibers (green arrows) crossing the isthmus between the orifices of the left superior PV (LSPV) and left inferior PV (LIPV). (a) The fibers runs along the posterior wall of the superior PV crossing through the interpulmonary region to the anterior margin of the inferior PV; (b) a reverse orientation of the muscular connections.

were obtained [41] (Figure 1.18). The presence of collagenous septa between myocardial fibers may result in progressive electrical uncoupling of the side-to-side connections between groups of parallel atrial fibers. These findings are important, since they may be the basis for a non-uniform anisotropic conduction of a wavefront at a given area and for the development of reentry within smaller regions [97–99]. A recent postmortem morphological study found a higher incidence of myocardial sleeves with more severe discontinuity, hypertrophy, and fibrosis in patients with AF than in those without the latter arrhythmia [100]. Hocini et al. [101] correlated the conduction properties with the anatomic myofiber architecture of the canine pulmonary veins and showed zones of activation delay correlating with histological assessment of myofiber arrangement and distribution with sudden change in myocardial fiber orientation. These findings suggest that micro reentry could occur or promote the exit of activation from a focal source. In our series of structurally normal human hearts, we did not observe node-like cells or discrete tract of specialized myocites as found by other studies in animals [102] and humans [103].

Muscular myoarchitecture of the left posterior atrial wall

It is still unclear whether the initiation and maintenance of human AF depends on automatic focal or reentrant mechanisms. Initial catheter ablation approaches were aimed at obtaining an electrical disconnection of the PVs so as to isolate the LA from the venous triggers. Additional linear lesions targeting the region of the posterior left atrial wall have been shown to increase the success rate of catheter ablation in paroxysmal, persistent, and chronic AF. Recent reports have shown the contribution of different atrial regions on the fibrillatory process and to the maintenance of AF, emphasizing the role of structural discontinuities and heterogeneous fiber orientation favoring anatomic reentry or anchoring rotors [17–23]. Modification of the

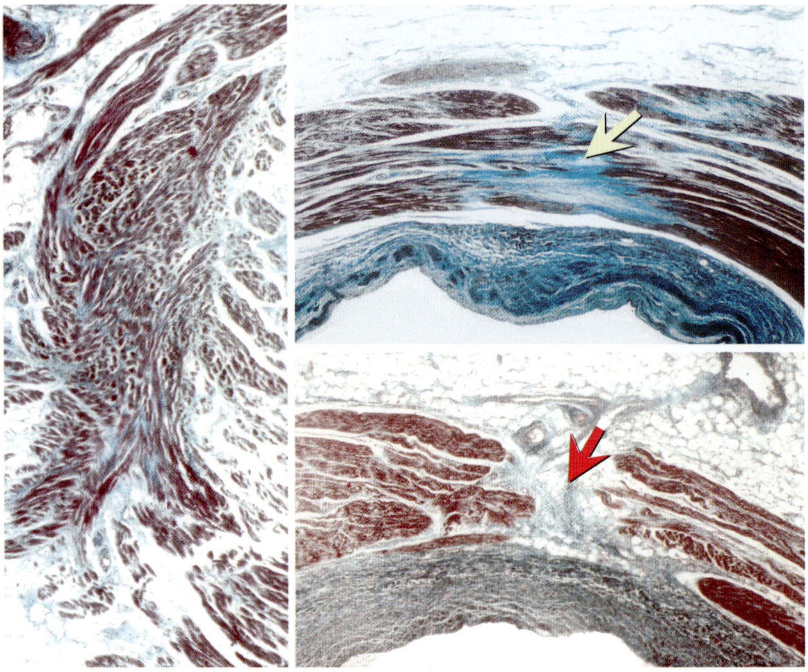

Figure 1.18 (a) Histological longitudinal section of the myocardial sleeve of the right superior PV at the venoatrial junction. Note the mixed arrangement of myocardial fibers making up the myocardial sleeves. (b, c) Cross-sections illustrating a small area of myocardial degeneration with fibrous replacement (yellow arrow, b) and the presence of gaps of connective tissue bridges between the myocardial fibers (red arrow, c)

atrial substrate by targeting structures of the LA that are thought to maintain AF appears to increase success rates. The posterior wall of the LA, for example, seems to play an important role in maintaining AF. Morillo et al. reported in a canine model of AF that cryoablation at sites of short cycle length activity in the posterior LA resulted in the interruption of this arrhythmia [104]. Observations from the laboratory of Jalife and co-workers [105–107] demonstrated in the isolated sheep heart the presence of a small number of stable ongoing circuits generating high frequency waves and providing a base to generate fibrillatory conduction. Data derived from high resolution optical mapping in this animal model also showed that the focal sources correspond to single or a small number of reentrant rotors discharging at a high frequency and that these are localized in the PV orifices or at the contiguous posterior left atrial region. Postmortem examination in human specimens, showed in most hearts an abrupt change of subendocardial fiber orientation (circumferential, oblique, and longitudinal) in the posterior wall of the LA at the venoatrial junctions (Figure 1.19). In these areas the subendocardial fibers are usually looplike extensions from the longitudinal fibers encircling the venoatrial junctions [40]. Also relevant is the finding of changes in myoarchitecture transmurally. Histology confirmed the changes in fiber orientation in the subendocardium and also revealed crossover arrangements deeper in the wall. The most obvious broad band or linear anatomic barrier of longitudinal and oblique fibers was formed by the "septopulmonary bundle" that also marked a change in LA wall thickness. This was thicker toward the septum (1.4 ± 0.5 mm) and thinner laterally (0.7 ± 0.4 mm). Left atrial endocardial activation was mapped in 19 patients with a percutaneous non-contact mapping system during episodes of focal initiation of AF [108]. In this study Markides et al. observed that the pattern of LA activation was predominantly determined by a principal line of conduction block [108]. It appears to be related to the linear anatomic barrier identified by the examination of fiber orientation. Another area of change in subendocardial fiber orientation was observed adjacent to the anterior mitral valve annulus in seven of 10 hearts, whereas abundant

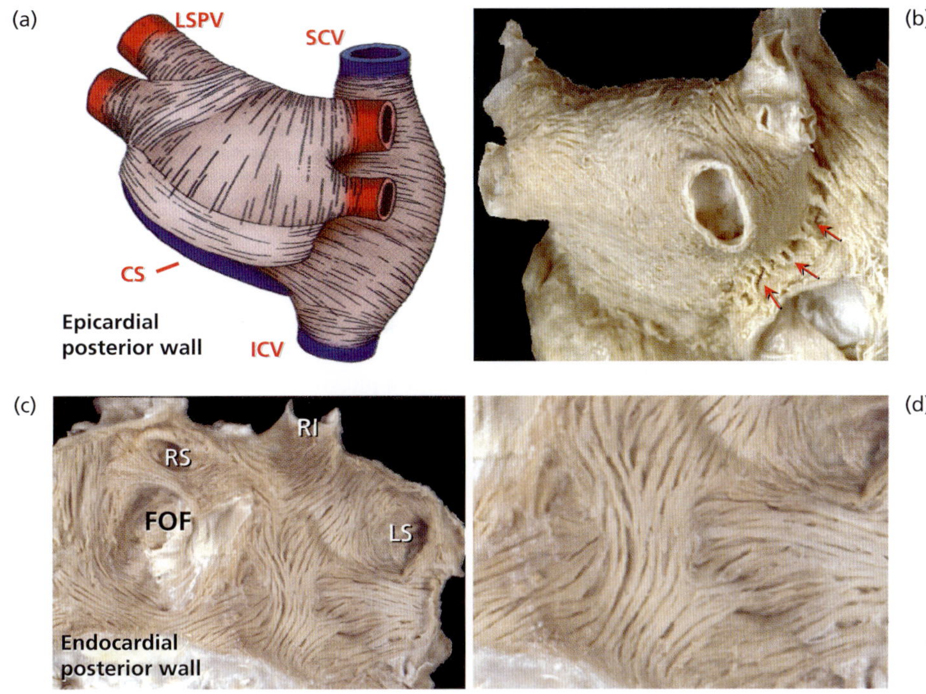

Figure 1.19 Schematic representation of the general arrangement of myocardial fibers (a) and subepicardial dissection seen from the postero-epicardial aspect (b). Note in (b) the interatrial muscular bridges (arrows) crossing the septal raphe. (c, d) Dissection of the subendocardium showing the abrupt change of subendocardial fiber orientation in the posterior region of the LA. (d) Enlarged figure showing the predominantly longitudinal orientation of the myocardial fibers of the posterior left atrial wall encircling the orifice of the PV subendocardially. CS, coronary sinus inferior; FOF, flap oval fossa; ICV, inferior caval vein; LS, left superior pulmonary vein; LSPV, left superior pulmonary vein; RI, right inferior pulmonary vein; RS, right superior pulmonary vein; SCV, superior caval vein.

fatty tissue was observed above the posterior mitral valve annulus in six of 10 hearts [108].

The coronary sinus

The topic of early recurrence of AF after catheter ablation is far from being settled. It has been said that early recurrence is due to recovery of conduction of previously isolated PVs and in some cases to the existence of non-PV foci that were not properly identified at the initial ablation session. Non-PV foci can be located at the posterior LA wall close to the orifices of the PVs or be related to non-pulmonary thoracic veins such as caval veins, the oblique vein of Marshall, or the musculature lining of the coronary sinus [27–32].

The coronary sinus runs along the inferior aspect of the LA and opens into the right atrium through an ostium. The oblique vein of Marshall and the valve of Vieussens (found in 87% of patients) can been used as anatomic landmarks to define the distal limits of the coronary sinus from the ostium of the coronary venous system [109] (see Figure 1.13). The inferior portion of the vestibular component of the LA (smooth circumferential area surrounding the orifice of the mitral valve) directly apposes the wall of the coronary sinus. Here, posteriorly and parietally, the atrial wall is thin and overlies the great cardiac vein. The coronary sinus, and its continuation into the great cardiac vein, has it own muscular wall that increases in thickness the closer it is to its ostium in the right atrium. These muscular sleeves extend from the ostium to 25–52 mm distally along the wall of the coronary sinus [109]. Frequently, small tongues of myocardial fibers extend from the coronary sinus to insert into the posterior and inferior wall of the left atrium (Figure 1.19).

Electrophysiological studies have also demonstrated the electrical connection between the right atrium and LA through the musculature of the coronary sinus [110,111]. Recent observations have identified focal sources of premature depolarizations originating within the coronary sinus that may trigger AF [29]. It has been suggested that electrical disconnection of the two atria targeting the interatrial connections diminishes the electrophysiological substrate for perpetuation of AF [29,112].

The esophagus and other extracardiac structures

As repeatedly stated, catheter ablation techniques in patients with AF have progressively evolved to more extensive procedures. Two of the most widely used approaches involve not only circumferential ablation around the PVs but also the performance of linear lesions between the encircled PV orifices and between the left lower PV and the mitral annulus. These linear lesions involve the posterior wall of the LA. In addition, catheter ablation tools capable of creating larger and deeper lesions are increasingly used to reduce the number of pulses and the duration of the procedure and to assure transmurality of the ablation. The current approaches creating linear lesions on the posterior LA wall, in combination with tools capable of generating deeper lesions, has resulted in new, albeit rare, complications for catheter ablation of AF: atrioesophageal fistula, vagal injury resulting in gastric hypomotility, and phrenic nerve injury resulting in diaphragmatic paralysis [34–36].

Morphological relation between the esophagus and posterior left atrial wall

The development of an atrioesophageal fistula after catheter ablation in the posterior wall of the LA is probably the most severe complication that has been encountered in patients subjected to an ablation procedure. Understanding the spatial relations between the esophagus and the LA is essential to reduce risk.

The esophagus descends in virtual contact with the posterior LA. In its upper course, the esophagus is situated slightly to the left between the trachea and the vertebral column (see Figure 1.7). It then passes behind the LA and to the right of the aortic arch to descend to the posterior mediastinum along the right side of the descending thoracic aorta. In a recent anatomic study we examined the course of the esophagus in 15 cadavers [52]. The length of the esophagus in contact with the posterior LA ranged between 30 and 53 mm (mean 42 ± 7 mm). Transversely, the width of the esophagus in contact with the posterior LA wall was 13. ± 5 mm (range 9–15.5 mm) (Figures 1.20 and 1.21). It is important to recognize that the esophagus follows a variable course along the posterior aspect of the LA. It was < 5 mm from the endocardium in 40% of specimens. In 40% of cases it passed along the middle portion of the posterior LA wall (Figure 1.20). In 20% of specimens it descended close to the right venoatrial junction; in the remaining cases it had a leftward course close to the left venoatrial junction [52]. However, the esophagus coursed obliquely from left superior to right inferior in 36% of patients, and can move during the ablation procedure from one side to the other [113]. Being able to image the esophagus during the procedure can reduce the risk of damaging it.

Behind the posterior left atrial wall is a layer of fibrous pericardium and fibro-fatty tissue of irregular thickness that contains esophageal arteries and

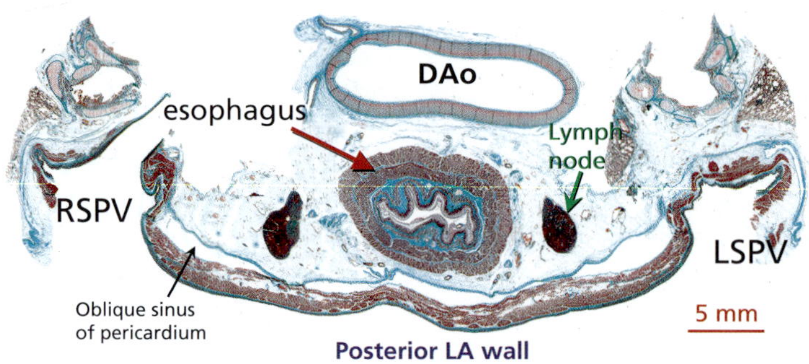

Figure 1.20 Transverse histological sections (Masson's trichrome stain) showing the proximity of the esophagus to the middle of the posterior wall of the left atrium (LA). DAo, descending aorta; LSPV, left superior pulmonary vein; RSPV, right superior pulmonary vein.

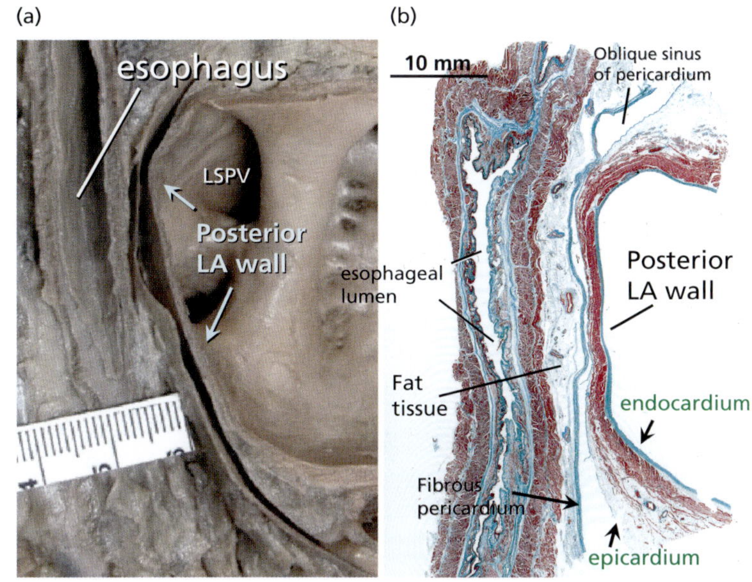

Figure 1.21 (a) Sagittal section through the left atrium (LA) and esophagus showing how the esophagus is related to the middle of the posterior wall of the LA. (b) Histological section (Masson's trichrome stain) in similar orientation showing the fibrous pericardium between the posterior left atrial wall and the esophageal wall and the fatty tissue plane immediately behind that. LSPV, left superior pulmonary vein.

the vagus nerve plexus (Figures 1.20–1.22). These anatomic structures may be affected by ablative procedures. It has been shown that radiofrequency may substantially elevate the temperature within the esophageal lumen and that atrioesophageal fistulae may result from this thermal injury. The heat from the probe may also result in subacute inflammatory reaction of the esophageal wall. Overlapping lines in the posterior wall may have been responsible for esophageal injury. Thus, the investigators recommend avoiding excessively deep lesions by decreasing the power, temperature, and duration of radiofrequency energy application. The posterior left atrial wall is significantly thinner at the superior part of the LA (2.2 ± 0.5 mm in the left venoatrial junction) [52] (Figure 1.21). The esophagus is not in direct contact with the roof of the LA, thus some investigators also suggest that the posterior ablation line should be placed at the LA roof to avoid esophageal injury.

Anatomic risk of phrenic nerve injury

A few instances of phrenic nerve injury have been reported after catheter ablation. The incidence of this complication seems to depend on the type of ablation source: 0.1% using radiofrequency energy, 0.6% utilizing cryothermal ablation, 6% with ultrasound approaches, and 5% using laser energy [37,38]. The right phrenic nerve has a close anatomic relationship with the superior caval vein (minimum distance 0.3 ± 0.5 mm) and the right superior pulmonary vein (minimum distance 2.1 ± 0.4 mm) as it runs through the lateral and posterolateral wall of the right atrium [114,115] (Figure 1.23). In 32% of our unselected human heart specimens the anterior wall of the right superior PV was < 2 mm from the right phrenic nerve [115]. Consequently, catheter ablation techniques aimed at modifying the sinus node function at the lateral right atrium and catheter ablation for AF at the orifice and adjacent area of the right superior PV carry a certain risk of injuring the right phrenic nerve [37].

On the other hand, the left phrenic nerve is in the vicinity of the lateral vein of the heart, the great cardiac vein, the left atrial appendage, and the lateral wall of the left ventricle. We observed that the left phrenic nerve passed over the left atrial appendage and descended along the obtuse cardiac margin in relation with the left obtuse marginal vein (minimum distance 3.5 ± 0.5 mm) in 79% of our specimens (Figure 1.24). In the remaining specimens, its course was anterosuperior, passing over the main

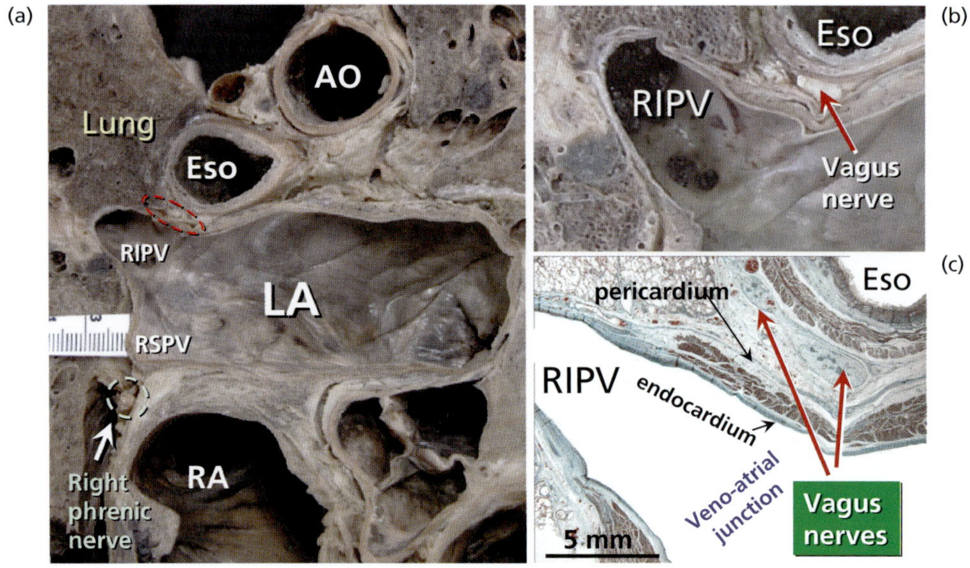

Figure 1.22 An overview of a transthoracic section through the mediastinum showing the locations of the vagus nerves (red dashed circle) and the phrenic nerve (green dashed circle) relative to the PVs and left atrium (LA). (b) A close-up of the right inferior venoatrial junction. (c) A corresponding histological section (trichrome stain). AO, aorta; Eso, esophagus; RA, right atrium; RIPV, right inferior pulmonar vein; RSPV, right superior pulmonary vein.

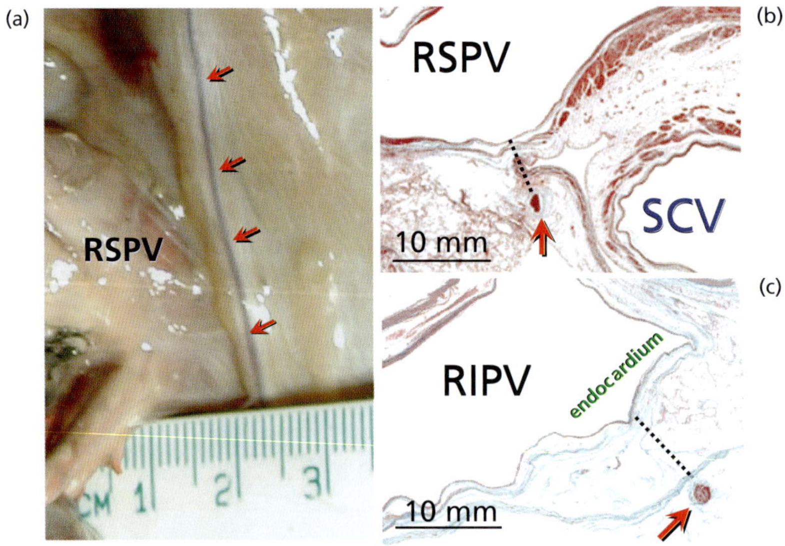

Figure 1.23 (a) Dissection of the right superior pulmonary vein (RSPV) close to the right phrenic nerve (red arrows). (b, c) Histological sections through the RSPV and right inferior pulmonary vein (RIPV), respectively. The right phrenic nerve (red arrows) is adherent to the fibrous pericardium (stained green). The broken lines indicate the distance between the endocardium of the right PVs and the right phrenic nerve. (Masson's trichrome stain.) SCV, superior caval vein.

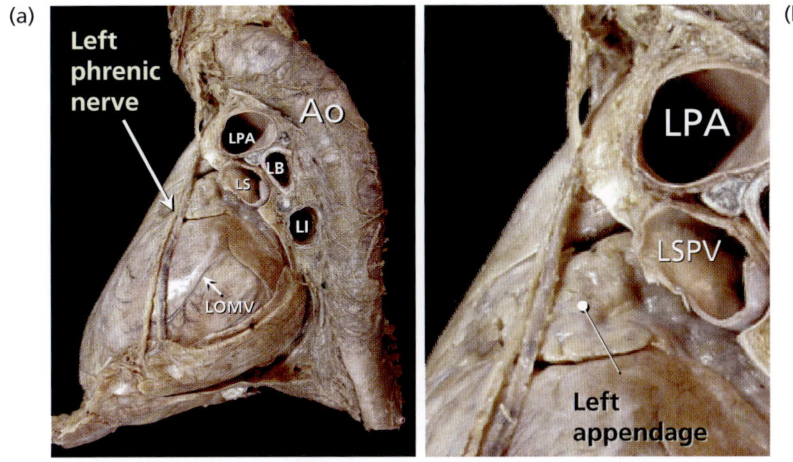

Figure 1.24 (a, b) Left lateral view of the heart showing the close anatomic relation of the left phrenic nerve with the LAA and the left obtuse marginal vein (LOMV). Ao, aorta; LB, left bronchus; LI, left inferior pulmonary vein; LPA, left pulmonary artery; LS, left superior pulmonary vein; LSPV, left superior pulmonary vein.

stem of the left coronary artery or the anterior descending artery and the great cardiac vein (minimum distance 1.4 ± 0.3 mm). Catheter ablation or pacing close to these areas may cause injury of the left phrenic nerve [116]. In the human clinical setting, transient phrenic nerve paresis has been observed during cryoablation of the right superior pulmonary vein in 2% of patients [117]; others [116] have reported functional recovery from phrenic nerve injury, although two of 17 patients developed pulmonary complications, with one needing a recovery period of up to 28 months. Recurrent pneumonia and dependence on mechanical ventilation are serious complications that can lead to a vicious circle.

Anatomic relations between the left atrium and the neighboring vagus nerves

Thermal injury may involve the periesophageal vagal nerves, resulting in acute pyloric spasm and gastric hypomotility [39]. The vagus nerves pass behind the root of the lungs and form the right and left posterior pulmonary plexuses [40]. From the caudal part of the left pulmonary plexus two branches descend on the anterior surface of the esophagus, joining with a branch from the right pulmonary plexus to form the anterior esophageal plexus. The anterior esophageal plexus passes external to the pericardial sac but in very close proximity to the posterior and the right and left venoatrial junctions (Figure 1.25). The posterior and anterior esophageal plexuses enter the abdomen through the diaphragm to become the posterior and anterior vagal trunks that innervate the pyloric sphincter and the gastric antrum. Shah et al. [39] recently reported four patients who underwent ablation of the ostial PVs and posterior LA who experienced an acute delayed gastric emptying syndrome 3–48 h after the procedure. Our observation on seven normal cadavers revealed a mean distance between the bundles of the anterior esophageal plexus and the posterior left atrial endocardium of 4.1 ± 1.4 mm (range 2.5–6.5 mm) [118] (see Figure 1.22).

Left atrial autonomic nervous system content

Experimental studies have shown that initiation and maintenance of AF can be enhanced by both parasympathetic and sympathetic stimulation [119–127]. Elvan et al. [120] in an animal model of AF by atrial and cervical vagal stimulation abolished induction of sustained AF by circumferential ablation of the PVs. Schauerte et al. [122] also demonstrated in dogs that selective vagal denervation along the right pulmonary artery prevents vagal-induced AF. In patients with AF, Pappone et al. [24] have shown that complete vein denervation is an additional predictor of long-term benefit

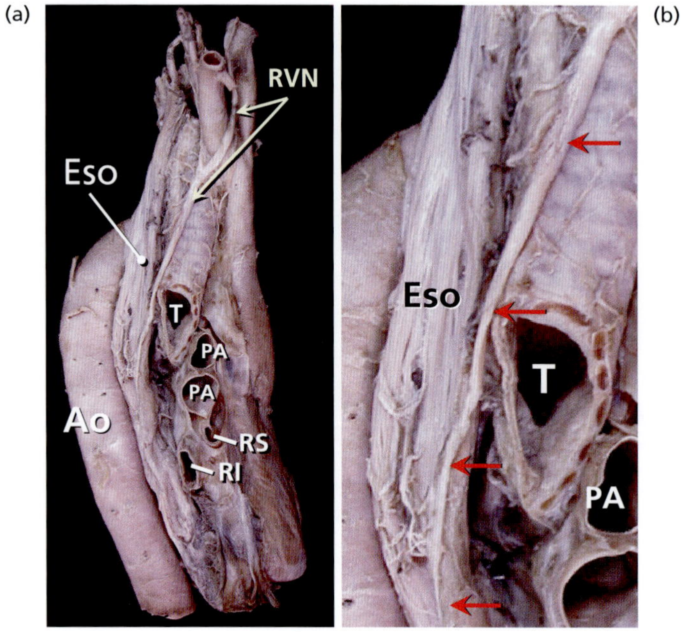

Figure 1.25 (a) Posterior view of the esophagus (Eso), descending thoracic aorta (Ao), and trachea (T) to show the course of the esophagus and its relationship with the right vagus nerve (RVN). (b) Enlarged figure with the right vagus nerve indicated (red arrows). PA, pulmonary artery; RI, right inferior pulmonary vein; RS, right superior pulmonary vein.

after circumferential PV ablation of AF. More recently, Scanavacca et al. [25] have demonstrated that catheter ablation of selected atrial sites where high frequency stimulation induced vagal reflexes, may prevent AF recurrence in patients with vagal-induced paroxysmal AF. The above studies represent an additional piece of the complex and still unassembled puzzle that is the pathophysiology of AF, and reinforce the need of revisiting the anatomy of the autonomic nervous system elements of the LA.

Abundant nerves and ganglions of the autonomic nervous system are present at the junction between the PVs and the LA, and some more distally inside the vein. A regional distribution of the cardiac nerves and differential patterns of innervation have been observed in mammalian hearts. In the human LA, ganglionated plexuses were observed in the superior surface between the PVs and in the posterior aspect of the LA. Preganglionic parasympathetic fibers and postganglionic sympathetic fibers come together in the fat pads on the epicardial surface of the posterior LA wall [123]. Histochemical studies for acetylcholinesterase have shown epicardial ganglionated nerves that extend through three neural pathways or subplexuses in the LA: the left ventral, left dorsal, and middle dorsal. Interestingly the left dorsal subplexus extends over the area of the vein of Marshall along the epicardial aspect of the left posterolateral ridge [124].

Chiou et al. [125] showed that transmural lesions were needed to denervate the atria, and it was felt that the autonomic nervous system elements were mainly present subepicardially rather than endocardially. However, the presence of innervation within the myocardium of the LA suggests that non-transmural lesions may have an impact on atrial innervation. A quantitative histological evaluation identified gradients of innervation in the LA and in the PVs [126]. This study showed that the greatest nerve densities were found in the left and posterior parts of the LA and at the antrum of the PVs. Left-sided PVs had a more dense content of nervous system elements than the right-sided veins, and the density of innervation was higher at the orifices of the PVs than in their distal segments. In a recent immunohistochemical study, Tan et al. [127] have demonstrated that adrenergic and cholinergic nerve densities are highest within 5 mm of the junction between the PVs and the LA and that because both sympathetic and parasympathetic elements are highly co-located, it is impossible to define areas for a selective vagal or sympathetic ablation.

Conclusion

In one and a half decades catheter ablation has been shown to be an increasingly important therapeutic option for patients with paroxysmal, persistent, and chronic atrial fibrillation. Ablation techniques have evolved from rather limited initial approaches to quite extensive atrial interventions. In spite of more or less substantial differences among the various techniques that are currently utilized worldwide, results seem to be uniformly similar with success rates in the range of 70–90%. Because the amount of myocardium that is ablated at the present time is more extensive, the rate and type of complications of ablation in AF might also be larger. The time has come to ascertain if some of these approaches are unnecessarily extensive. We are far from being able to answer this question but we believe that the refinement and tuning of catheter ablation techniques for atrial fibrillation has to come from a better understanding of the anatomo-functional substrate of the arrhythmia. In this chapter we have reviewed the gross morphological details of the PV orifices and their neighboring left atrial landmarks and the myocardial architecture of the venoatrial junction and the posterior atrial wall. In addition, we described the anatomy and architecture of the left atrial appendage, the left posterolateral ridge, the vein of Marshall, and the coronary sinus. Finally, the autonomic innervation of the atria, as well as the relations between the left atrium and the pulmonary veins with the extracardiac structures, are also described.

References

1 Jais P, Haissaguerre M, Shah DC, et al. A focal source of atrial fibrillation treated by discrete radiofrequency ablation. *Circulation* 1997;**95**:572–6.
2 Haïssaguerre M, Jais P, Shah DC, et al. Spontaneous initiation of atrial fibrillation by ectopic beats originating in the pulmonary veins. *N Engl J Med* 1998;**339**: 659–66.
3 Chen SA, Hsieh MH, Tai CT et al. Initiation of atrial fibrillation by ectopic beats originating from the pulmonary veins: electrophysiological characteristics, pharmacologic responses and effects of radiofrequency ablation. *Circulation* 1999;**100**:1879–86.
4 Haissaguerre M, Jais P, Shah DC, et al. Catheter ablation of chronic atrial fibrillation targeting the reinitiating triggers. *J Cardiovasc Electrophysiol* 2000;**11**:2–10.
5 Chen SA, Tai CT, Tsai CF, et al. Radiofrequency catheter ablation of atrial fibrillation initiated by pulmonary vein ectopic beats. *J Cardiovasc Electrophysiol* 2000;**11**:218–27.
6 Haissaguerre M, Shah DC, Jais P, et al. Electrophysiological breakthroughs from the left atrium to the pulmonary veins. *Circulation* 2000;**102**:2463–5.
7 Haissaguerre M, Jais P, Shah DC, et al. Electrophysiological end point for catheter ablation of atrial fibrillation initiated from multiple pulmonary venous foci. *Circulation* 2000;**101**:1409–17.
8 Oral H, Knight BP, Tada H, et al. Pulmonary vein isolation for paroxysmal and persistent atrial fibrillation. *Circulation* 2002;**105**:1077–81.
9 Ernst S, Schluter M, Ouyang F, et al. Modification of the substrate for maintenance of idiopathic human atrial fibrillation: efficacy of radiofrequency ablation using nonfluoroscopic catheter guidance. *Circulation* 1999; **100**:2085–92.
10 Pappone C, Rosanio S, Oreto G, et al. Circumferential radiofrequency ablation of pulmonary vein ostia. *Circulation* 2000;**102**:2619–28.
11 Pappone C, Oreto G, Rosanio S, et al. Atrial electroanatomic remodeling after circumferential radiofrequency pulmonary vein ablation: efficacy of an anatomic approach in a large cohort of patients with atrial fibrillation. *Circulation* 2001;**104**(21):2539–44.
12 Oral H, Sharf C, Chugh A, et al. Catheter ablation for paroxysmal atrial fibrillation. Segmental pulmonary vein ostial ablation versus left atrial ablation. *Circulation* 2003;**108**:2355–60.
13 Jais P, Hocini M, Sanders P, et al. Technique and results of linear ablation at the mitral isthmus. *Circulation* 2004;**110**:2996–3002.
14 Ernst S, Ouyan F, Lober F, et al. Catheter-induced linear lesions in the left atrium in patients with atrial fibrillation: an electroanatomic study. *J Am Coll Cardiol* 2003;**42**:1271–82.
15 Ouyang F, Bansch D, Ernst S, et al. Complete isolation of left atrium surrounding the pulmonary veins. New insights from the double-lasso technique in paroxysmal atrial fibrillation. *Circulation* 2004;**110**:2090–6.
16 Jais P, Haisaguerre M, Shah DC, et al. Regional disparities of endocardial atrial activation in paroxysmal atrial fibrillation. *Pacing Clin Electrophysiol* 1996;**19**:1998–2003.
17 Todd DM, Skanes AC, Guiraudon G, et al. Role of the posterior left atrium and pulmonary veins in human lone atrial fibrillation: electrophysiological and pathological data from patients undergoing atrial fibrillation surgery. *Circulation* 2003;**108**:3108–14.
18 Nademanee K, McKenzie J, Kosar E, et al. A new approach for catheter ablation of atrial fibrillation:

mapping of the electrophysiological substrate. *J Am Coll Cardiol* 2004;**43**:2044–53.

19 Haissaguerre M, Sanders P, Hocini M, et al. Catheter ablation of long-lasting persistent atrial fibrillation: critical structures for termination. *J Cardiovasc Electrophysiol* 2005;**16**:1125–37.

20 Sanders P, Berenfeld O, Hocini M, et al. Spectral analysis identifies sites of high frequency activity maintaining atrial fibrillation in humans. *Circulation* 2005;**112**: 789–97.

21 Haissaguerre M, Hocini M, Sanders P, et al. Localized fibrillatory sources maintaining atrial fibrillation. *Heart Rhythm* 2005;2:S20.

22 Rostock T, Rotter M, Sanders P, et al. Fibrillating areas isolated within the left atrium after radiofrequency liner catheter ablation. *J Cardiovasc Electrophysiol* 2006;**17**: 1–6.

23 Haisaguerre M, Hocini M, Sanders P, et al. Localized sources maintaining atrial fibrillation organized by prior ablation. *Circulation* 2006;**113**:616–25.

24 Pappone C, Santinelli V, Manguso F, et al. Pulmonary vein denervation enhances long-term benefit after circumferential ablation for paroxysmal atrial fibrillation. *Circulation* 2004;**109**:327–34.

25 Scanavacca M, Pisani C, Hachul D, et al. Selective atrial vagal denervation guided by evoked vagal reflex to treat patients with paroxysmal atrial fibrillation. *Circulation* 2006;**114**:876–85.

26 Jais P, Shah DC, Haisaguerre M, et al. Efficacy and safety of septal and left-atrial linear ablation for atrial fibrillation. *Am J Cardiol* 1999;**84**:139R–146R.

27 Chen PS, Wu TJ, Hwang C, et al. Thoracic veins and the mechanism on non-paroxysmal atrial fibrillation. *Cardiovas Res* 2002;**54**:295–301.

28 Tsai CF, Tai CT, Hsieh MH, et al. Initiation of atrial fibrillation by ectopic beats originating from the superior vena cava: electrophysiological characteristic and results of radiofrequency ablation. *Circulation* 2000; **102**:67–74.

29 Oral H, Ozaydin M, Chugh A, et al. Role of the coronary sinus in maintenance of atrial fibrillation. *Cardiovasc Electrophysiol* 2003;**14**:1329–36.

30 Hwang C, Wu TJ, Doshi RN, et al. Vein of Marshall cannulation for the analysis of electrical activity in patients with focal atrial fibrillation. *Circulation* 2000;**101**: 1503–5.

31 Katritsis D, Ioannidis JPA, Anagnostopoulos CE, et al. Identification and catheter ablation of extracardiac and intracardiac components of ligaments of Marshall tissue for treatment of paroxysmal atrial fibrillation. *J Cardiovasc Electrophysiol* 2001;**12**:750–8.

32 Takahashi Y, Sanders P, Rotter M, et al. Disconnection of the left atrial appendage for elimination of foci maintaining atrial fibrillation. *J Cardiovasc Electrophysiol* 2005;**16**:917–19.

33 Cappato R, Clakins H, Chen SA, et al. Worldwide survey on the methods, efficacy, and safety of catheter ablation for human atrial fibrillation. *Circulation* 2005;**111**: 1100–5.

34 Scanavacca MI, Dávila A, Parga J, et al. Left atrial-esophageal fistula following radiofrequency ablation of atrial fibrillation. *Cardiovasc Electrophysiol* 2004;**15**: 960–2.

35 Pappone C, Oral H, Santinelli V, et al. Atrio-esophageal fistula as a complication of percutaneous transcatheter ablation of atrial fibrillation. *Circulation* 2004;**109**: 2724–6.

36 Cummings JE, Schweikert RA, Saliba W, et al. Brief communication: atrial-esophageal fistulas after radiofrequency ablation. Ann Intern Med 2006;**144**:572–4.

37 Lee BK, Choi KJ, Kim J, et al. Right phrenic nerve injury following electrical disconnection of the right superior pulmonary vein. *Pacing Clin Electrophysiol* 2004;**27**: 1444–6.

38 Sacher F, Monahan K, Thomas S, et al. Phrenic nerve injury after atrial fibrillation catheter ablation. *J Am Coll Cardiol* 2006;**47**:2498–503.

39 Shah D, Dumonceau JM, Burri H, et al. Acute pyloric spasm and gastric hypomotility: an extracardiac adverse effect of percutaneous radiofrequency ablation for atrial fibrillation. *J Am Coll Cardiol* 2005;**46**:327–30.

40 Pai R, Boyle N, Child J, et al. Transient left recurrent laryngeal nerve palsy following catheter ablation of atrial fibrillation. *Heart Rhythm* 2005;**2**:182–4.

41 Ho SY, Sánchez-Quintana D, Cabrera JA, et al. Anatomy of the left atrium: implication for radiofrequency ablation of atrial fibrillation. *J Cardiovasc Electrophysiol* 1999;**10**:1525–33.

42 Ho SY, Cabrera JA, Tran VH, et al. Architecture of the pulmonary veins: relevance to radiofrequency ablation. *Heart* 2001;**86**:265–70.

43 Farré J, Anderson RH, Cabrera JA, et al. Fluoroscopic cardiac anatomy for catheter ablation of tachycardia. *Pacing Clin Electrophysiol* 2002;**25**:79–94.

44 Ho SY, Cabrera JA, Sánchez-Quintana D. Anatomy of the pulmonary vein-atrium junction. In: Chen SA, Haissaguerre M, Zipes D, eds. *Throracic Vein Arrhythmias. Mechanism and Treatment*. Blackwell Futura, Massachusetts, 2004:42–53.

45 Farré J, Cabrera JA, Sánchez-Quintana D, et al. Fluoroscopic and angiographic heart anatomy for catheter mapping and ablation of arrhythmias. In: Huan ST, Wood MA, eds. *Catheter Ablation of Cardiac Arrhythmias*. Saunder Elsevier, Philadelphia, 2006:85–106.

46 Visible Human Slice and Surface Server. Available at http://visiblehuman.epfl.ch.

47 Sánchez-Quintana D, Ho SY, Cabrera JA, et al. Topograhic anatomy of the inferior pyramidal space: relevante to radiofrequency catheter ablation. *J Cardiovasc Electrophysiol* 2001;**2**:210–17.
48 Anderson RH, Webb S, Brown NA. Clinical anatomy of the atrial septum with reference to its developmental components. *Clin Anat* 1999;**12**:362–74.
49 De Ponti R, Zardini M, Storti C, et al. Trans-septal catheterization for radiofrequency catheter ablation of cardiac arrhythmias. Results and safety of a simplified method. *Eur Heart J* 1998;**19**:943–50.
50 Schwinger ME, Tunick PA, Freedberg RS, Kronzon I. Vegetations on endocardial surfaces struck by regurgitant jets: diagnosis by transesophageal echocardiography. *Am Heart J* 1990;**119**:1212–15.
51 Ho SY, Anderson RH, Sánchez-Quintana D. Atrial structure and fibres: morphological basis of atrial conduction. *Cardiovasc Res* 2002;**54**:325–36.
52 Sánchez-Quintana D, Cabrera JA, Climent V, et al. Anatomic relations between the esophagus and left atrium and relevance for ablation of atrial fibrillation. *Circulation* 2005;**112**:1400–5.
53 Cabrera JA, Sánchez-Quintana D, Farré J, et al. Ultrasonic characterization of the pulmonary venous wall. Echographic and histological correlation. *Circulation* 2002;**106**:968–73.
54 Bachmann G. The inter-auricular time interval. *Am J Physiol* 1916;**41**:309–20.
55 Papez JW. Heart musculature of the atria. *Am J Anat* 1920;**27**:255–85.
56 Wittkampf FH, Vonken EJ, Derksen R, et al. Pulmonary vein ostium geometry: analysis by magnetic resonance angiography. *Circulation* 2003;**107**:21–3.
57 Kato R, Lickfett L, Meininger G, et al. Pulmonary vein anatomy in patients undergoing catheter ablation of atrial fibrillation: lessons learned by use of magnetic resonance imaging. *Circulation* 2003;**107**:2004–10.
58 Tsao HM, Yu WC, Cheng HC, et al. Pulmonary vein dilation in patients with atrial fibrillation: detection by magnetic resonance imaging. *J Cardiovasc Electrophysiol* 2001;**12**:809–13.
59 Scharf C, Sneider M, Case I, et al. Anatomy of the pulmonary veins in patients with atrial fibrillation and effects of segmental ostial ablation analysed by computed tomography. *J Cardiovasc Electrophysiol* 2003;**14**:150–5.
60 Lin WS, Prakash VS, Tai CT, et al. Pulmonary vein morphology in patients with paroxysmal atrial fibrillation initiated by ectopic beats originating from the pulmonary veins: implications for catheter ablation. *Circulation* 2000;**101**:1274–81.
61 Mansour M, Refaat M, Heist EK, et al. Three-dimensional anatomy of the left atrium by magnetic resonance angiography: implication for catheter ablation for atrial fibrillation. *J Cardiovasc Electrophysiol* 2006;**17**: 719–23.
62 Schmidt B, Ernst S, Ouyang F, et al. External and endoluminal analysis of left atrial anatomy and the pulmonary veins in three-dimensional reconstruction of magnetic resonance angiography: the full insight from inside. *J Cardiovasc Electrophysiol* 2006;**17**:957–64.
63 Wongcharoen W, Tsao HM, Wu MH, et al. Morphologic characteristics of the left atrial appendage, roof, and septum: implication. *J Cardiovasc Electrophysiol* 2006;**17**:951–6.
64 Cosio FG, Anderson RH, Kuck KH, et al. Living anatomy of the atrioventricular junctions: a guide to electrophysiologic mapping. A consensus from the Cardiac Nomenclature Study Group, Working Group of Arrhythmias, European Society of Cardiology, and the Task Force on Cardiac Nomenclature from NASPE. *Circulation* 1999;**100**:e31.
65 Petersen P, Kastrup J, Brinch K, et al. Relation between left atrial dimension and duration of atrial fibrillation. *Am J Cardiol* 1987;**60**:382–4.
66 Yamane T, Shah DC, Jais P, et al. Dilatation as a marker of pulmonary veins initiating atrial fibrillation. *J Interv Cardiac Electrophysiol* 2002;**6**:245–9.
67 Keith A. An account of the structures concerned in the production of the jugular pulse. *J Anat Physiol* 1907;**42**:1–25.
68 Sharma S, Devine W, Anderson RH. The determination of atrial arrangement by examination of appendage morphology in 1842 heart specimens. *Br Heart J* 1988;**60**:227–31.
69 Veinot J, Harrity P, Gentile F, et al. Anatomy of the normal left atrial appendage. A quantitative study of age-related changes in 500 autopsy hearts: implications for echocardiographic examination. *Circulation* 1997;**96**: 3112–15.
70 Shadevan J, Ryu K, Peltz L, et al. Epicardial mapping of chronic atrial fibrillation in patients: preliminary observations. *Circulation* 2004;**110**:3293–9.
71 Harada A, Konishi T, Fukata M, et al. Intraoperative map guided operation for atrial fibrillation due to mitral valve disease. *Ann Thoracic Surg* 2000;**69**:446–51.
72 Wu TJ, Doshi RN, Huan HL. Simultaneous biatrial computerized mapping during permanent atrial fibrillation in patients with organic heart disease. *J Cardiovasc Electrophysiol* 2002;**13**:571–7.
73 Marshall J. On the development of the great anterior veins in man and mammalian including an account of certain remnants of foetal structure found in the adult, a comparative view of these great veins in the different mammalian, and an analysis of their occasional

peculiarities in the human subject. *Phil Trans Roy Soc Lond* 1850;**140**:133–69.

74 Sherlag BJ, Yeh BK, Robinson MJ. Inferior interatrial pathway in the dog. *Circ Res* 1972;**31**:18–35.

75 Tai CT, Hsieh MH, Tsai CF, et al. Differentiating the ligament of Marshall from the pulmonary vein musculature potentials in patients with paroxysmal atrial fibrillation: electrophysiological characteristics and results of radiofrequency ablation. *Pacing Clin Electrophysiol* 2000;**23**: 1493–501.

76 Hwang C, Wu TJ, Doshi RN, et al. Vein of Marshall cannulation for the analysis of electrical activity in patients with focal atrial fibrillation. *Circulation* 2000; **101**:1503–5.

77 Lin WS, Tai CT, Hsieh MH, et al. Catheter ablation of paroxysmal atrial fibrillation initiated by non-pulmonary vein ectopy. *Circulation* 2003;**107**:3176–83.

78 Doshi RN, Wu T-J, Yashmina M, et al. Relation between ligament of Marshall and adrenergic atrial tachyarrhythmia. *Circulation* 1999;**100**:876–83.

79 Kurotobi T, Ito H, Inoue K, et al. Marshall vein as arrhythmogenic source in patients with atrial fibrillation: correlation between its anatomy and electrophysiological findings. *J Cardiovasc Electrophysiol* 2006;**17**: 1062–7.

80 Kim DT, Lai AC, Hwang C, et al. The ligament of Marshall: a structural analysis in human hearts with implications for atrial arrythmias. *J Am Coll Cardiol* 2000;**36**:1324–7.

81 Makino M, Inoue S, Matsuyama TA, et al. Diverse myocardial extension and autonomic innervation on ligament of Marshall in humans. *J Cardiovasc Electrophysiol* 2006;**17**:594–9.

82 Roithinger FX, Cheng J, SippensGroenewegen A, Lee RJ, Saxon LA, Scheinman MM, Lesh MD. Use of electroanatomic mapping to delineate transseptal atrial conduction in humans. *Circulation* 1999;**100**:1791–7.

83 Schilling RJ, Kadish AH, Peters NS, Goldberger J, Davies DW. Endocardial mapping of atrial fibrillation in the human right atrium using a non-contact catheter. *Eur Heart J* 2000;**21**:550–64.

84 Villacastin J, Pérez-Castellano N, Moreno J, et al. Left atrial flutter after radiofrequency catheter ablation of focal atrial fibrillation. *J Cardiovasc Electrophysiol* 2003;**14**:417–21.

85 Becker A. Left atrial isthmus: anatomic aspects relevant for linear catheter ablation procedures in humans. *J Cardiovasc Electrophysiol* 2004;**15**:809–12.

86 Wittkampf F, Oosterhout M, Loh P, et al. Where to draw the mitral isthmus line in catheter ablation of atrial fibrillation: histological analysis. *Eur Heart J* 2005;**26**: 689–95.

87 Burch GE, Romey RB. Functional anatomy and "throttle valve" action of the pulmonary veins. *Am Heart J* 1954;**47**:58–66.

88 Nathan H, Eliakim M. The junction between the left atrium and the pulmonary veins. An anatomic study of human hearts. *Circulation* 1966;**34**:412–22.

89 DeAlmeida OA, Bohm GM, De Paulo, et al. The cardiac muscles in pulmonary vein of the rat: a morphological and electrophysiological study. *J Morphol* 1975;**145**: 409–34.

90 Cheung DW. Electrical activity of the pulmonary vein and its interaction with the right atrium in the guinea-pig. *J Physiol* 1981;**314**:445–56.

91 Zipes DP, Knope RF. Electrical properties of the thoracic veins. *Am J Cardiol* 1972;**29**:372–6.

92 Yamane T, Shah DC, Jais P, et al. Electrogram polarity reversal as an additional indicator of breakthroughs from the left atrium to the pulmonary veins. *J Am Coll Cardiol* 2002;**39**:1337–44.

93 Moubarak JB, Rozwadowski JV, Strzalka CT, et al. Pulmonary veins–left atrial junction: anatomic and histological study. *PACE* 2000;**23**:1836–8.

94 Sanchez J, Plumb VJ, Epstein AE, et al. Evidence for longitudinal and transverse fiber conduction in human pulmonary veins. *Circulation* 2003;**108**:590–7.

95 Tritto M, De Ponti R, Zardini M, Spadacini G, Oliveira M, Salerno-Uriarte JA. Electrical connection between pulmonary veins in humans. Evidence after radiofrequency ablation of the venoatrial junction. *Circulation* 2001;**104**:e30–e31.

96 Takahashi A, Iesaka Y, Takahashi Y, et al. Electrical connections between pulmonary veins. Implication for ostial ablation of pulmonary veins in patients with paroxysmal atrial fibrillation. *Circulation* 2002;**105**:2998–3003.

97 Saito T, Waki K, Becker AE. Left atrial myocardial extension onto pulmonary veins in humans: anatomic observations relevant for atrial arrhythmias. *J Cardiovasc Electrophysiol* 2000;**11**:888–94.

98 Spach MS, Barr RC, Jewett PH. Spread of excitation from the atrium into the thoracic veins in human beings and dogs. *Am J Cardiol* 1972;**30**:844–54.

99 Spach MS, Dolber PC. Relating extracellular potentials and their derivatives in anisotropic propagation at a microscopic level in human cardiac muscle. Evidence for electrical uncoupling of side-to-side fiber connection with increasing age. *Circ Res* 1986;**58**:356–71.

100 Hassink RJ, Aretz T, Ruskin J, et al. Morphology of atrial myocardium in human pulmonary veins. A post-mortem analysis in patients with and without atrial fibrillation. *J Am Coll Cardiol* 2003;**42**:108–14.

101 Hocini M, Ho SY, Kawara T, et al. Electrical conduction in canine pulmonary veins. Electrophysiological and anatomical correlation. *Circulation* 2002;**105**:2442–8.

102 Masani F. Node-like cells in the myocardial layer of the pulmonary vein of rats: an ultrastructural study. *J Anat* 1986;**145**:133–42.

103 Pérez-Lugones A, McMahon JT, Ratliff NB, et al. Evidence of specialized conduction cells in human pulmonary veins of patients with atrial fibrillation. *J Cardiovasc Electrophysiol* 2002;**14**:803–9.

104 Morillo CA, Klein GJ, Jones DL, et al. Chronic rapid atrial pacing. Structural, functional and electrophysiological characteristics of a new model of sustained atrial fibrillation. *Circulation* 1995:**91**:1588–95.

105 Jalife J, Berenfeld O, Mansour M. Mother rotors and fibrillatory conduction: a mechanism of atrial fibrillation. *Cardiovasc Res* 2002;**54**:59–70.

106 Mandapati R, Skanes A, Chen J, et al. Stable microreentrant sources as mechanism of atrial fibrillation in the isolated sheep heart. *Circulation* 2000;**101**:194–9.

107 Kalifa J, Tanaka K, Zaitsev A, et al. Mechanism of wave fractionation at boundaries of high-frequency excitation in the posterior left atrium of the isolated sheep heart during atrial fibrillation. *Circulation* 2006;**113**: 626–33.

108 Markides V, Shilling RJ, Ho SY, et al. Characterization of the left atrial activation in the intact human heart. *Circulation* 2003;**107**:733–9.

109 Chauvin M, Shah DC, Haissaguerre M, et al. The anatomic basis of connection between the coronary sinus musculature and the left atrium in humans. *Circulation* 2000;**101**:647–52.

110 Antz M, Otomo K, Arruda M, et al. Electrical conduction between the right atrium and the left atrium via the musculature of the coronary sinus. *Circulation* 1998: **98**:1790–5.

111 Betts TR, Ho SY, Sánchez-Quintana D, et al. Characterization of right atrial activation during coronary sinus pacing. *J Cardiovasc Electrophysiol* 2002;**13**:794–800.

112 Chen SA, Tai CT, Yu WC, et al. Right atrial focal atrial fibrillation: electrophysiologic characteristics and radiofrequency catheter ablation. *J Cardiovasc Electrophysiol* 1999;**10**:328–35.

113 Han J, Good E, Morady F, et al. Esophageal migration during left atrial catheter ablation for atrial fibrillation. *Circulation* 2004;**110**:e528.

114 Lowe MD, Peterson LA, Monahan KH, Asivatham SJ, Packer DL. Electroanatomical mapping to assess phrenic nerve proximity to superior vena cava and pulmonary vein ostia. *Heart* 2004;**90**:24.

115 Sanchez-Quintana D, Cabrera JA, Climent V, et al. How close are the phrenic nerves to cardiac structures? Implications for cardiac interventionalists. *J Cardiovasc Electrophysiol* 2005;**16**:309–13.

116 Bai R, Patel D, di Biase L, et al. Phrenic nerve injury after catheter ablation: should we worry about this complication? *J Cardiovasc Electrophysiol* 2006;**17**:944–8.

117 Tse H-F, Reek S, Timmermans C, et al. Pulmonary vein isolation using transvenous catheter cryoablation for treatment of atrial fibrillation without risk of pulmonary vein stenosis. *J Am Coll Cardiol* 2003;**42**:752–8.

118 Ho SY, Cabrera JA, Sánchez-Quintana D, et al. Vagaries of the vagus nerve: relevance to ablationist. *J Cardiovasc Electrophysiol* 2006;**17**:330–1.

119 Zipes DP, Mihalick MJ, Robbins GT. Effects of selective vagal and stellate ganglion stimulation of atrial refractoriness. *Cardiovasc Res* 1974;**8**:647–55

120 Elvan A, Pride HP, Eble JN, Zipes DP. Radiofrequency catheter ablation of the atria reduces inducibility and duration of atrial fibrillation in dogs. *Circulation* 1995; **81**:2235–44.

121 Liu L, Nattel S. Differing sympathetic and vagal effects on atrial fibrillation in dogs: role of refractoriness heterogeneity. *Am J Physiol* 1997;**273**:H805–H816.

122 Schauerte P, Scherlag BJ, Pitha J, Scherlag MA, Reynolds D, Lazzara R, Jackman WM. Catheter ablation of cardiac autonomic nerves for prevention of vagal atrial fibrillation. *Circulation* 200;**102**:2774–80.

123 Armour JA, Murphy DA, Yuan BX, Macdonald S, Hopkins DA. Gross and microscopic anatomy of the human intrinsic cardiac nervous system. *Anat Rec* 1997;**247**:289–98.

124 Pauza DH, Skripka V, Pauziene N, Stropus R. Morphology, distribution, and variability of the epicardiac neural ganglionated subplexuses in the human heart. *Anat Rec* 2000;**259**:353–82.

125 Chiou CW, Eble JN, Zipes DP. Efferent vagal innervation of the canine atria and sinus and atrioventricular nodes. The third fat pad. *Circulation* 1997;**95**:2573–84.

126 Chevalier P, Tabib A, Meyronnet D, et al. Quantitative study of nerves of the human left atrium. *Heart Rhythm* 2005;**2**: 518–22.

127 Tan AY, Li H, Wachsmann-Hogiu S, Chen LS, Chen PS, Fishbein MC. Autonomic innervation and segmental muscular disconnections at the human pulmonary vein–atrial junction: implications for catheter ablation of atrial–pulmonary vein junction. *J Am Coll Cardiol* 2006;**48**:132–43.

2

CHAPTER 2

Mechanisms and significance of fractionated electrograms recorded during atrial fibrillation

Sander Verheule, Els Tuyls, Natasja de Groot, & Maurits Allessie

An unfractionated unipolar electrogram has a single negative deflection with a maximal negative rate of rise (dV/dt) at the local time point of activation. By contrast, a fractionated unipolar electrogram (FE) is composed of multiple negative deflections during one cycle (Figure 2.1). The simplest form of an FE is a "double potential" with two deflections, but many more deflections may be discernible. The most complex FEs display "continuous electrical activity" throughout the whole cycle length. In this chapter, we will first present a brief historical perspective on the recording of FEs; after a review of the physiological mechanisms and regional distribution of FEs, we will discuss some practical applications of FE recordings, particularly with respect to atrial fibrillation (AF).

Historical perspective

Durrer et al. were the first to report FEs recorded both with unipolar and bipolar electrodes in human hearts after chronic myocardial infarction [1]. They ascribed these FEs to local fractionation of the excitation wave in the infarcted region. Others showed that FEs appeared within hours after coronary artery ligation in dog hearts. Ventricular arrhythmias often occurred when these fractionated potentials extended into the diastole [2,3]. In healed infarcts, the presence of local "continuous electrical activity" has been equated with "local reentry" or "local fibrillation", which was proposed to be pivotal for the mechanism of the arrhythmia [4,5]. Although complex FEs, especially low amplitude signals with continuous activity may be due to conduction disturbances, there has been some concern that they could also be caused by electrode movement. For example, electrograms with continuous activity could be recorded during sinus rhythm from a sponge sutured to the ventricles [6] and even from electrodes in a bowl of Jell-O [7]. However, ventricular complex FEs recorded in vivo are specifically associated with infarct zones, where motion is weaker than in healthy myocardium. In addition, in studies of perfused and superfused preparations, where electrode movement could be controlled, complex FEs were also observed (see, for example [8–10]). Under these circumstances, the occurrence of FEs was specifically correlated to the underlying tissue structure.

Spach et al. originally hypothesized that FEs may result either from intracellular action potentials with multiphasic upstrokes or from superposition of potentials from asynchronously activated strands of myocytes [11]. Subsequently, in a seminal study on canine ventricular infarcts, Gardner et al. showed that even in areas with highly fractionated electro-

Catheter Ablation of Atrial Fibrillation Edited by Etienne Aliot, Michel Haïssaguerre and Warren M. Jackman

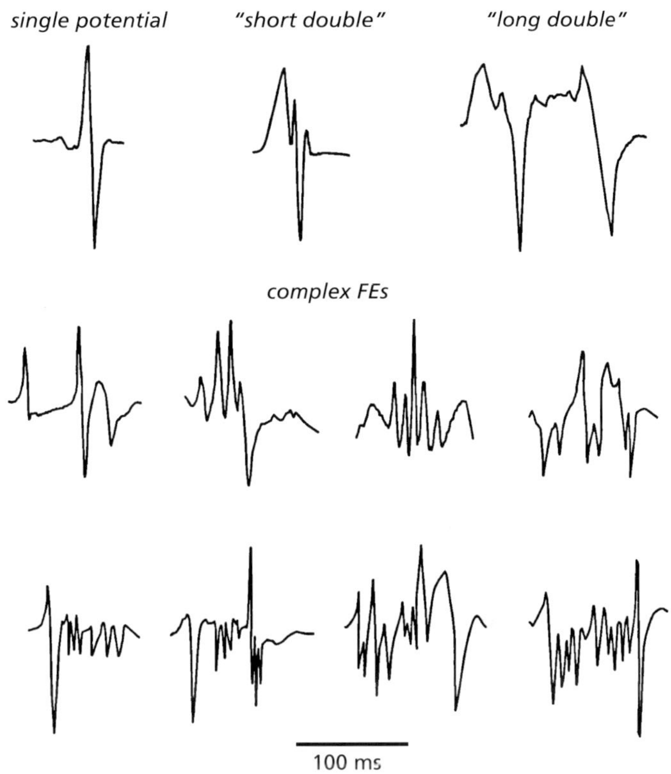

Figure 2.1 Morphology of fractionated unipolar electrograms (FEs) recorded during atrial fibrillation (AF) in patients with chronic AF. A normal electrogram is characterized by a single sharp deflection. A "short double" has a biphasic deflection, whereas a "long double" displays two separate deflections. Complex FEs can have a varying number of deflections within one cycle length.

grams, intracellular action potentials still displayed single rapid upstrokes [9] (Figure 2.2). Although these authors demonstrated the presence of muscle bundles separated by fibrous tissue, there was not a one-to-one relationship between the number of strands of surviving myocytes observed histologically and the number of deflections in the recorded FEs. Based on this and other evidence, they postulated that these strands were not completely isolated electrically, but that remaining transverse connections led to a zigzag pattern of conduction. Around the same time, Spach et al. investigated highly fractionated electrograms in atrial trabeculae [8]. In one example, they reconstructed the complex fiber arrangement that best explained the recorded FE [8] (Figure 2.3). The computed structure in Figure 2.3c is rather complex, indicating that an exact correlation of the FE morphology with the underlying tissue structure will often not be feasible. However, these studies do demonstrate that fractionation is the result of dissociated activation between myocyte fibers sensed by a single electrode.

Electrogram fractionation reflects both the tissue structure in the vicinity of the recording electrode and the extent to which this structure is unmasked by the way the activation waves are propagating in that area. As such, there are two requirements for electrogram fractionation:

1 The presence of myocyte bundles close to the recording electrode with poor electrical coupling, making activation at distinctly different time points possible.

2 Activation wavefronts entering the area sensed by the recording electrode that do actually cause asynchronous activation of these bundles.

In the following two sections, we will discuss these two conditions for fractionation in more detail.

Electrogram fractionation and discontinuous conduction

In the working myocardium, conduction velocity is larger in the longitudinal direction than in the

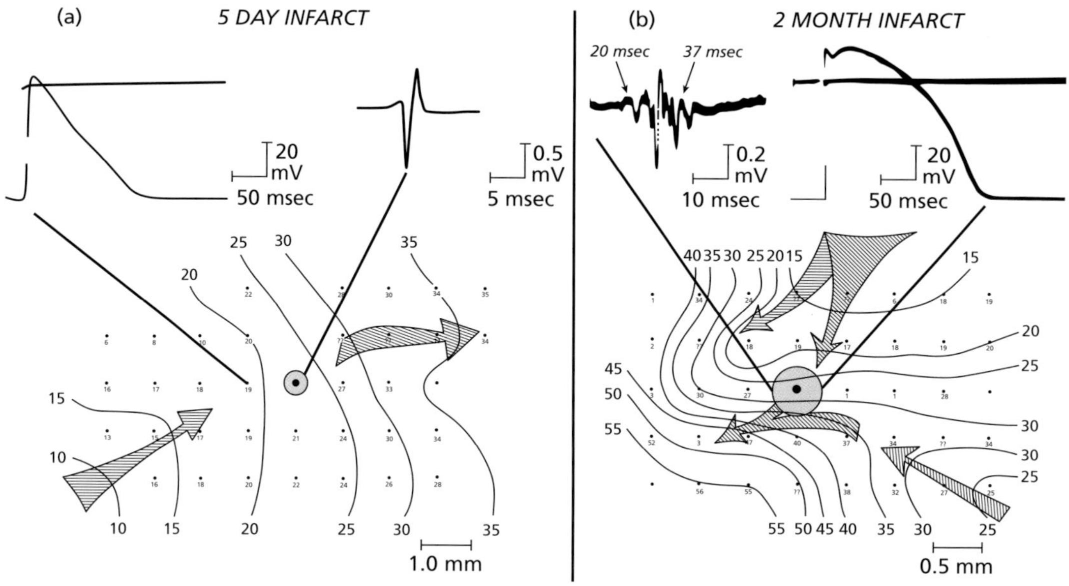

Figure 2.2 Relationship between closely spaced bipolar electrograms and intracellular action potentials. (a) In 5-day-old infarcts, conduction was still homogeneous. Extracellular electrograms (bipole spacing 0.5 mm) showed single deflections and intracellular action potentials had a single fast upstroke and a shortened action potential duration. (b) In a healed 2-month-old infarct, crowded isochrones show that regions of slow conduction had developed. In such regions, bipolar electrograms showed multiple deflections with an increased total duration of the electrogram complex. However, intracellular action potentials recorded at the same site still showed a single fast upstroke and had a normal time course of repolarization. Thus, fractionation in a closely spaced bipolar electrogram can exist in the absence of cellular abnormalities. (Adapted from [9].)

transverse direction. In the transverse direction, a propagating wavefront has to cross more cell-to-cell boundaries within a given distance. In addition, the smaller and sparser gap junctional plaques at side-to-side connections represent a higher resistance than the larger intercalated discs at end-to-end connections [12]. With age, gap junctions also become increasingly localized at end-to-end connections between myocytes, thus further increasing anisotropy [13–15]. Furthermore, myocytes are organized in bundles, separated by perimysial fibrous tissue. Within these bundles, strands of myocytes can be separated from each other by endomysial fibrous tissue. Structural remodeling due to heart disease is often associated with fibrosis and an increased transverse fiber separation. In healed ventricular infarcts, thin strands of surviving myocytes have been demonstrated to be separated by fibrosis [9]. In ventricular cardiomyopathy [16] as well as in the atria of animal models of atrial dilation [17,18] and congestive heart failure [19], the amount of fibrosis between myocyte bundles is increased. In the atria, collagenous septa between myofibers also increase in volume during normal aging [8,15]. Spach and coworkers have demonstrated that the non-uniform anisotropic arrangement in cell-to-cell connections leads to discontinuous conduction at a microscopic scale; while longitudinal conduction may still be fast, transverse conduction may show discrete time delays in the activation of adjoining myocytes or myocyte bundles [20]. During such delays due to poor electrical coupling, propagation becomes increasingly dependent on the slow calcium current rather than on the fast sodium current [21,22]. Discontinuities in conduction can become more apparent at short cycle lengths or during extrastimulation with short coupling intervals due to incomplete recovery of the sodium and calcium channels [21]. Discontinuous conduction between poorly coupled myocytes forms the basis of dissociated activation during AF and is reflected by fractionated electrograms.

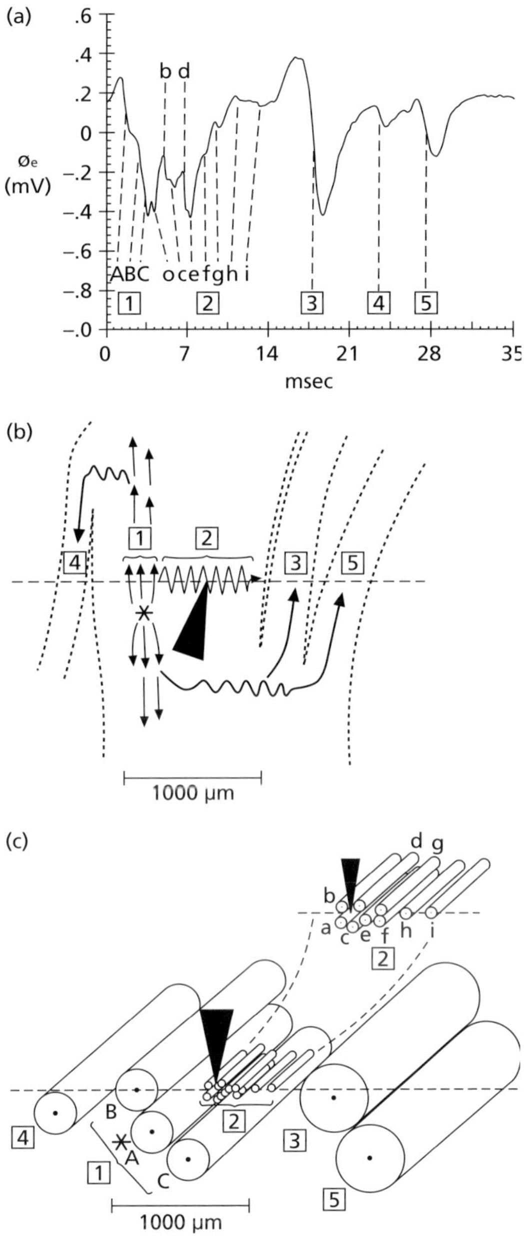

Figure 2.3 Reconstruction of the fiber arrangment leading to a complex FE. (a) A single unipolar complex recorded from a superfused atrial trabecula from a 62-year-old male, recorded at the site indicated by the solid black triangle in (b). (b) The anatomy of the trabeculated structure of the preparation is outlined with dashed lines and the asterisk indicates the stimulation site. Parallel to the fiber orientation, conduction was fast (straight arrows), but in the transverse direction conduction was markedly delayed and discontinuous (crumpled arrows). (c) From the electrogram in (a) and the anatomy in (b), a fiber arrangement (size of the bundles and their distance to the electrode) was computed that best explained the different components in the fractionated electrogram. The inset shows a magnification of the area closest to the recording electrode. The numbers 1–5 in each panel represent the main bundles within the trabecula. In the computed structure, bundle 1 was subdivided into three sub-bundles (A–C), whereas bundle 2 was subdivided into nine sub-bundles (a–i, see inset). (Adapted from [8].)

Relation between electrogram fractionation and activation pattern

With high density mapping of propagation, it became clear that FEs were associated with certain types of activation patterns. The best-studied example of an activation pattern associated with FEs is a line of block. In superfused canine papillary muscles, de Bakker et al. created an anatomic barrier by making a long incision parallel to the main fiber orientation [23]. During slow pacing with propagation perpendicular to the barrier, electrograms displayed double deflections corresponding to the activation time points at either side of the line of block (Figure 2.4a). However, when a number of smaller incisions were made, local FEs were recorded without the presence of lines of conduction block (Figure 2.4b). In this case, the anatomic obstacles were apparently too small to disturb the overall conduction pattern of the propagating wavefront, but they did cause dissociated activation of neighboring myocyte fibers. An earlier study had already shown that lines of block associated with FEs can also be functional (i.e. not present at long cycle lengths) [10]. In the epicardial border zone of 3–5-day-old myocardial infarcts, conduction was homogeneous during slow pacing, but long "functional" lines of block developed during ventricular tachycardia (Figure 2.4c). The FEs observed around these lines of functional block were often complex, showing numerous deflections. Interestingly, the activation wavefront continued to propagate parallel to the line of block at the distal side, indicating that the impulse actually propagated with delay through the line of block (pseudoblock), rather than around it. Slow, discontinuous transverse conduction between fibers partially separated

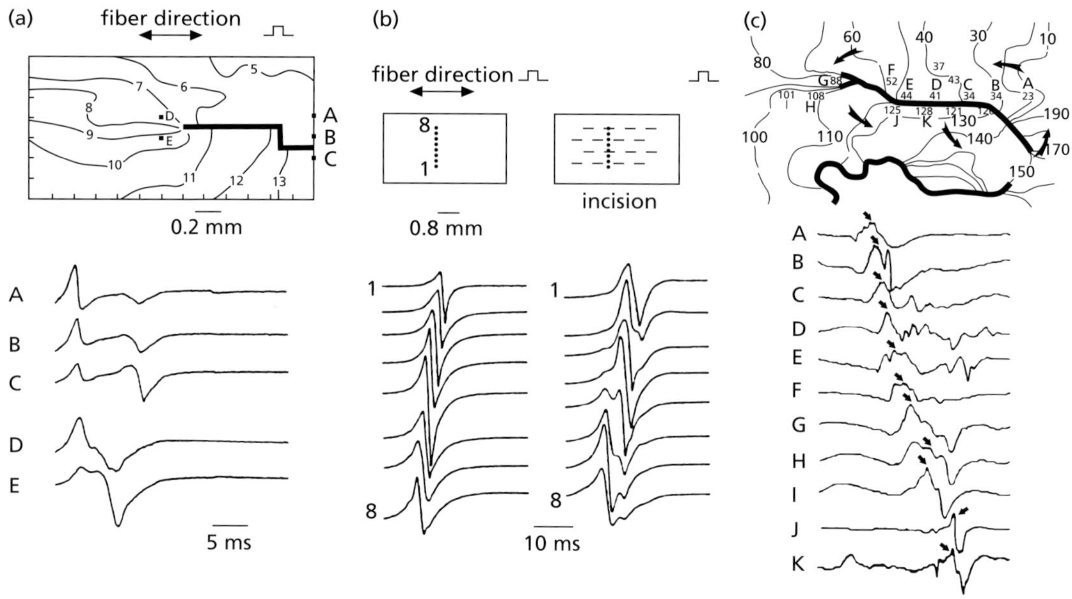

Figure 2.4 Effect of local conduction block on the fractionation of electrograms. (a) In a superfused canine papillary muscle, a long incision parallel to the fiber orientation caused the wavefront to turn around the line of block. Bipolar electrograms (spacing 0.2 mm) along this line showed double potentials corresponding to activation at either side of the incision (A–C). At the pivot point, crowding of isochrones with a short double potential (D) indicate functional block. (b) The left panel represents the control situation, in which eight electrograms (numbers 1–8) were recorded along a straight line, perpendicular to the fiber orientation. The right panel depicts the preparation after a number of small incisions was made, which led to FEs although no lines of block were apparent in the activation pattern (not shown). (c) In the ventricular epicardium of a dog with 5-day-old myocardial infarction, a functional line of block was present during an induced episode of counterclockwise reentrant ventricular tachycardia. The electrograms (bipoles with 1 mm spacing) recorded along this line (A–K) showed a varying degree of fractionation. Note the propagation of the wavefront distal to the line of block, indicating very slow conduction across this line. ((a, b) Adapted from [23]; (c) adapted from [10].)

by fibrous tissue may explain why the recorded FEs were more complex than in the case of a complete anatomic lesion (Figure 2.4a).

In recordings from human right atria during acute AF, fractionation of fibrillation electrograms was observed in areas of slow conduction, at lines of conduction block, around pivot points, and in regions where wavefronts collided [24] (Figure 2.5). This association does not imply that these types of activation pattern necessarily cause fractionation. For example, in ventricular trabeculae, head-on collision of homogeneously propagating wavefronts leads to electrograms with a single deflection and a high R : S ratio at the point of collision [25]. Also, homogeneous slowing of conduction is expected to lead to a widening of the electrogram with smaller dV/dt at the time point of activation. In old canine infarcts, homogeneous conduction slowing due to an elevated extracellular potassium concentration increased the intervals between deflections within FEs without affecting the number of deflections [9]. The observation that during AF, collision and slow conduction were associated with FEs indicates that these activation patterns were associated with dissociated activation in the atrial wall [24]. In this study of unipolar electrogram morphology in normal human atria, FEs were categorized as short double potentials, long double potentials, and complex FEs. Compared to sinus rhythm, the incidence of "long doubles" and complex FEs was increased during AF. In addition, the incidence of these electrogram morphologies was higher at shorter cycle lengths and during more complex AF patterns. By contrast, the incidence of "short doubles" was unaffected by AF. Of the activation patterns shown in Figure 2.5, short doubles were typical for the collision of fibrillation waves (Figure 2.5a), while long doubles were associated

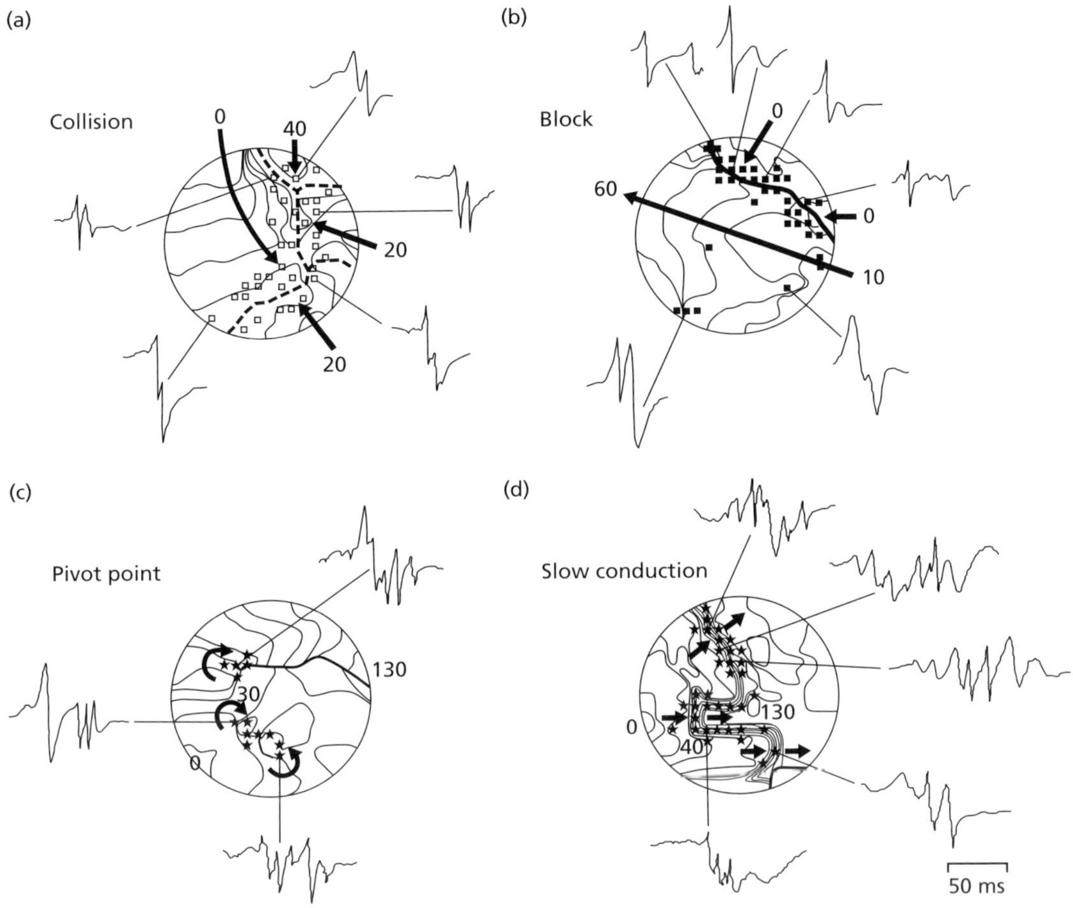

Figure 2.5 Unipolar electrograms and underlying activation patterns during acute AF in humans, recorded with a high density array of electrodes from the right atrial free wall. (a) Four wavefronts (arrows) collide at the dashed lines. FEs with short double potentials were recorded at sites of collision. (b) Long double potentials were recorded along a functional line of block (thick black line). Complex FEs were recorded at pivot points (curved arrows, (c)) and in regions of slow conduction (crowded isochrones, (d)). (Adapted from [24].)

with lines of block (Figure 2.5b). More complex FEs were typically observed around pivot points (Figure 2.5c) and in areas of slow conduction (Figure 2.5d). Overall, 23% of the fibrillation electrograms were fractionated, compared to 7% during sinus rhythm [24]. Of these FEs, approximately 0.2% displayed complex fractionation (more than two deflections) during sinus rhythm, as compared to 6% during AF. In chronic AF or atria of hearts with underlying heart disease, the slow process of structural remodeling may increase transverse fiber separation and may thus reduce the number of side-to-side connections throughout the free walls. As a result, FEs would become more frequent and more widespread. Indeed, activation patterns are more complex and dissociated in persistent AF than in paroxysmal AF [26] and we have recently found that the degree of electrogram fractionation in the free wall of the right and left atria is higher in chronic AF than in acute AF [27].

Regional distribution of atrial fractionated electrograms

Based on anatomic and histological studies of the atria, areas with inherently anisotropic properties include the crista terminalis, the bundle of Bachmann (BB), and the area around the pulmonary veins (PVs) [28–31]. Interestingly, examples of regional electrogram fractionation have

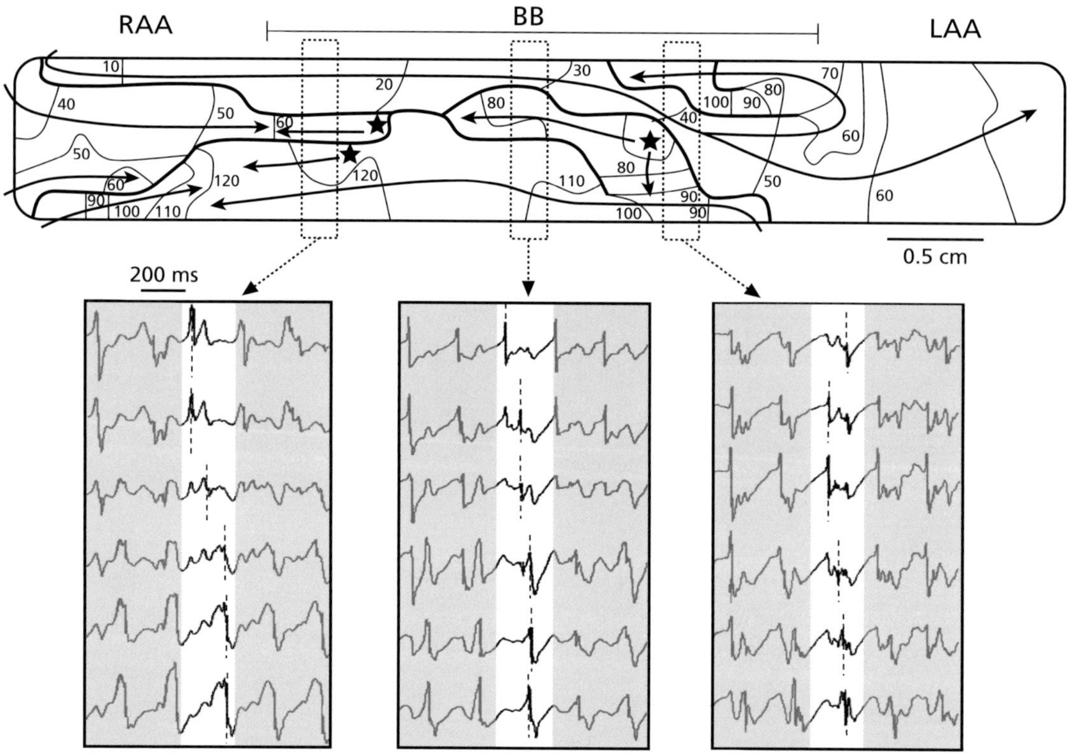

Figure 2.6 Fractionated unipolar electrograms in the bundle of Bachmann (BB) after 2.5 weeks of AF in the goat. A high density rectangular array of unipolar electrodes (interelectrode distance 1.4 mm) was inserted from the posterior side of the left atrial appendage (LAA) to the posterior side of the right atrial appendage (RAA), thus covering the entire epicardial aspect of the BB. In the upper panel, an activation map during one cycle of AF is displayed. This area was activated by narrow wavelets propagating mainly along the length axis of the BB. Asterisks indicate epicardial breakthroughs. The three lower panels display unipolar electrogram signals at three rows of electrodes (dashed boxes in the top panel) at right angles to the length axis of the BB. The beat displayed in the map is highlighted and the time points of activation (highest dV/dt) are indicated by dashed vertical lines. Each of the electrode rows was activated by three narrow fibrillation wavelets. This "longitudinal dissociation" apparent in the activation map was reflected in the FEs.

been reported for all these areas. Electrogram fractionation at the crista terminalis in humans increased with age [32], and was higher in patients with sick sinus syndrome [33,34] and congestive heart failure [35]. The BB forms the major conducting pathway between the right and left atrium and consists of parallel-oriented muscle bundles. In goats after 1 month of AF, this structure showed an incidence of complex FEs of 23%, compared to 5–6% in the atrial free walls [36]. We have recently studied the conduction properties of the BB in goats after 2.5 weeks of AF. At this point in time, atrial electrical remodeling (shortening of refractory period) is complete, but structural changes are not yet apparent. During electrically induced AF episodes, the BB showed pronounced lines of transverse conduction block. This "longitudinal dissociation" of the activation process led to several narrow wavelets propagating out of phase along the long axis of the BB (Figure 2.6). A detailed analysis showed that the individual deflections of the FEs were caused by desynchronized propagation of narrow neighboring waves. The long distances over which these wavelets remained dissociated indicate that side-to-side connections between these parallel bundles were quite sparse.

Fractionated electrograms are often recorded in the PV area, which has been shown to be the source of rapid electrical activity in patients with paroxysmal AF (see, for example [37]). In 1972, Spach et al. had already recorded unipolar electrograms in human and canine PVs. They reported the presence

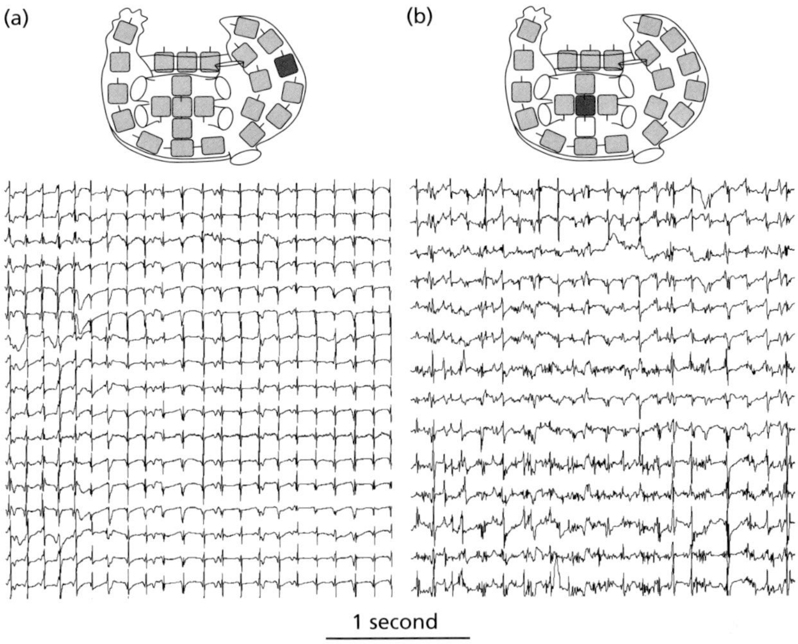

Figure 2.7 Regional variation in fractionation of fibrillation electrograms. Unipolar electrograms were recorded with a small mapping array (64 electrodes on 1 cm^2) in a patient with chronic AF. In the schematic representations of the atria, light gray squares indicate the recording locations. (a) Electrograms in the right atrial free wall showed temporal variability in cycle length and were polymorphic. However, there was a high degree of spatial coherence, leading to a minor degree of electrogram fractionation, mainly characterized by short double potentials. (b) In the area between the pulmonary veins, the electrograms showed a high degree of complex fractionation.

of double spikes, the first corresponding to the adjacent atrial myocardium and the second to the local PV myocardium [38]. Later, Hwang et al. observed double potentials in the PVs of patients with Wolff–Parkinson–White syndrome and patients with paroxysmal AF [39]. This fractionation was explained by slow conduction and/or conduction block between the myocardial sleeves of the PVs and the adjacent atrial myocardium. Histologically, zones of conduction delay and FEs in normal canine PVs were associated with abrupt changes in fiber orientation [40]. Electrogram characteristics of the PV area are more complex in patients with AF [41], but a comprehensive study comparing the morphology of PV electrograms in patients with and without paroxysmal AF is not yet available. FEs have not only been observed in myocardial sleeves, but also in the area between the PVs. In Figure 2.7, an example is provided of intraoperative mapping with a small high density epicardial array of 64 unipolar electrodes (spatial resolution 1.5 mm) in a patient with chronic AF and mitral valve disease. Compared to the right atrium, the area between the PVs displayed highly fractionated electrograms with periods of continuous electrical activity. Analysis of the activation pattern in this relatively small area revealed a multitude of narrow fibrillation wavelets (not shown), indicating that, as in the BB, longitudinal dissociation of muscle bundles was responsible for the fractionation.

Practical applications of fractionated electrogram recording

Because FEs occur in regions with disturbed conduction that may be pivotal in the maintenance of reentrant arrhythmias, it is an attractive idea to use FEs as a guide for targeted ablation strategies. Wiener et al. showed that FEs can be used to direct surgical resection of an infarcted area in drug-refractory post-ischemic ventricular tachycardia

(VT) [42]. However, this approach was never widely adopted and has been superseded by less invasive catheter ablation. Fractionated diastolic potentials during VT can arise from surviving myocardial fibers embedded within scar tissue that may form the central common pathway of a reentry circuit [43]. However, because fractionated diastolic potentials may also be recorded at bystander sites [44], a number of additional criteria or detailed activation mappings are required to increase the efficacy of electrogram-guided VT ablation strategies [45].

In typical atrial flutter, double potentials or more complex FEs are frequently observed. Double potentials are mainly associated with a functional line of block or area of slow conduction along the crista terminalis with opposing activation sequences on either side [46–48]. The inferior right atrium is another region in which FEs were recorded during atrial flutter. Mapping studies have revealed that this area contains a zone of slow conduction between the tricuspid annulus and the inferior caval vein [48–50]. As this area is also the narrowest part of the flutter circuit, ablation of atrial flutter can be performed by the creation of a linear lesion between these two anatomic structures [51,52]. In atypical flutter in patients with congenital heart disease, FEs may arise from surviving myocyte fibers within scar tissue forming a critical part of the reentrant circuit, but determination of the activation sequence is again required to determine the suitability of these sites as a target for ablation [53].

During AF, mapping of electrogram fractionation may allow identification of regions with structural conduction disturbances that are involved in perpetuation of AF. Nademanee et al. have studied FEs in patients with paroxysmal and chronic AF and frequently localized complex FEs in the interatrial septum, PVs, and the roof of the left atrium [54,55]. The authors defined complex FEs as electrograms with either complex fractionated potentials or a short activation cycle length (< 120 ms). Ablation of areas with complex FEs under this definition resulted in restoration of sinus rhythm in 91% of the patients after a follow-up of 1 year. The concept of targeting the local substrate by ablation of fractionated areas represents a novel strategy in the treatment of AF and there are a number of factors worth considering with respect to this new approach. First, FEs may not be specific for AF patients. In patients without a history of AF, Centurion et al. have reported a high incidence of FEs, which increased with age [56]. Konings et al. showed that in patients with Wolff–Parkinson–White syndrome, the occurrence of FEs was not related to a documented history of AF [24]. Regardless of their specificity, sites with complex FEs may be important in the maintenance of the arrhythmia in AF patients. In the study of Nademanee et al., the number of radiofrequency applications was considerable (mean 64 ± 36; range 7–168) [54]. Although the degree of fractionation at any given site may vary in time, due to variation in AF cycle length, degree of dissociation of fibrillation waves, and direction of propagation [24,57], Nademanee et al. reported that areas with complex FEs were quite stationary in time [54]. While some of these fractionated areas may only be "bystanders", measurement of the nature and degree of electrogram fractionation is a relatively simple way to detect areas of abnormal conduction and may provide vital clues for the diagnosis of the substrate responsible for perpetuation of AF.

References

1 Durrer D, Formijne P, van DR, et al. The electrocardiogram in normal and some abnormal conditions; in revived human fetal heart and in acute and chronic coronary occlusion. *Am Heart J* 1961;**61**:303–16.

2 Boineau JP, Cox JL. Slow ventricular activation in acute myocardial infarction. A source of re-entrant premature ventricular contractions. *Circulation* 1973;**48**:702–13.

3 Waldo AL, Kaiser GA. A study of ventricular arrhythmias associated with acute myocardial infarction in the canine heart. *Circulation* 1973;**47**:1222–8.

4 Josephson ME, Wit AL. Fractionated electrical activity and continuous electrical activity: fact or artifact? *Circulation* 1984;**70**:529–32.

5 Josephson ME, Horowitz LN, Farshidi A. Continuous local electrical activity. A mechanism of recurrent ventricular tachycardia. *Circulation* 1978;**57**:659–65.

6 Ideker RE, Lofland GK, Bardy GH, et al. Late fractionated potentials and continuous electrical activity caused by electrode motion. *Pacing Clin Electrophysiol* 1983;**6**:908–14.

7 Gallagher JJ, Kasell JH, Cox JL, et al. Techniques of intraoperative electrophysiologic mapping. *Am J Cardiol* 1982;**49**:221–40.

8 Spach MS, Dolber PC. Relating extracellular potentials and their derivatives to anisotropic propagation at a

microscopic level in human cardiac muscle. Evidence for electrical uncoupling of side-to-side fiber connections with increasing age. *Circ Res* 1986;**58**:356–71.

9 Gardner PI, Ursell PC, Fenoglio JJ, Jr., et al. Electrophysiologic and anatomic basis for fractionated electrograms recorded from healed myocardial infarcts. *Circulation* 1985;**72**:596–611.

10 Dillon SM, Allessie MA, Ursell PC, et al. Influences of anisotropic tissue structure on reentrant circuits in the epicardial border zone of subacute canine infarcts. *Circ Res* 1988;**63**:182–206.

11 Spach MS, Barr RC, Johnson EA, et al. Cardiac extracellular potentials. Analysis of complex wave forms about the Purkinje networks in dogs. *Circ Res* 1973;**33**:465–73.

12 Spach MS, Heidlage JF. The stochastic nature of cardiac propagation at a microscopic level. Electrical description of myocardial architecture and its application to conduction. *Circ Res* 1995;**76**:366–80.

13 Gourdie RG, Green CR, Severs NJ, et al. Immunolabelling patterns of gap junction connexins in the developing and mature rat heart. *Anat Embryol (Berl)* 1992;**185**:363–78.

14 Peters NS, Severs NJ, Rothery SM, et al. Spatiotemporal relation between gap junctions and fascia adherens junctions during postnatal development of human ventricular myocardium. *Circulation* 1994;**90**:713–25.

15 Koura T, Hara M, Takeuchi S, et al. Anisotropic conduction properties in canine atria analyzed by highresolution optical mapping: preferential direction of conduction block changes from longitudinal to transverse with increasing age. *Circulation* 2002;**105**:2092–8.

16 Kawara T, Derksen R, de Groot JR, et al. Activation delay after premature stimulation in chronically diseased human myocardium relates to the architecture of interstitial fibrosis. *Circulation* 2001;**104**:3069–75.

17 Boyden PA, Hoffman BF. The effects on atrial electrophysiology and structure of surgically induced right atrial enlargement in dogs. *Circ Res* 1981;**49**:1319–31.

18 Verheule S, Wilson E, Everett T, et al. Alterations in atrial electrophysiology and tissue structure in a canine model of chronic atrial dilatation due to mitral regurgitation. *Circulation* 2003;**107**:2615–22.

19 Li D, Fareh S, Leung TK, et al. Promotion of atrial fibrillation by heart failure in dogs: atrial remodeling of a different sort. *Circulation* 1999;**100**:87–95.

20 Spach MS, Boineau JP. Microfibrosis produces electrical load variations due to loss of side-to-side cell connections: a major mechanism of structural heart disease arrhythmias. *Pacing Clin Electrophysiol* 1997;**20**:397–413.

21 Sugiura H, Joyner RW. Action potential conduction between guinea pig ventricular cells can be modulated by calcium current. *Am J Physiol* 1992;**263**:H1591–H1604.

22 Shaw RM, Rudy Y. Ionic mechanisms of propagation in cardiac tissue. Roles of the sodium and L-type calcium currents during reduced excitability and decreased gap junction coupling. *Circ Res* 1997;**81**:727–41.

23 de Bakker JM, van Capelle FJ, Janse MJ, et al. Fractionated electrograms in dilated cardiomyopathy: origin and relation to abnormal conduction. *J Am Coll Cardiol* 1996;**27**:1071–8.

24 Konings KT, Smeets JL, Penn OC, et al. Configuration of unipolar atrial electrograms during electrically induced atrial fibrillation in humans. *Circulation* 1997;**95**:1231–41.

25 Spach MS, Barr RC, Serwer GS, et al. Collision of excitation waves in the dog Purkinje system. Extracellular identification. *Circ Res* 1971;**29**:499–511.

26 Ndrepepa G, Weber S, Karch MR, et al. Electrophysiologic characteristics of the spontaneous onset and termination of atrial fibrillation. *Am J Cardiol* 2002; **90**:1215–20.

27 de Groot NMS, Houben RM, Klautz R, et al. *Degree of fractionation of atrial fibrillation electrograms during acute and chronic AF.* Thesis, Leiden University, the Netherlands, 2006:169–94.

28 Ho SY, Cabrera JA, Tran VH, et al. Architecture of the pulmonary veins: relevance to radiofrequency ablation. *Heart* 2001;**86**:265–70.

29 Ho SY, Anderson RH, Sanchez-Quintana D. Atrial structure and fibres: morphologic bases of atrial conduction. *Cardiovasc Res* 2002;**54**:325–36.

30 Verheule S, Wilson EE, Arora R, et al. Tissue structure and connexin expression of canine pulmonary veins. *Cardiovasc Res* 2002;**55**:727–38.

31 Sanchez-Quintana D, Anderson RH, Cabrera JA, et al. The terminal crest: morphological features relevant to electrophysiology. *Heart* 2002;**88**:406–11.

32 Kistler PM, Sanders P, Fynn SP, et al. Electrophysiologic and electroanatomic changes in the human atrium associated with age. *J Am Coll Cardiol* 2004;**44**:109–16.

33 Centurion OA, Fukatani M, Konoe A, et al. Different distribution of abnormal endocardial electrograms within the right atrium in patients with sick sinus syndrome. *Br Heart J* 1992;**68**:596–600.

34 Sanders P, Morton JB, Kistler PM, et al. Electrophysiological and electroanatomic characterization of the atria in sinus node disease: evidence of diffuse atrial remodeling. *Circulation* 2004;**109**:1514–22.

35 Sanders P, Morton JB, Davidson NC, et al. Electrical remodeling of the atria in congestive heart failure: electrophysiological and electroanatomic mapping in humans. *Circulation* 2003;**108**:1461–8.

36 Shan Z, Van Der Voort PH, Blaauw Y, et al. Fractionation of electrograms and linking of activation during pharmacologic cardioversion of persistent atrial fibrillation in the goat. *J Cardiovasc Electrophysiol* 2004;**15**:572–80.

37 Haissaguerre M, Jais P, Shah DC, et al. Spontaneous initiation of atrial fibrillation by ectopic beats originating in the pulmonary veins. *N Engl J Med* 1998;**339**:659–66.

38 Spach MS, Barr RC, Jewett PH. Spread of excitation from the atrium into thoracic veins in human beings and dogs. *Am J Cardiol* 1972;**30**:844–54.

39 Hwang C, Karagueuzian HS, Chen PS. Idiopathic paroxysmal atrial fibrillation induced by a focal discharge mechanism in the left superior pulmonary vein: possible roles of the ligament of Marshall. *J Cardiovasc Electrophysiol* 1999;**10**:636–48.

40 Hocini M, Ho SY, Kawara T, et al. Electrical conduction in canine pulmonary veins: electrophysiological and anatomic correlation. *Circulation* 2002;**105**:2442–8.

41 Hsieh MH, Tai CT, Tsai CF, et al. Pulmonary vein electrogram characteristics in patients with focal sources of paroxysmal atrial fibrillation. *J Cardiovasc Electrophysiol* 2000;**11**:953–9.

42 Wiener I, Mindich B, Pitchon R. Fragmented endocardial electrical activity in patients with ventricular tachycardia: a new guide to surgical therapy. *Am Heart J* 1984;**107**: 86–90.

43 Stevenson WG, Weiss JN, Wiener I, et al. Fractionated endocardial electrograms are associated with slow conduction in humans: evidence from pace-mapping. *J Am Coll Cardiol* 1989;**13**:369–76.

44 Cabo C, Schmitt H, Masters G, et al. Location of diastolic potentials in reentrant circuits causing sustained ventricular tachycardia in the infarcted canine heart: relationship to predicted critical ablation sites. *Circulation* 1998;**98**:2598–607.

45 El-Shalakany A, Hadjis T, Papageorgiou P, et al. Entrainment/mapping criteria for the prediction of termination of ventricular tachycardia by single radiofrequency lesion in patients with coronary artery disease. *Circulation* 1999;**99**:2283–9.

46 Cosio FG, Arribas F, Barbero JM, et al. Validation of double-spike electrograms as markers of conduction delay or block in atrial flutter. *Am J Cardiol* 1988;**61**: 775–80.

47 Shimizu A, Nozaki A, Rudy Y, et al. Characterization of double potentials in a functionally determined reentrant circuit. Multiplexing studies during interruption of atrial flutter in the canine pericarditis model. *J Am Coll Cardiol* 1993;**22**:2022–32.

48 Okumura K, Plumb VJ, Page PL, et al. Atrial activation sequence during atrial flutter in the canine pericarditis model and its effects on the polarity of the flutter wave in the electrocardiogram. *J Am Coll Cardiol* 1991;**17**:509–18.

49 Olshansky B, Okumura K, Hess PG, et al. Demonstration of an area of slow conduction in human atrial flutter. *J Am Coll Cardiol* 1990;**16**:1639–48.

50 Olgin JE, Kalman JM, Lesh MD. Conduction barriers in human atrial flutter: correlation of electrophysiology and anatomy. *J Cardiovasc Electrophysiol* 1996;**7**:1112–6.

51 Nakagawa H, Lazzara R, Khastgir T, et al. Role of the tricuspid annulus and the eustachian valve/ridge on atrial flutter. Relevance to catheter ablation of the septal isthmus and a new technique for rapid identification of ablation success. *Circulation* 1996;**94**:407–24.

52 Morady F. Catheter ablation of supraventricular arrhythmias: state of the art. *J Cardiovasc Electrophysiol* 2004;**15**: 124–39.

53 de Groot NM, Kuijper AF, Blom NA, et al. Three-dimensional distribution of bipolar atrial electrogram voltages in patients with congenital heart disease. *Pacing Clin Electrophysiol* 2001;**24**:1334–42.

54 Nademanee K, McKenzie J, Kosar E, et al. A new approach for catheter ablation of atrial fibrillation: mapping of the electrophysiologic substrate. *J Am Coll Cardiol* 2004;**43**:2044–53.

55 Nademanee K, Schwab M, Porath J, et al. How to perform electrogram-guided atrial fibrillation ablation. *Heart Rhythm* 2006;**3**:981–4.

56 Centurion OA, Shimizu A, Isomoto S, et al. Influence of advancing age on fractionated right atrial endocardial electrograms. *Am J Cardiol* 2005;**96**:239–42.

57 Rostock T, Rotter M, Sanders P, et al. High-density activation mapping of fractionated electrograms in the atria of patients with paroxysmal atrial fibrillation. *Heart Rhythm* 2006;**3**:27–34.

CHAPTER 3

Computer simulation studies of atrial fibrillation

Nathalie Virag, Lam Dang, Patrick Ruchat, Juerg Schlaepfer, & Lukas Kappenberger

Introduction

Computer modeling is a rapidly growing field that aims at providing a better understanding of the mechanisms underlying cardiac arrhythmias such as atrial fibrillation (AF) as well as of their therapies. Several computer models of atria have been developed over the last decades. Moe et al. developed the first model of AF using cellular automata [1]. Later, more sophisticated models taking into account several aspects of the complex atrial anatomy have been put forward [2–7]. Existing models differ in the tradeoff made between accuracy of the anatomic representation and the computational load. In most cases, these models have been developed to improve our insight into the electrical propagation during normal activation and in particular during arrhythmias such as atrial flutter or fibrillation. Some of these models are now being used to evaluate the effect of atrial therapies such as termination with antiarrhythmic drugs [8] or non-pharmacological ablation procedures [9].

This chapter describes how a biophysical model of human atria can be used to evaluate different surgical/catheter ablation patterns in a real-size virtual human atria. Modeling of ablation procedures requires simulations of long periods of AF on a computer modeling scale (several minutes instead of several seconds). The heavy computational demand of the advanced available atrial models precludes their use in this type of analysis. Therefore, a simpler model requiring far less computation effort was designed such that sufficient realism for the particular application was retained [9].

In the presented computer simulations, the gold standard Cox's maze III surgical procedure was evaluated and taken as a basic reference [10]. This complex ablation procedure has proven to be effective in treating chronic AF [11] but is time-consuming and associated with a risk of serious complications. Therefore, less invasive radiofrequency (RF) catheter ablation alternatives were investigated clinically. Alongside, simulations were performed in the biophysical model to evaluate simpler catheter ablations patterns involving lines in the right and/or left atrium and to compare these to the reference maze III procedure. The advantage of a computer modeling study over a clinical procedure is that it allows a systematic evaluation, under controlled conditions, of the respective importance of ablation lines in the right and left atrium. Furthermore, computer simulations allow access to the whole human atria at any time during a (simulated) ablation intervention.

While cut-and-sew techniques offer a real transmural barrier lesion to electrical propagation, other physical media of ablation could lead to non-transmural ablation lines. Computer modeling can easily mimic this occurrence by introducing gaps in the ablation lines and can assess the effect of non-transmurality, generally manifested by residual

Catheter Ablation of Atrial Fibrillation Edited by Etienne Aliot, Michel Haïssaguerre and Warren M. Jackman

atrial flutter. Finally, hybrid therapies such as the combined effect of therapeutical pacing and AF ablation can also be tested.

From magnetic resonance images to a computer model of atrial fibrillation

An anatomy-based biophysical model of AF with an atrial membrane kinetics model was used in this study. Existing models extract the information about anatomy from several sources: commercial/published atrial datasets [4,7] or basic considerations from the literature on atrial dimensions, atrial muscle bundles, and propagation velocities [4,5]. The geometry used in our model was derived from magnetic resonance (MR) images of the human atria segmented slice by slice, with 1 mm spacing (Figure 3.1). These formed the basis for the atrial surface in three-dimensional space. Surface smoothing was applied to construct a suitable mesh of triangular elements. Like in all computer models of electrical propagation, this atrial surface consists of a grid of nodes representing atrial cells interconnected via resistors representing the interconnections of the myocytes at the gap junctions. The mathematical formulation of this model has been described previously [6].

Several simplifications were made in order to maintain computational load within a tractable range. The model used for our study was given a realistic size and geometry but the thickness of the atrial wall was taken to be infinitesimal (monolayer model). The resistors connecting the cells were all given an equal value, resulting in a surface with intrinsic homogeneous and isotropic properties. For each atrial cell, an ionic model based on membrane channel kinetics was implemented. In the study reported on, we chose a variant of the ventricular model described by the Luo and Rudy model [12]. This was modified to mimic atrial cellular properties [13]. It was used instead of one of the dedicated atrial cell models [14] because of its significantly reduced computational demand.

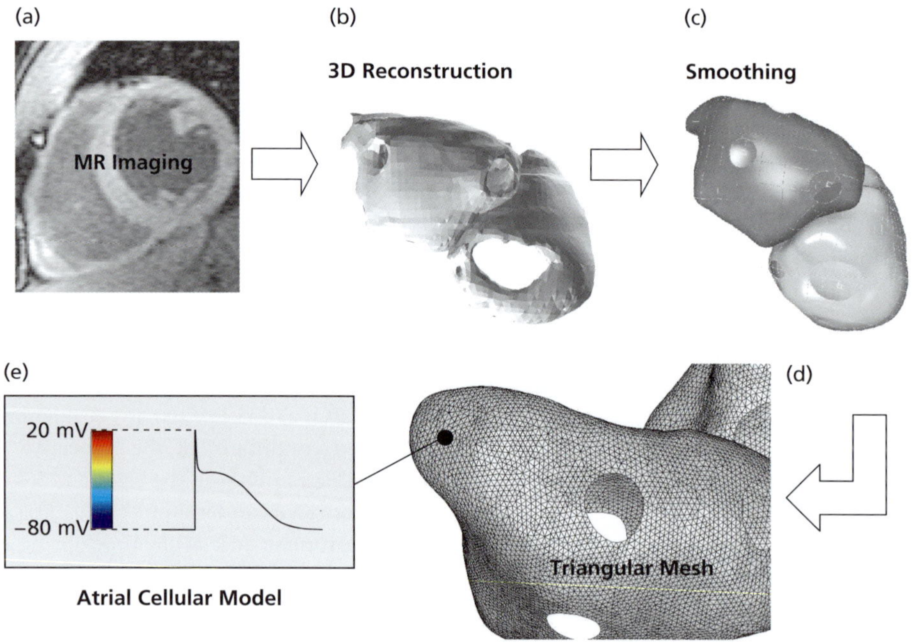

Figure 3.1 From MR images to computer model of human atria. (a) MR imaging and segmentation of atrial contours slice by slice. (b) Reconstruction of a three-dimensional atrial structure. (c) Surface smoothing and correction of the contours of veins and valves. (d) Meshing of the atrial surface using triangular elements. (e) For each node in the mesh, an atrial membrane cellular model is computed generating an action potential, which is then color coded (red for potentials greater than 20 mV and dark blue for the resting potential at –80 mV). This representation corresponds to isopotential maps.

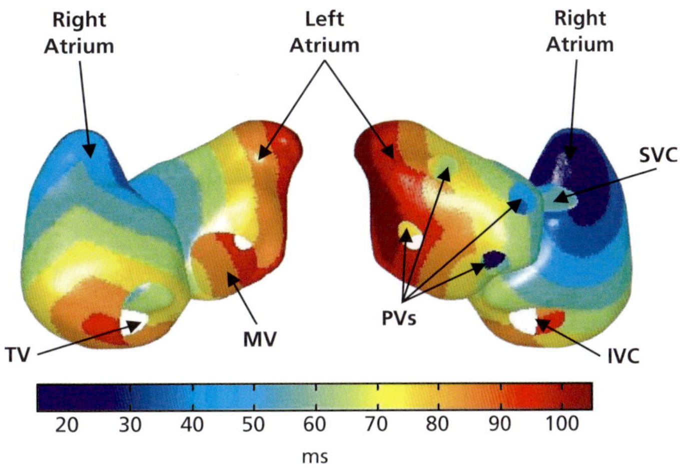

Figure 3.2 Biophysical model of human atria: anterior and posterior view of atrial geometry and propagation of normal sinus rhythm. The major valves and vessels are included: tricuspid valve (TV), mitral valve (MV), pulmonary veins (PVs), and superior and inferior vena cava (SVC and IVC). Isoactivation areas are shown in color, from earliest in dark blue to latest in dark red.

The entire model as used for our study on ablation consisted of 100,000 triangular elements, corresponding to 50,000 nodes spaced at a resolution of 400 μm. The resulting computational load is 1 h/s of simulation on a standard PC (Pentium III 1.4 GHz). This is significantly less than the time required by more complete but complex models. For example, almost 16 h of CPU (central processing unit) time on 28 simultaneously active processors were required to simulate 1 s of atrial activation for the atrial model by Harrild and Henriquez [4]. The simpler model by Vigmond et al. required about 5 h on three processors for 1 s of AF [5].

Besides the simplified model used in this study, we have developed more sophisticated versions with atrial membrane kinetics including anisotropy, heterogeneities, and the computation of electrograms [15,16]. Recently, the model has been extended by including multilayers of cells representing the thickness of the atrial walls [17]. However, these improvements are at the expense of an increased computational load and render these models difficult for use in large-scale evaluations such as the ones presented here.

Propagation of atrial activation

In our biophysical model of human atria, left and right atria are connected through the atrial septum. The propagation of a normal sinus beat was initiated by injecting an intracellular current with a strength of 80 $\mu A/cm^2$ into the cells of the sinoatrial node region, located anatomically on the anterolateral portion of the right atrium, near the border of the superior vena cava orifice. The atrial geometry and the isochrones of a normal sinus beat are shown in Figure 3.2. Atrial activation terminated in the left lateral wall below the appendage, where three wavefronts converged. Despite homogeneous tissue properties, the global behavior of the activation maps is comparable to the ones from experimental data [18] or other anatomic computer models specifically aimed at simulating normal atrial conduction [4]. The main differences are found in the left atrium close to the mitral valve, which is activated somewhat too early compared to the left atrial appendage due to the absence of any bundles of preferential conduction in this simplified model.

Simulation of atrial fibrillation

Atrial arrhythmias are initiated in a computer model in a similar way as in clinical experiments: using a programmed stimulation protocol or a burst-pacing protocol. Burst pacing at 20 Hz near the sinoatrial node was eventually chosen here because it does not require any adjustment of timing or stimulus location. In our baseline atrial model, most of the attempts to initiate arrhythmias either failed or initiated unstable reentrant waves terminating after a few seconds due to mutual interactions. Consequently, most AF episodes spontaneously converted to sinus rhythm after a few seconds, as was found in biological models [18].

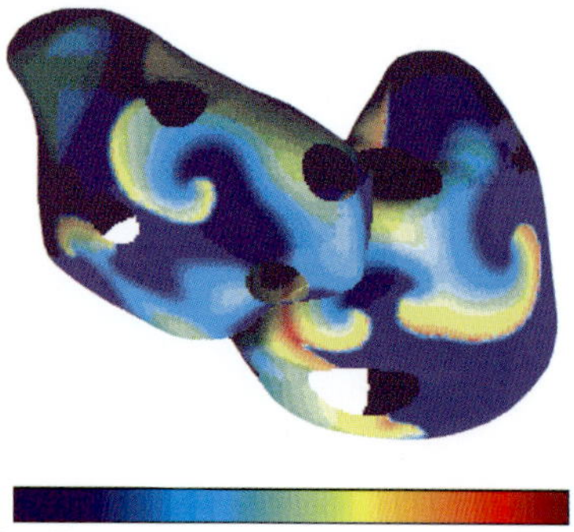

Figure 3.3 Example of atrial activation pattern during sustained chronic AF.

Conditions for sustained arrhythmias in computer models can be based on different factors, such as the introduction of heterogeneities in refractoriness [8,19] or in atrial structures [5]. In our study, sustained arrhythmias could be realized by including in the model mechanisms mimicking electrical remodeling as observed in patients suffering from permanent AF, such as shortening of action potential duration and a flattening of the action potential restitution curve [13]. The various conditions for the initiation and perpetuation of AF in this model have been studied and compared to clinical mapping data [6,15,16]. Figure 3.3 shows an example of an atrial activation map during simulated chronic AF involving multiple reentrant wavelets (three to eight), continuously changing in size and direction due to functional and anatomic reentries. In this model of chronic AF, simulated sustained AF lasting longer than 7 min could be observed, which is the longest simulation ever performed in a biophysical model of the atria.

Simulation of therapies for atrial fibrillation

A computer model able to simulate sustained AF with realistic properties offers the possibility to evaluate different therapies for AF. The simulation of pharmacological interventions can be performed in models with a detailed description of atrial myocyte membrane kinetics [14] even with simpler geometries such as two-dimensional rectangles of atrial tissue [8]. In addition to pharmacological therapies, electrical interventions such as pacing or defibrillation can also be tested, although defibrillation simulations have been developed mostly in ventricular models [20]. Therapeutical pacing is simulated by injecting intracellular current at any location on the atria.

Our study focused on the ablation therapy. Ablation lines were implemented by making the cardiac cells located on the ablation lines non-propagating (infinite resistivity). This process resulted in the creation of continuous lesions that were transmural since we were using a monolayer model. This is equivalent to a surgical ablation or a continuous RF ablation on both the epicardial and endocardial sides. In order to reproduce the effect of incomplete RF ablation lines (for example when applied only on the endocardial side) in this monolayer model, a gap (or gaps) in an ablation line could be created at any desired location. Gap widths from 1.3 to 3 mm were tested; gaps shorter than 1.3 mm did not allow the wavefront to travel through it [9].

The different ablation patterns studied were evaluated during simulated chronic AF. Patterns were applied instantaneously and the ablation was considered successful if AF termination was observed within 30 s. Simulations were arbitrarily stopped after this time interval since analysis of the simulations showed that termination occurring after 30 s were generally due to spontaneous termination of AF. For each pattern evaluated, a group of 10–40 simulations of AF ablation were performed by applying the ablation lines at different time instants of the simulated AF. The results obtained in these groups of simulations based on different AF states were then averaged. Success rate, time to AF termination, and AF reinitiation capacities were assessed for each pattern studied.

Each ablation pattern required a simulation of a total of a minimum of 5 min of AF. In the research described here we studied about 20 different patterns, tested the effect of a gap in most of the lines, and evaluated the combined effect of these patterns with pacing from different sites. This represents a total time of several hours of simulated AF.

This type of study of ablation lines by means of computer simulation has some intrinsic limitations that sometimes make a direct comparison between computer simulations and clinical data difficult. Firstly, we used the geometry of only one patient (MR images from a male with a heart of average size), whereas atrial anatomy differs from patient to patient. Secondly, we applied the ablation lines instantaneously instead of one by one as is done during the clinical procedure of RF ablation. Thirdly, in these experiments of chronic AF, our model is based on multiple reentrant wavelets and does not take into account rapid foci originating from the area of the pulmonary veins [21], which may create differences in the success rate obtained with lines in the left atrium. Finally, the timescales between computer simulations and clinical data is different: simulations last only a few minutes while permanent AF can be present over days, months, or years. This is partly taken into account in the model by the use of electrically remodeled cells [13] and the comparison is only performed during the AF termination phase initiated by ablation.

Systematic evaluation of ablation patterns

Several published ablation patterns involving right and/or left ablation lines were implemented in the computer model with the objective to compare their results to clinical data. The best results and the shortest time to AF termination were obtained in the computer model with the standard maze III procedure, which is in agreement with clinical data for the complete maze III pattern showing a long-term success rate ranging from 80% to 99% [10,11]. Figure 3.4a shows an example of simulation of AF termination with the maze III ablation pattern: the ablation pattern was instantaneously applied during an episode of chronic AF at time = 0 s, and we can observe a gradual decrease in the number of wavelets and a reorganization of electrical activity towards one reentrant wavelet that eventually dies. Reinitiation of AF after this ablation procedure was not possible.

Our simulation studies were directed at finding possible ways of reproducing the success of the complete maze procedure while using a minimum number of lesions. Therefore, a systematic study was performed by combining the following basic ablation lines:

- right isthmus line between the inferior vena cava and tricuspid valve (RAI);
- line between the superior and inferior vena cava (SIVC);
- right atrial appendage line (RAA);
- left atrial isthmus line between the left inferior pulmonary vein and mitral valve (LAI);
- connection of three pulmonary veins (CPV);
- isolation of four pulmonary veins (IPV);
- left atrial appendage line (LAA).

Our systematic evaluation confirms that the most complex ablation patterns lead both to the best success rate and shortest time to AF termination. Figure 3.5 presents some of the combinations of lesions tested in this systematic study. Ablation patterns involving lines in the right or left atrium led to success rates in the ranges 20–60% and 55–80%, respectively, while those combining lines in both atria showed an increased rate in the range 80–100%. A detailed study of the time to AF termination and the number of wavelets present in the tissue during ablation has been performed [9]. Some patterns tested in this study are used in clinical interventions. For the right atrium only, the success rate obtained in computer simulation with the pattern RAI + SIVC was 60%, which is comparable to the published results of a clinical study with lesions only in the right atrium and with a long-term success rate of right atrial compartmentalization of 67% [22]. For the left atrium only, the best simulated pattern led to a success rate of 80%, which is comparable to published results about ablation in the pulmonary veins region reporting a long-term success rate of 82% [23]. Interesting ablation patterns that led to a high success rate with a minimum number of lesions are either a connection or an isolation of the pulmonary veins, combined with a left atrial isthmus line and either a line between the vena cavae or a right atrial isthmus line.

Clinical validation is a crucial point when analyzing computer simulation results. Some of the results simulated in the computer model have been compared to clinical experiments. For example, we compared simulated and clinical data in the case of a minimized maze procedure represented by pattern J in Figure 3.5. In the clinical settings, the RF left atrial compartmentalization was performed during mitral valve repair or replacement [24]. In this simplified maze pattern, our simulations of ablation led to a success rate of 88% averaged over 26 simulations comparable to a success rate of 92% averaged over 26 patients in our clinical experience of using RF ablation [9]. No significant difference

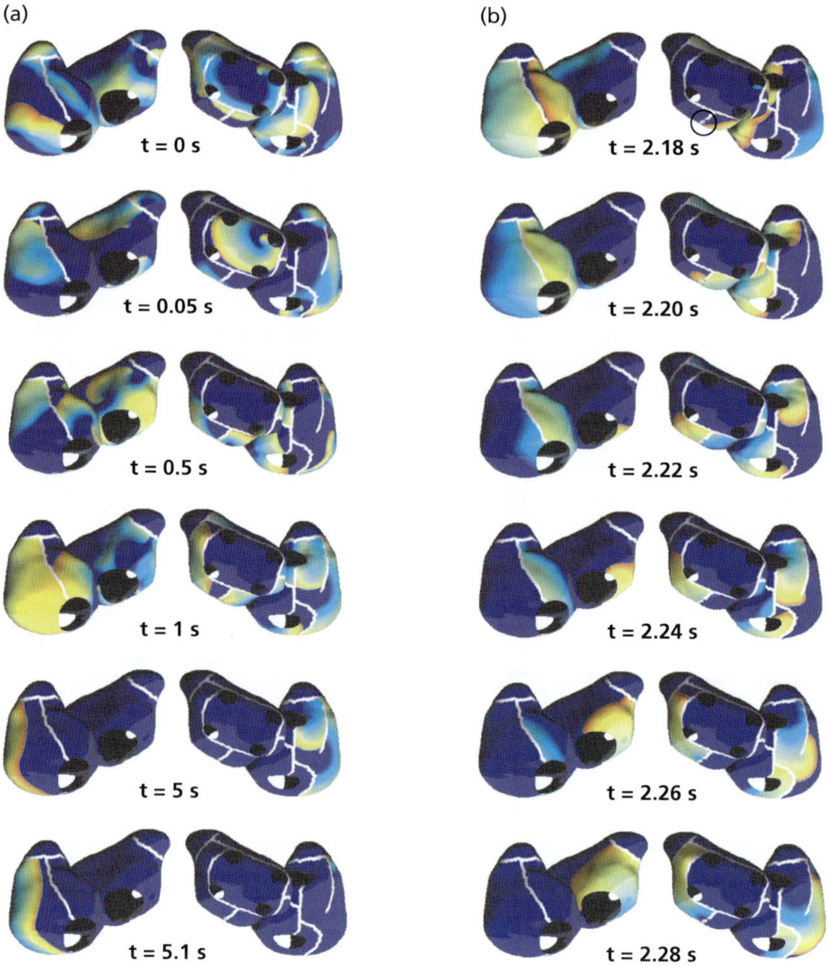

Figure 3.4 Example of computer simulation of ablation with a maze III pattern. (a) Simulation in the case of ideal transmural lesions. (b) Simulations of the effect of a gap of 2.4 mm in the ablation line connecting the pulmonary veins and the mitral valve (encircled).

was observed between the clinical data and the computer results.

The advantage of computer simulations over clinical experiments in this study is mainly that a detailed observation of the ablation process is possible during the whole procedure (Figure 3.5) and areas where reentrant waves are still present can be identified. It is also possible to test individually and systematically each lesion in a given ablation pattern, defining the relative importance of each of its components. Finally, patterns not generally performed in clinical experiments could also be evaluated.

Evaluation of the effect of non-transmural ablation lines

One important aspect in computer simulations of ablation is that it permits the study of the imperfections that may be present in the ablation lines. Several experiments were performed to assess which lesions in the set studied previously were more sensitive to non-transmurality in their effect on AF termination rate. Our simulations studies suggested that gaps in the ablation lines between the pulmonary veins and mitral valve annulus in the left atrium have a significant

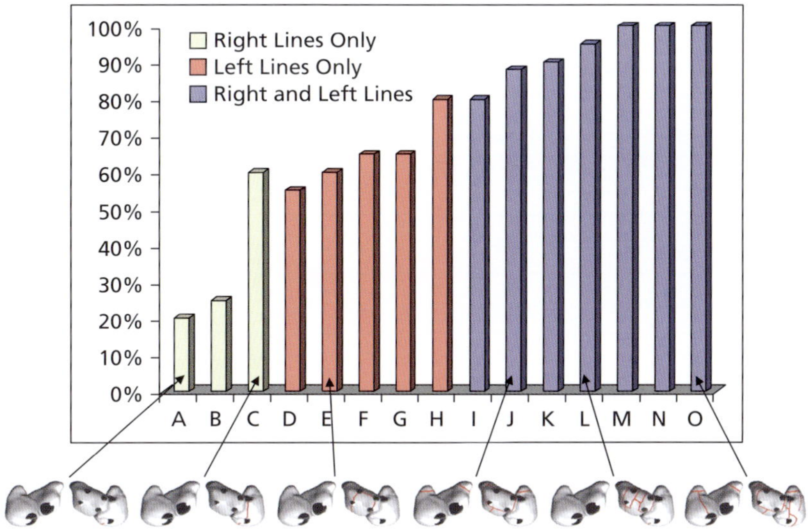

Figure 3.5 Percentage of successful AF termination for some of the ablation patterns evaluated in the computer model: (A) RAI, (B) SIVC, (C) RAI + SIVC, (D) IPV, (E) CPV + LAI, (F) IPV + LAA, (G) IPV + LAI, (H) IPV + LAI + LAA, (I) IPV + LAI + SIVC, (J) IPV + LAI + LAA + RAA, (K) CPV + LAI + RAI, (L) IPV + LAI + RAI, (M) CPV + LAI + SIVC, (N) IPV + LAI + RAI + SIVC, and (O) complete maze III. See the text for abbreviations.

impact on the AF termination success rate, with an increasing effect in wider gaps or in gaps located closer to the valve. This also holds true for the line between the vena cavae in the right atrium. The lower performance in these cases was due to the appearance of uncommon flutter after ablation. Figure 3.4b shows an example of the application of a complete maze III pattern with a gap in the lesion between the pulmonary veins lesion and the mitral valve. The effect in this case was a reduction of AF termination from 100% to 82.2% and a residual atypical atrial flutter around the mitral valve [9].

Evaluation of hybrid therapies for atrial fibrillation

One way to keep the number of ablation lines minimal, while having a high success rate in AF termination, would be to use a hybrid technique and combine ablation with another therapy. We chose to evaluate the combined effect of pacing and ablation. In our model, single-site pacing alone could not terminate AF but could capture an area of 4–6 cm in the right atrium, where wavefront propagation was uniform without wave breaks. The pacing frequency was determined based on the cycle length of the arrhythmias present in the tissue. However, once this regional control was achieved, a decrease in pacing rate led to a loss of capture due to the penetration of reentrant wavelets in the area under control. These results are consistent with clinical observation [25].

Therefore we investigated in our model if ablation lines could increase pacing capture and termination of AF. In the example shown in Figure 3.6, single-site pacing was initiated on chronic AF at eight different pacing sites indicated by the red dots. The seven different ablation patterns tested were applied at the beginning of pacing, and pacing was continued until capture was achieved (maximum 30 s). AF termination was considered successful if no reinitiation was observed after the pacing stopped. The increase in success rate obtained by adding an ablation line to the single-site pacing procedure was divided into three groups: (1) no improvement; (2) minor improvement; and (3) significant improvement.

Our simulations suggest that ablation patterns have little impact on AF termination by pacing if they included lines in the right atrium only. Isolation of the pulmonary veins seems to help

	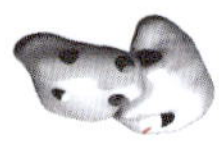	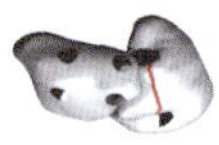	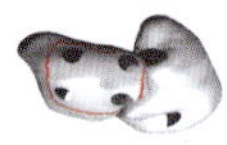	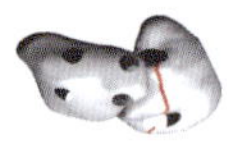	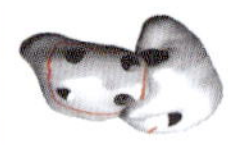	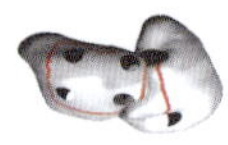	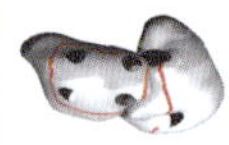
Pacing **LAA**	–	–	–	–	–	+	+
Pacing **LAFW**	–	–	–	–	–	+	–
Pacing **BB**	–	–	+	–	+	+	++
Pacing **RAI**	–	–	–	–	–	++	–
Pacing **RAFW**	–	–	–	+	+	++	++
Pacing **RAA**	–	–	–	–	+	–	++
Pacing **RAIF**	+	–	++	–	++	++	++
Pacing **RAVC**	–	–	++	–	++	++	++

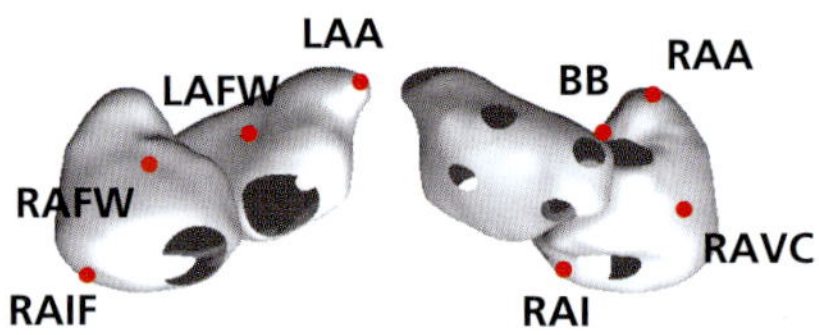

Figure 3.6 Evaluation of combined pacing and ablation of AF. The following seven ablation patterns were evaluated: RAI, SIVC, IPV, RAI + SIVC, IPV + RAI, IPV + SIVC, and IPV + RAI + SIVC (see text for abbreviations). Pacing at an optimal frequency was performed at eight different pacing sites in combination with the different ablation lines: left atrial appendage (LAA), left atrial free wall (LAFW), Bachmann's bundle (BB), right atrial isthmus (RAI), right atrial free wall (RAFW), right atrial appendage (RAA), right atrial inferior (RAIF), and right atrial between vena cavae (RAVC). The effect of the hybrid technique was evaluated by the improvement in AF termination obtained by adding the ablation line to pacing: –, no improvement (less than 15%); +, slight improvement (15–30%); ++, significant improvement (more than 30%).

pacing capture, probably because it avoids wave breaks often observed in that area. The best results were obtained for ablation lines involving both the right and left atria. Our simulations also suggest that the best pacing sites amongst those tested are located in the right atrium, probably because they allow a better control of the large uninterrupted areas of the right atrium where many wave breaks are usually observed during our simulations of AF. These preliminary results are encouraging and future simulations will work at a joint optimization of ablation and pacing therapies in this computer model. Besides the simulation of ablation presented here, computer modeling allows the study of a very wide range of different therapeutic pacing protocols: from single site to multisite at any location, with a fixed pacing frequency, with ramp pacing algorithms, or with an adaptive frequency in a closed-loop framework.

Conclusion

This chapter shows how a biophysical model of AF can be used to evaluate surgical and catheter ablation of AF. The results discussed confirm the good performance of the standard maze III procedure in treating chronic AF. They suggest that less invasive patterns need to include ablation lines in both atria and that discontinuities in specifically designated ablation lines lead to a decrease in success rate. The model may also help to identify the ablation lines that are essential both in the right and left atria for successful, less invasive patterns. This method may be used to pre-evaluate new ablation strategies in estimating success rates and potential proarrhythmic effects like atrial flutter. This tool also permits the evaluation of hybrid therapies for AF, such as combined pacing and ablation.

Acknowledgments

This study was made possible through grants from the Theo-Rossi-Di-Montelera Foundation, Medtronic Europe, and the Swiss Governmental Commission of Innovative Technologies (CTI). The authors wish to thank Ryan Lahm, Dr Josée Morisette, and Dr Arthur Stillman who kindly furnished the atrial geometry surface model. The authors also would like to thank Professor Adriaan van Oosterom for helpful discussions and suggestions regarding the manuscript.

References

1 Moe G, Rheinbold W, Abildskov J. A computer model of atrial fibrillation. *Am Heart J* 1964;**67**:200–20.

2 Gray RA, Jalife J. Ventricular fibrillation and atrial fibrillation are two different beasts. *Chaos* 1998;**8**:65–78.

3 Ellis WS, SippensGroenewegen A, Auslander DM, Lesh M. The role of crista terminalis in atrial flutter and fibrillation: A computer modeling study. *Ann Biomed Eng* 2000;**28**:742–754.

4 Harrild D, Henriquez C. A computer model of normal conduction in the human atria. *Circ Res* 2000;**87**:e25–e36.

5 Vigmond EJ, Ruckdeschel R, Trayanova N. Reentry in a morphologically realistic atrial model. *J. Cardiovasc Electrophysiol* 2001;**12**:1046–54.

6 Virag N, Jacquemet V, Henriquez CS, et al. Study of atrial arrhythmias in a computer model based on magnetic resonance images of human atria. *Chaos* 2002;**12**:754–63.

7 Seeman G, Hoper C, Sachse FB, Dossel O, Holden AV, Zhang H. Heterogeneous three-dimensional anatomical and electrophysiological model of human atria. *Phil Trans A Math Phys Eng Sci* 2006;**364**:1465–81.

8 Kneller J, Kalifa J, Zou R, et al. Mechanims of atrial fibrillation termination by pure sodium channel blockade in an ionically-realistic mathematical model. *Circ Res* 2005;**96**:35–47.

9 Dang L, Virag N, Ihara Z, et al. Evaluation of ablation patterns using a biophysical model of atrial fibrillation. *Ann Biomed Eng* 2005;**33**:465–74.

10 Cox JL, Schuessler RB, D'Agostino HJ, Jr., et al. The surgical treatment of atrial fibrillation: III. Development of a definitive surgical procedure. *J Thoracic Cardiovasc Surg* 1991;**101**:569–83.

11 Cox JL. Atrial transport function after the maze procedure for atrial fibrillation: a 10 year clinical experience. *Am Heart J* 1998;**136**:934–6.

12 Luo C-H, Rudy Y. A model of the ventricular cardiac action potential. *Circ Res* 1991;**68**:1501–26.

13 Li D, Zhang L, Knellet J, Nattel S. Potential ionic mechanism for repolarization differences between canine right and left atrium. *Circ Res* 2001;**88**:1168–75.

14 Courtemanche M, Ranirez RJ, Nattel S. Ionic mechanisms underlying human atrial action potential properties: insights from a mathematical model. *Am J Physiol* 1998;**275**:H301–H321.

15 Jacquemet V, Virag N, Ihara Z, et al. Study of unipolar electrogram morphology in a computer model of atrial fibrillation. *J Cardiovasc Electrophysiol* 2003;**14**:S172–S179.

16 Jacquemet V, Virag N, Kappenberger L. Wavelength and vulnerability to atrial fibrillation: insights from a computer model of human atria. *Europace* 2005;**7**:S83–S92.

17 Van Oosterom A, Jacquemet V. Genesis of the P wave: atrial signal as generated by the equivalent double layer source model. *Europace* 2005;**7**:S21–S29.

18 Allessie MA, Rensma PL, Brugada J, et al. Pathophysiology of atrial fibrillation. In: Zipes DP, Jalife J, eds. *Cardiac Electrophysiology from Cell to Bedside.* WB Saunders, Philadelphia, 1990:548–59.

19 Vigmond EJ, Tsoi V, Kuo S, Arvalo H, Kneller J, Nattel S, Trayanova N. The effect of vagally induced dispersion of action potential duration on atrial arrhythmogenesis. *Heart Rhythm* 2004;**1**:334–44.

20 Skouibine K, Trayanova NA, Moore P. Success and failure of the defibrillation shocks: insights from a simulation study. *J Cardiovasc Electrophysiol* 2000;**11**:785–96.

21 Haissaguerre M, Jais P, Shah S, et al. Spontaneous initiation of atrial fibrillation by ectopic beats originating in the pulmonary veins. *N Engl J Med* 1998;**339**:649–66.

22 Garg A, Finneran W, Mollerus M, Birgersdotter-Green O, Fujimura O, Time L, Fled GK. Right atrial compartmentalization using radiofrequency catheter ablation for management of patients with refractory atrial fibrillation. *J Thoracic Cardiovasc Surg* 1999;**10**:763–71.

23 Kottkamp H, Hindricks G, Hammel D, et al. Intraoperative radiofrequency ablation of chronic atrial fibrillation: a left curative approach by elimination of anatomic "anchor" reentrant circuit. *J Cardiovasc Electrophysiol* 1999;**10**:772–80.

24 Ruchat P, Schlaepfer J, Delabays A, Hurni M, Milne J, von Segesser LK. Left atrial radiofrequency compartmentalization for chronic atrial fibrillation during heart surgery. *Thoracic Cardiovasc Surg* 2002;**50**:155–9.

25 Allessie M, Kirchof C, Scheffer GJ, Chorro F, Brugada J. Regional control of atrial fibrillation by rapid pacing in conscious dogs. *Circulation* 1991;**84**:1689–97.

4

CHAPTER 4

Experimental and theoretical insights into fundamental mechanisms of antiarrhythmic drug actions on atrial fibrillation: prospects for improved pharmacotherapy

Stanley Nattel

Introduction

Atrial fibrillation (AF) is a problem of large and growing proportions. It is estimated that between 12 and 16 million Americans will suffer from AF by 2050 [1], so that irrespective of the great efficacy and increasing safety of AF ablation, drugs will likely remain part of our approach to AF for a long time to come. This chapter reviews the principles of antiarrhythmic therapy for sinus rhythm maintenance, dealing with presently available antiarrhythmic drugs, ideas about how they work, and new avenues for drug therapy of AF currently under investigation.

Classical antiarrhythmic drug therapy for sinus rhythm maintenance

What is classical antiarrhythmic drug therapy and how good is it?

Antiarrhythmic drugs have been used to keep AF patients in sinus rhythm for nearly 100 years [2]. A wide range of agents is presently available, and the list of drugs approved for AF can differ significantly from one country to another. Japan and France have the largest number of approved AF drugs: seven each (Figure 4.1). All the available drugs for sinus rhythm maintenance block K^+ channels, Na^+ channels, or a combination of the two.

Overall, antiarrhythmic drug efficacy for sinus rhythm maintenance is poor. Although there is wide variability in sinus rhythm maintenance without drug therapy, a range of published studies shows that ~40% of AF patients will remain in sinus rhythm for approximately 6–12 months after cardioversion and that chronic administration of antiarrhythmic drugs like quinidine, sotalol, and flecainide can increase the sinus rhythm maintenance rate to ~55–60% [3]. Amiodarone is significantly more effective, improving sinus rhythm maintenance to ~80% [4–6].

The adverse effect profile of currently available antiarrhythmic agents is the greatest factor limiting their use. Of largest concern is their proarrhythmic potential, which can increase sudden death mortality [2,3]. Amiodarone has a reduced proarrhythmic potential compared to other available sinus rhythm maintenance drugs, but is fraught with difficult

Catheter Ablation of Atrial Fibrillation Edited by Etienne Aliot, Michel Haïssaguerre and Warren M. Jackman
© 2008 Blackwell Publishing, ISBN: 978-1-4501-6349-1.

	Japan	USA	France	Gmny	England	Holland
Procainamide	O	X	–	–	–	–
Disopyramide	O	X	O	O	O	O
Quinidine	O	O	X	O	O	–
Propafenone	O	X	O	O	O	O
Aprindine	O	–	O	–	–	O
Cibenzoline	O	–	O	–	–	–
Pirmenol	X	–	–	–	–	–
Flecainide	X	O	O	O	O	O
Pilsicainide	O	–	–	–	–	–
Bepridil	X	X	X	–	–	–
Sotalol	X	O	O	O	O	O
Amiodarone	△	X	O	O	O	O
Dofetilide	–	O	–	–	–	–

O : Approved X : Not approved – : Not available △ : Amiodarone for AF complicating HCM

Figure 4.1 Antiarrhythmic drugs available in different countries as of November 2006. Grmny, Germany; HCM, hypertrophic cardiomyopathy. (Courtesy of Dr Hideo Mitamura, Tokyo, Japan.)

pharmacokinetics and a host of troublesome potential long-term side effects [2,3].

How do antiarrhythmic drugs prevent AF?

Figure 4.2 presents the classical notions regarding AF maintenance and antiarrhythmic drug action. AF was classically thought to be maintained by multiple circuit reentry. The ability of a functional reentry circuit to maintain itself is classically understood by the leading circle mechanism [7], as a result of the time taken to traverse a functional reentrant circuit in relation to circuit dimensions. In order for reentry to be sustained, the circuit time has to be greater than the refractory period (RP). The minimal circuit time is therefore equal to the RP, and the size of the smallest possible circuit is the distance traveled by the impulse in one RP, or RP × conduction velocity (CV). This minimum circuit size (RP × CV) is called the wavelength. When the wavelength is large (as is the case in most normal hearts), the atria can only contain a small number of functional reentrant waves and AF does not persist very long. However, if the wavelength is reduced, for example by reducing RP, more waves can be accommodated and AF persists. The same is true if the atria are enlarged. The classical notion was that drugs suppress AF by increasing the RP (e.g. by delaying repolarization with a K^+ channel blocker).

Problems with classical ideas and the development of newer theories

An important problem with the classical notion of AF is that it does not explain how certain antiarrhythmic drugs work. According to classical ideas, a Na^+ channel blocker, which slows conduction (i.e. decreases CV, and consequently wavelength), should promote AF by allowing more simultaneous reentry circuits. However, it turns out that Na^+ channel blockers are just about as good anti-AF agents as K^+ channel blockers [2,3]. One possible explanation for this is that AF is not, in fact, a reentrant arrhythmia at all in many patients, and that

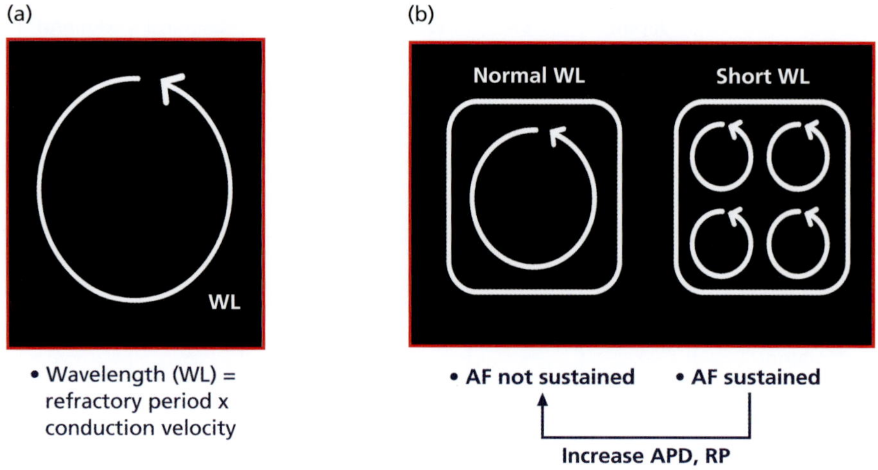

Figure 4.2 Classical notions of AF mechanisms and therapy. (a) The wavelength (WL), a product of conduction velocity and the refractory period (RP), is the size of the smallest possible reentry circuit. (b) When the wavelength is normal, the atria cannot accommodate many waves simultaneously and AF tends to die out spontaneously (left). When the wavelength is reduced, multiple waves can coexist, making AF more stable and much less likely to terminate (right). APD, action potential duration.

atrial ectopic activity plays a major role in AF maintenance [8,9]. Another possibility, however, is that the classical notion of reentry may be faulty. Advances in our understanding of cardiac electrical activity and in computer simulation methods have permitted the creation of very realistic cell and tissue models of atrial electrical function and AF [10,11]. When these are applied, reentrant activity does not look like a "leading circle", but rather like a "spiral wave" (for a detailed review of these concepts, see [12]). In fact, the differences between leading circles and spiral waves are in some senses related to how one looks at things; however, spiral wave theory fits better with biophysical reality, and the predictions about arrhythmic activity that result from spiral wave theory differ in subtle but important ways from those of the leading circle model [12]. One notable difference is that the persistence of spiral waves depends on their ability to remain stable in a tissue substrate. By enlarging spiral waves and making them drift to regions where they can no longer sustain themselves, Na^+ channel-blocking drugs extinguish atrial fibrillatory activity [13]. These theoretical considerations fit well with experimental evidence that Na^+ channel blockers effectively terminate AF without altering the reentry wavelength [13–15].

Present status of antiarrhythmic drug therapy

The drugs that are now on the market for sinus rhythm maintenance are simply not very satisfactory [16]. Perhaps as a result, sinus rhythm maintenance with presently available antiarrhythmic drugs is not a superior strategy to merely leaving patients in AF and controlling the ventricular response rate; in fact, there is evidence of greater risk with a rhythm control strategy [17,18]. That this may be a problem not with the strategy but with the available drugs is suggested by an analysis of the results of patients who did, versus those that did not, maintain sinus rhythm in the AFFIRM trial [19]. Patients that maintained sinus rhythm had a much better prognosis. One response to this information is to say that we should simply abandon the notion of using drug therapy to maintain sinus rhythm in AF patients and opt instead for non-pharmacological approaches – much as we have largely abandoned drugs to prevent atrioventricular (AV) nodal reentrant tachycardias.

The rest of this book is about ablation procedures for AF, and illustrates how quickly such procedures have developed and how effective they have become. Nevertheless, the complexity of the AF substrate, the variability in its clinical and mechanistic determinants, and the sheer size of the AF population suggest that AF ablation, no matter how much it improves, may not provide a universal solution for sinus rhythm maintenance. It therefore remains reasonable to pursue efforts to identify new and potentially superior pharmacological approaches for AF prevention, and this is an area in rapid development [20].

Approaches to developing new anti-atrial fibrillation drugs

Atrial-selective agents

The drugs that have in the past been used to prolong the RP (e.g. quinidine, sotalol, and dofetilide) targeted the rapid delayed rectifier current I_{Kr}. The problem with I_{Kr} is that this current is crucial for repolarization in other parts of the heart, particularly the ventricles and Purkinje system, and in predisposed patients I_{Kr} blockers destabilize ventricular repolarization, resulting in potentially lethal, acquired long QT syndromes and torsades de pointes arrhythmias [21]. Agents with atrial-selective RP prolonging actions could effectively prevent AF without a risk of torsades de pointes.

Atrial-selective ion-channel targets

One interesting potential target is the ultrarapid delayed rectifier K^+ current I_{Kur}, which in humans is important in the atria [22,23] but absent in the ventricles [23–25]. I_{Kur} inhibition should delay atrial repolarization and increase atrial RP without affecting ventricular tissue. Many I_{Kur} blockers have been developed [26] and some are presently in clinical trials. Another potentially interesting target is the acetylcholine-gated K^+ current, I_{KACh}. I_{KACh} is responsible for vagal effects on the atria, which cause strong, spatially heterogeneous atrial action potential and RP shortening, as well as clear AF promotion. Recent studies show that AF alters I_{KACh} properties, causing the channel to open even in the absence of acetylcholine [27,28] and producing action potential abbreviation that promotes AF [29]. I_{KACh} is absent in the ventricles: blocking I_{KACh} has no effect on ventricular cell currents or action potentials [29]. I_{KACh} blockers may therefore suppress AF without causing ventricular proarrhythmia.

Na^+ channel blockade is very effective in AF termination, by causing primary reentry waves to extinguish [13]. RSD1235 is an atrial-selective agent [30] that terminates recent-onset AF in about half of patients [31]. The drug produces Na^+ channel block with rapid unblocking kinetics [32], and would be expected to selectively affect Na^+ current during AF because of its rapid rates and the relatively less negative resting potentials of atrial cells.

Drugs that target stretch-operated and pacemaker channels

Atrial fibrillation classically occurs in contexts that involve atrial dilation and stretch. A variety of cardiac membrane channels are opened by cell stretch and could contribute to AF development [33]. The targeting of stretch-activated channels for antiarrhythmic therapy has been hampered by a lack of specific blockers or modulators. GsMTx4, a peptide from the tarantula spider, is a potent inhibitor of stretch-activated cation channels and has been found effective in experimental AF [34]. Dietary fish oil also acts against AF in a rabbit atrial-stretch model, and this property may contribute to the efficacy of fish oils in AF prevention [35].

Cardiac pacemaking activity depends on the balance among a number of cardiac channels, but a particularly important one is the hyperpolarization-gated cyclic nucleotide-binding (HCN) channel that underlies the "funny" current I_f. Atrial HCN subunits are upregulated in some AF-associated conditions like heart failure [36], and may contribute to AF-initiating ectopic activity by enhancing atrial automaticity. The recently introduced I_f channel-blocking drugs like ivabradine may therefore have a place in AF therapy, although this remains to be explored.

Atrial Ca^{2+} handling as a target

Ca^{2+} handling is a complex and essential heart cell function. Contraction requires a rapid systolic increase in free cytoplasmic Ca^{2+} concentration, but relaxation requires restoration of low Ca^{2+} concentrations in diastole. Efficient Ca^{2+} handling is afforded by a complex group of intracellular Ca^{2+}

sarcoplasmic reticulum stores, transporters, and ion channels. Abnormalities in cellular Ca^{2+} handling are associated with a variety of AF-associated conditions like congestive heart failure, ischemic heart disease, and myocardial hypertrophy. Spontaneous diastolic Ca^{2+} leaks from the sarcoplasmic reticulum are handled by exchange across the cell membrane for extracellular Na^+ through the Na^+, Ca^{2+} exchanger. The inward movement of positively charged Na^+ ions depolarizes the cell, causing delayed after-depolarizations. Abnormal diastolic Ca^{2+}-release events have been recorded in heart cells from AF patients [37,38] and in experimental AF models [38]. Calstabin2 binds to the Ca^{2+}-release channels (ryanodine receptors) of the sarcoplasmic reticulum and is a critical modulator of Ca^{2+}-release function. AF-inducing conditions like congestive heart failure deplete calstabin2 from ryanodine receptors, leading to abnormal function and Ca^{2+} leak [39,40]. JTV519 is an organic compound that promotes calstabin2–ryanodine receptor binding, reducing diastolic Ca^{2+} leak [41]. JTV519 also reduces AF inducibility in dogs with sterile pericarditis [42], and may serve as a prototype for newer drugs that act to restore normal Ca^{2+} handling in AF and AF-related conditions.

Targeting intercellular coupling mechanisms

Gap junctions connect cardiomyocytes through closely packed hemichannel subunits that allow intercellular electrical communication, making the heart into a functional syncytium. The conducting ion-channel protein subunits are named connexins, six of which constitute an individual connexon. Connexin 43 and connexin 40 are expressed in working atrial cardiomyocytes. There is evidence for connexin abnormalities in experimental models of AF [43–45], as well as in AF patient samples [46–48], although the results of different studies show a great deal of variability [49]. Increasing gap–junctional coupling could suppress AF by improving cell-to-cell communication and reversing spatially disparate conduction abnormalities. Rotigaptide is an intravenously administered agent that has evolved from a complex program to develop gap–junction conductance enhancing antiarrhythmic agents based on initial observations with peptide compounds [20]. This drug has been studied in various canine models of AF [50,51]. The results show efficacy that is very substrate-dependent, with no effectiveness against AF associated with atrial tachycardia remodeling or heart failure, but value in AF related to myocardial ischemia and mitral regurgitation. Because the class of compounds exemplified by rotigaptide is quite novel and the spectrum of action is still unknown, further work will be needed to determine its role in AF.

Prevention of arrhythmogenic remodeling: "upstream therapy"

Over the past 10 years, we have learned a lot about the arrhythmogenic alterations in cardiac structure and function, called "arrhythmogenic remodeling", that lead to acquired cardiac arrhythmias [49,52,53]. It is hoped that more direct targeting of arrhythmia substrate development will produce novel therapies that are safer and more effective. This approach is sometimes called "upstream therapy" because it acts upstream of the final electrical disturbances that actually generate arrhythmias.

Atrial structural remodeling

Many clinical conditions associated with AF show prominent atrial fibrosis. In congestive heart failure, atrial fibrosis causes local conduction abnormalities that are critical to AF maintenance [54,55]. Atrial rennin–angiotensin systems are strongly engaged by congestive heart failure [56,57], and their inhibition by angiotensin-converting enzyme inhibitors or angiotensin-receptor blockers prevents atrial fibrosis and AF maintenance [56–58]. There is emerging evidence for similar benefit from rennin–angiotensin axis inhibitors in humans [59]. In addition, statin drugs prevent the development of structural remodeling, possibly through anti-inflammatory and/or antioxidant properties [60]. In a retrospective study of patients with heart failure, lipid-lowering drugs, primarily statins, were associated with a reduced risk of AF [61].

Atrial tachycardia remodeling

Rapid atrial firing alters atrial ion channel function and electrophysiology, increasing susceptibility to AF induction and maintenance [62,63]. This phenomenon, called "atrial tachycardia remodeling", is believed to be an important contributor to early recurrences after AF cardioversion and the development of resistance to antiarrhythmic drug therapy with longer duration AF [62,64]. A variety of drugs have been tested in the prevention of atrial tachycardia remodeling, and several classes of agents have shown promise. Drugs that block T-type Ca^{2+} channels, including mibefradil, amiodarone, and efonidipine, are effective in dog models of tachycardia remodeling [65–67]. Antioxidant interventions may also prevent atrial remodeling [68,69]. Anti-inflammatory agents like glucocorticoids can prevent atrial tachycardia remodeling [70] and can also prevent AF recurrence in post-cardioversion patients [71]. The precise relevance of tachycardia remodeling prevention to AF therapeutics is not yet clear but is an area of active investigation.

Atrial inflammation

In addition to its potential role in atrial remodeling, inflammation appears to be particularly important in specific forms of AF. A striking example is postoperative AF, in which the evidence for a role of tissue inflammation is compelling [72,73]. Anti-inflammatory agents like glucocorticoids are quite effective in experimental and clinical post-cardiac surgery AF paradigms [73,74]. Statins show an anti-inflammatory and anti-AF action in a sterile pericarditis model of inflammation-associated AF, and show promise in the prevention of AF after cardiac surgical procedures [75,76].

Conclusion

Antiarrhythmic drug therapy for AF has many limitations but is likely to remain an important component of AF management for the foreseeable future. There is active interest in developing improved pharmacological approaches targeting novel ion channels, cellular Ca^{2+} handling, atrial remodeling, and the atrial inflammatory response. Hopefully, some of these efforts will bear fruit and lead to improvements in drug therapy that will complement the striking advances in AF ablation procedures that have occurred over the last 10 years.

References

1 Miyasaka Y, Barnes ME, Gersh BJ, et al. Secular trends in incidence of atrial fibrillation in Olmsted County, Minnesota, 1980 to 2000, and implications on the projections for future prevalence. *Circulation* 2006; **114**(2):119–25.

2 Nattel S, Khairy P, Roy D, Thibault B, Guerra P, Talajic M, Dubuc M. New approaches to atrial fibrillation management: a critical review of a rapidly evolving field. *Drugs* 2002;**62**(16):2377–97.

3 Nattel S, Hadjis T, Talajic M. The treatment of atrial fibrillation. An evaluation of drug therapy, electrical modalities and therapeutic considerations. *Drugs* 1994;**48**(3):345–71.

4 Singh BN, Singh SN, Reda DJ, et al. (Sotalol Amiodarone Atrial Fibrillation Efficacy Trial (SAFE-T) Investigators). Amiodarone versus sotalol for atrial fibrillation. *N Engl J Med* 2005;**352**(18):1861–72.

5 Kochiadakis GE, Igoumenidis NE, Marketou ME, Kaleboubas MD, Simantirakis EN, Vardas PE. Low dose amiodarone and sotalol in the treatment of recurrent, symptomatic atrial fibrillation: a comparative, placebo controlled study. *Heart* 2000;**84**(3):251–7.

6 Roy D, Talajic M, Dorian P, et al. Amiodarone to prevent recurrence of atrial fibrillation. Canadian Trial of Atrial Fibrillation Investigators. *N Engl J Med* 2000;**342**(13): 913–20.

7 Allessie MA, Bonke FI, Schopman FJ. Circus movement in rabbit atrial muscle as a mechanism of tachycardia. III. The "leading circle" concept: a new model of circus movement in cardiac tissue without the involvement of an anatomical obstacle. *Circ Res* 1977;**41**(1):9–18.

8 Nattel S, Li D, Yue L. Basic mechanisms of atrial fibrillation – very new insights into very old ideas. *Annu Rev Physiol* 2000;**62**:51–77.

9 Nattel S. New ideas about atrial fibrillation 50 years on. *Nature* 2002;**415**(6868):219–26.

10 Kneller J, Zou R, Vigmond EJ, Wang Z, Leon LJ, Nattel S. Cholinergic atrial fibrillation in a computer model of a two-dimensional sheet of canine atrial cells with realistic ionic properties. *Circ Res* 2002;**90**(9):E73–E87.

11 Zou R, Kneller J, Leon LJ, Nattel S. Substrate size as a determinant of fibrillatory activity maintenance in a mathematical model of canine atrium. *Am J Physiol Heart Circ Physiol* 2005;**289**(3):H1002–H1012.

12 Comtois P, Kneller J, Nattel S. Of circles and spirals: bridging the gap between the leading circle and spiral wave concepts of cardiac reentry. *Europace* 2005;7 (Suppl 2):10–20.

13 Kneller J, Kalifa J, Zou R, et al. Mechanisms of atrial fibrillation termination by pure sodium channel blockade in an ionically-realistic mathematical model. *Circ Res* 2005;**96**(5):e35–e47.

14 Wijffels MC, Dorland R, Mast F, Allessie MA. Widening of the excitable gap during pharmacological cardioversion of atrial fibrillation in the goat: effects of cibenzoline, hydroquinidine, flecainide, and d-sotalol. *Circulation* 2000;**102**(2):260–7.

15 Kawase A, Ikeda T, Nakazawa K, et al. Widening of the excitable gap and enlargement of the core of reentry during atrial fibrillation with a pure sodium channel blocker in canine atria. *Circulation* 2003;**107**(6):905–10.

16 Nattel S, Opie LH. Controversies in atrial fibrillation. Lancet 2006;**367**(9506):262–72.

17 Wyse DG, Waldo AL, DiMarco JP, et al. (Atrial Fibrillation Follow-up Investigation of Rhythm Management (AFFIRM) Investigators). A comparison of rate control and rhythm control in patients with atrial fibrillation. *N Engl J Med* 2002;**347**(23):1825–33.

18 Van Gelder IC, Hagens VE, Bosker HA, et al. (Rate Control versus Electrical Cardioversion for Persistent Atrial Fibrillation Study Group). A comparison of rate control and rhythm control in patients with recurrent persistent atrial fibrillation. *N Engl J Med* 2002;**347**(23): 1834–40.

19 Corley SD, Epstein AE, DiMarco JP, et al. (AFFIRM Investigators). Relationships between sinus rhythm, treatment, and survival in the Atrial Fibrillation Follow-Up Investigation of Rhythm Management (AFFIRM) Study. *Circulation* 2004;**109**(12):1509–13.

20 Nattel S, Carlsson L. Innovative approaches to antiarrhythmic drug therapy. *Nat Rev Drug Discov* 2006;**5**(12):1034–49.

21 Roden DM. Taking the "idio" out of "idiosyncratic": predicting torsades de pointes. *Pacing Clin Electrophysiol* 1998;**21**:1029–34.

22 Wang Z, Fermini B, Nattel S. Sustained depolarization-induced outward current in human atrial myocytes. Evidence for a novel delayed rectifier K^+ current similar to Kv1.5 cloned channel currents. *Circ Res* 1993;**73**:1061–6.

23 Feng J, Wible B, Li G-R, Wang Z, Nattel S. Antisense oligodeoxynucleotides directed against Kv1.5 mRNA specifically inhibit ultrarapid delayed rectifier K^+ current in cultured adult human atrial myocytes. *Circ Res* 1997; **80**:572–9.

24 Li G-R, Feng J, Yue L, Carrier M, Nattel S. Evidence for two components of delayed rectifier K^+ current in human ventricular myocytes. *Circ Res* 1996;78:689–96.

25 Han W, Zhang L, Schram G, Nattel S. Properties of potassium currents in human cardiac Purkinje cells of failing human hearts. *Am J Physiol (Heart Circ Physiol)* 2002;**283**:H2495–H2503.

26 Peukert S, Brendel J, Pirard B, Strubing C, Kleemann HW, Bohme T, Hemmerle H. Pharmacophore-based search, synthesis, and biological evaluation of anthranilic amides as novel blockers of the Kv1.5 channel. *Bioorg Med Chem Lett* 2004;**14**:2823–7.

27 Ehrlich JR, Cha TJ, Zhang L, Chartier D, Villeneuve L, Hebert TE, Nattel S. Characterization of a hyperpolarization-activated time-dependent potassium current in canine cardiomyocytes from pulmonary vein myocardial sleeves and left atrium. *J Physiol* 2004;**557**:583–97.

28 Dobrev D, Friedrich A, Voigt N, et al. The G protein-gated potassium current I(K,ACh) is constitutively active in patients with chronic atrial fibrillation. *Circulation* 2005;**112**:3697–706.

29 Cha TJ, Ehrlich JR, Chartier D, Xiao L, Nattel S. Kir3-based inward rectifier potassium current: potential role in atrial tachycardia remodeling effects on atrial repolarization and arrhythmias. *Circulation* 2006;**113**:1730–7.

30 Nattel S, De Blasio E, Wang W-Q, Beatch GN. RSD1235: a novel antiarrhythmic agent with a unique electrophysiological profile that terminates AF in dogs (abstract). *Eur Heart J* 2001;**22**(Suppl):448.

31 Roy D, Rowe BH, Stiell IG, et al. (CRAFT Investigators). A randomized, controlled trial of RSD1235, a novel antiarrhythmic agent, in the treatment of recent onset atrial fibrillation. *J Am Coll Cardiol* 2004;**44**:2355–61.

32 Fedida D, Orth PM, Chen JY, et al. The mechanism of atrial antiarrhythmic action of RSD1235. *J Cardiovasc Electrophysiol* 2005;**16**:1227–38.

33 Ravens U. Mechano-electric feedback and arrhythmias. *Prog Biophys Mol Biol* 2003;**82**(1–3):255–66.

34 Bode F, Sachs F, Franz MR. Tarantula peptide inhibits atrial fibrillation. *Nature* 2001;**409**:35–6.

35 Ninio DM, Murphy KJ, Howe PR, Saint DA. Dietary fish oil protects against stretch-induced vulnerability to atrial fibrillation in a rabbit model. *J Cardiovasc Electrophysiol* 2005;**16**:1–6.

36 Zicha S, Fernandez-Velasco M, Lonardo G, L'Heureux N, Nattel S. Sinus node dysfunction and hyperpolarization-activated (HCN) channel subunit remodeling in a canine heart failure model. *Cardiovasc Res* 2005;**66**(3):472–81.

37 Hove-Madsen L, Llach A, Bayes-Genis A, et al. Atrial fibrillation is associated with increased spontaneous calcium release from the sarcoplasmic reticulum in human atrial myocytes. *Circulation* 2004;**110**:1358–63.

38 Vest JA, Wehrens XH, Reiken SR, et al. Defective cardiac ryanodine receptor regulation during atrial fibrillation. *Circulation* 2005;**111**:2025–32.

39 Marx SO, Reiken S, Hisamatsu Y, Jayaraman T, Burkhoff D, Rosemblit N, Marks AR. PKA phosphorylation dissociates FKBP12.6 from the calcium release channel (ryanodine receptor): defective regulation in failing hearts. *Cell* 2000;**101**:365–76.

40 Lehnart SE, Wehrens XHT, Marks AR. Calstabin deficiency, ryanodine receptors, and sudden death. *Biochem Biophys Res Comm* 2004;**322**:1267–79.

41 Yano M, Kobayashi S, Kohno M, et al. FKBP12.6 mediated stabilization of calcium release channel (ryanodine receptors) as a novel therapeutic strategy against heart failure. *Circulation* 2003;**107**:477–84.

42 Kumagai K, Nakashima H, Gondo N, Saku K. Antiarrhythmic effects of JVT510, a novel cardioprotective drug, on atrial fibrillation/flutter in a canine sterile pericarditis model. *J Cardiovasc Electrophysiol* 2003;**14**:880–4.
43 Elvan A, Huang XD, Pressler ML, Zipes DP. Radiofrequency catheter ablation of the atria eliminates pacing-induced sustained atrial fibrillation and reduces connexin 43 in dogs. *Circulation* 1997;**96**(5):1675–85.
44 van der Velden HM, Ausma J, Rook MB, Hellemons AJ, van Veen TA, Allessie MA, Jongsma HJ. Gap junctional remodeling in relation to stabilization of atrial fibrillation in the goat. *Cardiovasc Res* 2000;**46**(3):476–86.
45 Hagendorff A, Schumacher B, Kirchhoff S, Luderitz B, Willecke K. Conduction disturbances and increased atrial vulnerability in Connexin40-deficient mice analyzed by transesophageal stimulation. *Circulation* 1999;**99**:1508–15.
46 Dupont E, Ko Y, Rothery S, Coppen SR, Baghai M, Haw M, Severs NJ. The gap–junctional protein connexin40 is elevated in patients susceptible to postoperative atrial fibrillation. *Circulation* 2001;**103**:842–9.
47 Nao T, Ohkusa T, Hisamatsu Y, et al. Comparison of expression of connexin in right atrial myocardium in patients with chronic atrial fibrillation versus those in sinus rhythm. *Am J Cardiol* 2003;**91**:678–83.
48 Wetzel U, Boldt A, Lauschke J, et al. Expression of connexins 40 and 43 in human left atrium in atrial fibrillation of different aetiologies. *Heart* 2005;**91**:166–70.
49 Nattel S, Maguy A, Le Bouter S, Yeh Y-H. Arrhythmogenic ion-channel remodeling in the heart: heart failure, myocardial infarction, and atrial fibrillation. *Physiol Rev* 2007;**87**:425–56.
50 Guerra JM, Everett TH, 4th, Lee KW, Wilson E, Olgin JE. Effects of the gap junction modifier rotigaptide (ZP123) on atrial conduction and vulnerability to atrial fibrillation. *Circulation* 2006;**114**(2):110–18.
51 Shiroshita-Takeshita A, Sakabe M, Haugan K, Hennan JK, Nattel S. Model-dependent effects of the gap junction conduction-enhancing antiarrhythmic peptide rotigaptide (ZP123) on experimental atrial fibrillation in dogs. *Circulation* 2007;**115**(3):310–18.
52 Nattel S. Therapeutic implications of atrial fibrillation mechanisms: can mechanistic insights be used to improve AF management? *Cardiovasc Res* 2002;**54**(2):347–60.
53 Nattel S, Shiroshita-Takeshita A, Cardin S, Pelletier P. Mechanisms of atrial remodeling and clinical relevance. *Curr Opin Cardiol* 2005;**20**:21–5.
54 Li D, Fareh S, Leung TK, Nattel S. Promotion of atrial fibrillation by heart failure in dogs: atrial remodeling of a different sort. *Circulation* 1999;**100**:87–95.
55 Cha TJ, Ehrlich JR, Zhang L, Shi YF, Tardif JC, Leung TK, Nattel S. Dissociation between ionic remodeling and ability to sustain atrial fibrillation during recovery from experimental congestive heart failure. *Circulation* 2004;**109**:412–18.
56 Li D, Shinagawa K, Pang L, Leung TK, Cardin S, Wang Z, Nattel S. Effects of angiotensin-converting enzyme inhibition on the development of the atrial fibrillation substrate in dogs with ventricular tachypacing-induced congestive heart failure. *Circulation* 2001;**104**:2608–14.
57 Cardin S, Li D, Thorin-Trescases N, Leung T-K, Thorin E, Nattel S. Evolution of the atrial fibrillation substrate in experimental congestive heart failure: angiotensin-dependent and independent pathways. *Cardiovasc Res* 2003;**60**:315–25.
58 Kumagai K, Nakashima H, Urata H, Gondo N, Arakawa K, Saku K. Effects of angiotensin II type 1 receptor antagonist on electrical and structural remodeling in atrial fibrillation. *J Am Coll Cardiol* 2003;**41**(12):2197–204.
59 Ehrlich JR, Hohnloser SH, Nattel S. Role of angiotensin system and effects of its inhibition in atrial fibrillation: clinical and experimental evidence. *Eur Heart J* 2006;**27**(5):512–18.
60 Shiroshita-Takeshita A, Brundel BJ, Burstein B, Leung TK, Mitamura H, Ogawa S, Nattel S. Effects of simvastatin on the development of the atrial fibrillation substrate in dogs with congestive heart failure. *Cardiovasc Res* 2007;**74**:75–84.
61 Hanna IR, Heeke B, Bush H, et al. Lipid-lowering drug use is associated with reduced prevalence of atrial fibrillation in patients with left ventricular systolic dysfunction. *Heart Rhythm* 2006;**3**(8):881–6.
62 Wijffels MC, Kirchhof CJ, Dorland R, et al. Atrial fibrillation begets atrial fibrillation. A study in awake chronically instrumented goats. *Circulation* 1995;**92**:1954–68.
63 Morillo CA, Klein GJ, Jones DL, Guiraudon CM. Chronic rapid atrial pacing. Structural, functional, and electrophysiological characteristics of a new model of sustained atrial fibrillation. *Circulation* 1995;**91**:1588–95.
64 Nattel S. Atrial electrophysiological remodeling caused by rapid atrial activation: underlying mechanisms and clinical relevance to atrial fibrillation. *Cardiovasc Res* 1999;**42**(2):298–308.
65 Fareh S, Bénardeau A, Thibault B, Nattel S. The T-type Ca^{2+} channel blocker mibefradil prevents the development of a substrate for atrial fibrillation by tachycardia-induced atrial remodeling in dogs. *Circulation* 1999;**100**:2191–7.
66 Shinagawa K, Shiroshita-Takeshita A, Schram G, Nattel S. Effects of antiarrhythmic drugs on fibrillation in the remodeled atrium: insights into the mechanism of the superior efficacy of amiodarone. *Circulation* 2003;**107**:1440–6.
67 Ohashi N, Mitamura H, Tanimoto K, et al. A comparison between calcium channel blocking drugs with different

potencies for T- and L-type channels in preventing atrial electrical remodeling. *J Cardiovasc Pharmacol* 2004;**44**(3):386–92.

68 Carnes CA, Chung MK, Nakayama T, et al. Ascorbate attenuates atrial pacing-induced peroxynitrite formation and electrical remodeling and decreases the incidence of postoperative atrial fibrillation. *Circ Res* 2001;**89**(6): E32–E38.

69 Shiroshita-Takeshita A, Schram G, Lavoie J, Nattel S. The effect of simvastatin and antioxidant vitamins on atrial fibrillation – promotion by atrial tachycardia remodeling in dogs. *Circulation* 2004;**110**:2313–19.

70 Shiroshita-Takeshita A, Brundel BJJM, Lavoie J, Nattel S. Prednisone prevents atrial fibrillation promotion by atrial tachycardia remodeling in dogs. *Cardiovasc Res* 2006;**69**:865–75.

71 Dernellis J, Panaretou M. Relationship between C-reactive protein concentrations during glucocorticoid therapy and recurrent atrial fibrillation. *Eur Heart J* 2004;**25**:1100–7.

72 Gaudino M, Andreotti F, Zamparelli R, et al. The-174G/C interleukin-6 polymorphism influences postoperative interleukin-6 levels and postoperative atrial fibrillation. Is atrial fibrillation an inflammatory complication? *Circulation* 2003;**108**(Suppl 1):II195–II199.

73 Ishii Y, Schuessler RB, Gaynor SL, Yamada K, Fu AS, Boineau JP, Damiano RJ, Jr. Inflammation of atrium after cardiac surgery is associated with inhomogeneity of atrial conduction and atrial fibrillation. *Circulation* 2005;**111**(22):2881–8.

74 Prasongsukarn K, Abel JG, Jamieson WR, Cheung A, Russell JA, Walley KR, Lichtenstein SV. The effects of steroids on the occurrence of postoperative atrial fibrillation after coronary artery bypass grafting surgery: a prospective randomized trial. *J Thoracic Cardiovasc Surg* 2005;**130**(1):93–8.

75 Kumagai K, Nakashima H, Saku K. The HMG-CoA reductase inhibitor atorvastatin prevents atrial fibrillation by inhibiting inflammation in a canine sterile pericarditis model. *Cardiovasc Res* 2004;**62**(1):105–11.

76 Patti G, Chello M, Candura D, Pasceri V, D'Ambrosio A, Covino E, Di Sciascio G. Randomized trial of atorvastatin for reduction of postoperative atrial fibrillation in patients undergoing cardiac surgery: results of the ARMYDA-3 (Atorvastatin for Reduction of MYocardial Dysrhythmia After cardiac surgery) Study. *Circulation* 2006;**114**(14): 1455–61.

5

CHAPTER 5

Mechanisms of atrial fibrillation in animals and humans

Omer Berenfeld, Jérôme Kalifa, & José Jalife

Introduction

The mechanisms underlying the initiation and maintenance of atrial fibrillation (AF) are not clearly understood. On the other hand, it has recently been demonstrated that paroxysmal AF in patients is initiated by focal triggers localized usually in one or more pulmonary veins (PVs) [1] and can be cured by a catheter-based ablation procedure [2]. However, in persistent AF, the prevailing theory is that multiple, random wavelets of activation coexist to create a chaotic cardiac rhythm [3], and therapy is more challenging [4–7].

Characterizing the rate and regularity of electrical activation has always been at the cornerstone of arrhythmia diagnostics. Early studies on regional differences in cycle length of activation during AF [8,9] were followed by work demonstrating how measurements of AF cycle length in patients can contribute to its treatment [10,11]. In our experimental and clinical studies of AF we have focused on the frequency domain analysis as an approach to investigate the mechanisms that underlie arrhythmia maintenance. As suggested by recent studies [12,13], high resolution dominant frequency (DF) analysis offers the unique opportunity of being able to translate concepts derived from research in animal and computer models toward the determination of AF mechanisms in patients. From the practical standpoint, DF mapping offers a new way to facilitate the systematic correlations between the spatial distribution of excitation frequencies and cardiac anatomy, with the dual goal of more effectively guiding RF ablation procedures and enhancing therapeutic success.

Acute atrial fibrillation: the sheep heart model

The general working hypothesis that acute AF results from the activity of a small number of high frequency reentrant sources localized in one atrium, with fibrillatory conduction to the other atrium, is based primarily on results obtained in our experimental model of the isolated, Langendorff-perfused, sheep heart where we have studied the mechanism of acute AF induced by burst pacing in the presence of acetylcholine (ACh). Our initial work focused on the localization of the high frequency sources thought to be responsible for maintaining AF in this model [14–17]. We induced AF by rapid pacing in the presence of 0.1–0.6 μM ACh. In many cases our optical mapping studies demonstrated self-sustaining, high frequency rotors in the left atrium (LA) giving rise to periodic electrical waves [15] and strongly suggested that such rotors were the underlying mechanism of AF in the sheep heart model.

Simultaneous optical mapping of the LA and right atrium (RA) was done in combination with bipolar electrode recordings along the bundle of Bachmann (BB), the inferoposterior pathway along the coronary sinus, the RA free wall, the left atrial appendage and the PV region. Power spectral analysis (fast Fourier transform, FFT) of all signals was

Catheter Ablation of Atrial Fibrillation Edited by Etienne Aliot, Michel Haïssaguerre and Warren M. Jackman

performed [16]. A left-to-right decrease in the DFs occurred in all cases along the BB and the inferoposterior pathway, resulting in a LA–RA frequency gradient. This is illustrated in Figure 5.1, which shows data obtained from a representative experiment [17]. Panels (a) and (d) show, on the left, single pixel optical recordings obtained from the LA and RA during a 3 s episode of AF. Panels (b) and (c) show electrograms obtained, respectively, on the left and right portions of the BB. On the right are the corresponding power spectra, demonstrating a gradual decrease in DF from the LA through the BB to the RA. In (e) the color DF map illustrates the distribution of DF domains, demonstrating a gradient from the LA to RA. The mean gradient, calculated as the difference between the mean LA and RA DFs, was 5.7 ± 1.4 Hz. In these experiments left-to-right impulse propagation was present in 81 ± 5% and 80 ± 10% of cases along the BB and the inferoposterior pathway, respectively. Overall, our results strongly supported the hypothesis that AF in the sheep heart is the result of high frequency periodic sources located in the LA, with fibrillatory conduction toward the RA [14,15,17].

Fibrillatory propagation and the atrial structure

Studies in animals suggested that the intricate three-dimensional anatomic structure of the atria is an essential component that contributes to the complexity of propagation patterns identified by high resolution mapping during AF [18,19]. However, the information about how heterogeneous electrophysiology and heterogeneous anatomy interact to lead to AF initiation, maintenance, or perpetuation is incomplete at best. Advances have occurred in the understanding of geometric factors, such as wavefront curvature [20], non-uniform anisotropic coupling [21], sink-source relationships at areas of tissue expansion [22], and in the application of non-linear dynamics theory to the spatial and temporal organization underlying complex cardiac arrhythmias, particularly during ventricular fibrillation [23,24]. Such advances may be relevant to the ultimate understanding of the mechanisms of AF initiation by the interaction of the propagating wavefronts with anatomic or functional obstacles [25]. In addition, computer modeling may provide useful tools for research aimed at the study of the manner in which electrical "fibrillatory" waves interact with the highly complex three-dimensional structure of the atria [26,27].

A recent study from our laboratory provides detailed analysis of the manner in which propagating waves initiated by high frequency pacing in the BB interact with the RA and result in fibrillatory conduction [28]. Our goal was to determine the underlying basis of the complex patterns of propagation that characterize AF. In other words, we wanted to answer the following question: what is the mechanism of fibrillatory conduction in this model in which activation by a high frequency rotor in the LA is highly periodic? We hypothesized that the left-to-right frequency gradient and fibrillatory conduction observed in our previous studies resulted from breakdown of waves traveling from the LA across interatrial pathways, into the pectinate muscle network of the RA. Thus, we expected to demonstrate that periodic repetitive input to the RA at increasing frequencies should result in increased complexity and decreased organization of wave propagation, compatible with fibrillatory conduction. To this aim, we used simultaneous high resolution endocardial and epicardial optical mapping (di-4-ANEPPS) in isolated, coronary perfused sheep RA preparations [28]. Rhythmic pacing at the BB allowed well-controlled and realistic conditions at the LA-driven RA. Pacing at increasingly higher frequencies (2.0–6.7 Hz) led to increasing delays in activation distal to major branching sites of the crista terminalis and pectinate muscles (PMs) [28]. As shown by the frequency maps presented in Figure 5.2a, stimulation of the BB at 5.0 Hz resulted in 1 : 1 activation of the entire preparation at 5.0 Hz. However, at 7.7 Hz, there was spatially distributed intermittent blockade with the establishment of well-demarcated frequency domains (compare the color DF maps on the left and right in Figure 5.2a), and significant discordance between the epicardium and endocardium. In fact, as illustrated in Figure 5.2b, stimulation at frequencies between 2 and 6.7 Hz, resulted in rhythmic flutter-like activation of both the epicardium and endocardium. However, above the "breakdown frequency" of ~6.7 Hz, RA activity

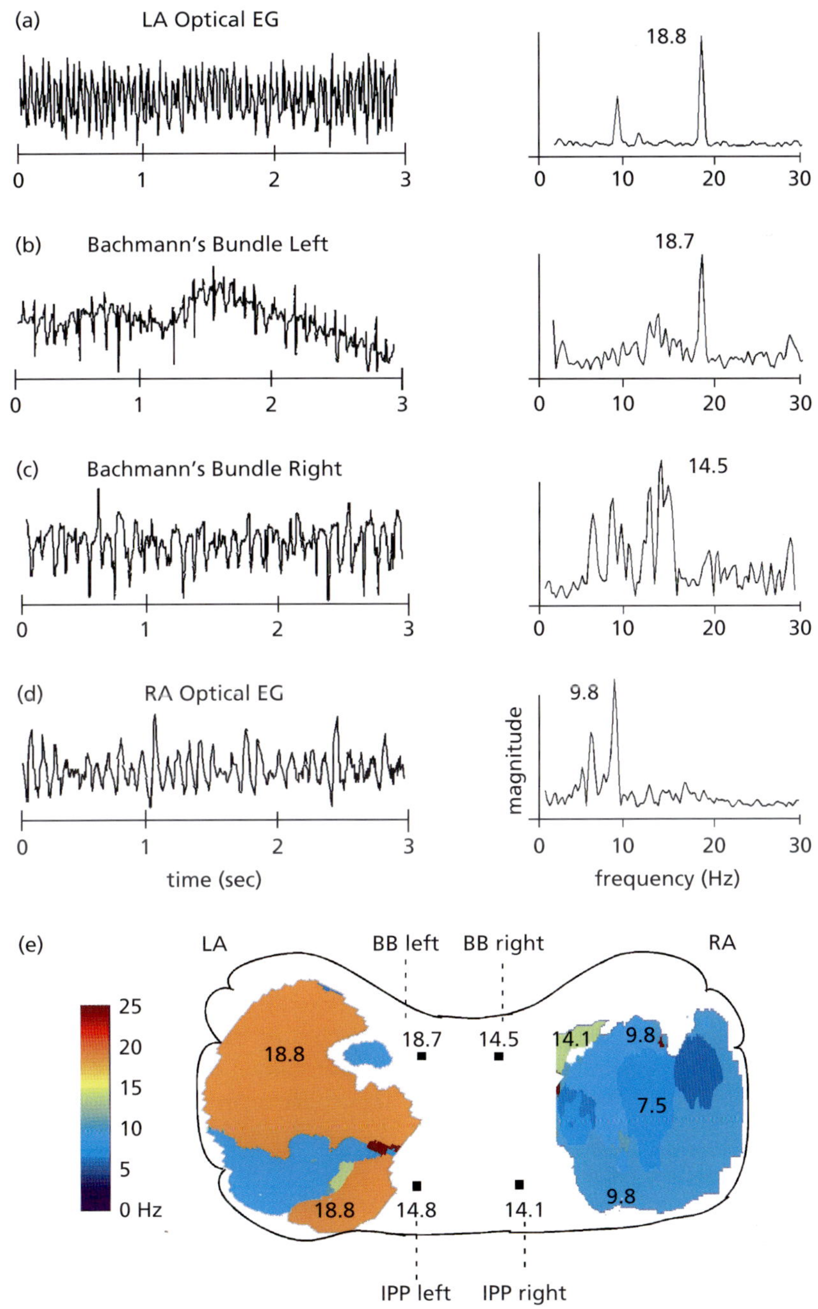

Figure 5.1 (a) Optical "electrogram" (EG) and FFT from the left atrium (LA). (b, c) True EGs and FFT from the bundle of Brachmann (BB), left and right. (d) Right atrium (RA) optical EG and FFT. (e) Color DF map of the RA and LA including the BB and inferoposterior pathway (IPP). Note the LA–RA frequency gradient. (Reproduced from [17] with permission.)

underwent a significant loss of consistency in the direction of propagation, and thus transformed into fibrillatory conduction [28]. Such frequency-dependent changes were independent of action potential duration. Rather, the spatial boundaries between proximal and distal frequencies correlated well with branch sites of the pectinate musculature. From these experiments we concluded that there

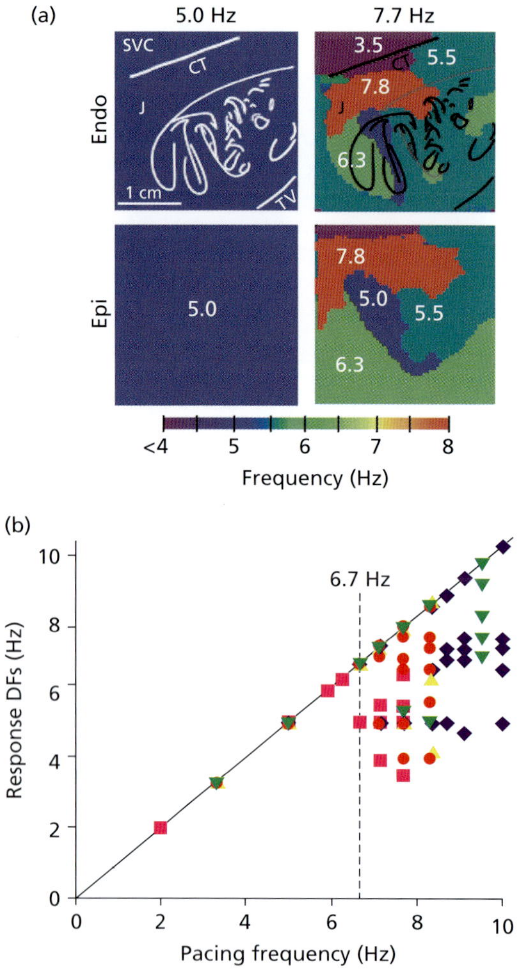

Figure 5.2 The "breakdown frequency" in a sheep heart. (a) Endocardial and epicardial dominant frequency (DF) maps of the same isolated RA preparation paced at 5.0 and 7.7 Hz. Note the appearance of heterogeneous DF domains at 7.7 Hz. (b) Response DFs versus the pacing rate ($n = 5$). Each symbol represents one experiment. Pacing the BB at rates below ~6.7 Hz results in 1 : 1 activation. At higher rates, the number of domains increases but the value of the DFs decreases. (Reproduced from [28] with permission.)

exists a "breakdown frequency" in the sheep RA below which activity is flutter-like and above which it is fibrillation-like. The data strongly supported the idea that, during AF, high frequency activation initiated in the LA undergoes fibrillatory conduction toward the RA and that branching points at the crista terminalis and PMs play a major role in increasing the complexity of the arrhythmia.

Fibrillatory propagation and dispersion of action potential duration

Spatial dispersion in action potential duration (APD) and refractoriness, measured at relatively slow stimulation rates, are usually invoked to explain complex wave propagation during AF [29]. Wang et al. found that at a cycle length of 250 ms in dogs susceptible to sustained AF, the dispersion of refractoriness in the RA epicardium was 19 ± 3 ms, with the longest refractoriness being ~120 ms at the free wall [30]. Satoh and Zipes reported that refractoriness was shortest at the lower portion of the crista terminalis relative to the superior vena cava [31]. However, none of the above seemingly conflicting studies measured refractoriness in the PM region and their data are therefore difficult to compare with our results. We constructed high resolution APD maps at a cycle length of 300 ms (3.3 Hz; not shown here) to assess indirectly the degree of spatial dispersion of refractoriness [32]. In agreement with the results of Feng et al., our data indicate that the crista terminalis has the longest APD during pacing at slow rates (3.3 Hz) [33]. Spach et al. [34] also reported that, at 1.7 Hz, APD in the crista terminalis is longer than in the PMs. In single cells, Yamashita et al. [35] showed that APD in the rabbit crista terminalis was longer than in the PMs at 1 Hz. In our experiments, however, the crista terminalis consistently showed the largest DF when the BB is paced at a rate comparable to the frequency of the LA during AF (> 7 Hz). Thus, the distribution of APD under normal conditions seems different from the distribution of DF domains during AF, which leads us to suggest that dispersion of refractoriness at normal frequencies is a poor predictor of the spatial distribution of intermittent block patterns that characterize AF.

Fibrillatory conduction and fractionation

DF mapping allowed accurate identification of sites of periodic activity and the demonstration that stable, localized, high frequency sources were responsible for AF maintenance in the isolated sheep heart [14,15,17]. The highest DF was most often (80%) localized to the posterior LA, near or at one of the PV ostia [15]. In addition, using high resolution video imaging we demonstrated that such sources corresponded to fast vortex-like reentry around minuscule cores (microreentry) [15] that resulted in a large dispersion of frequencies throughout the atria during AF [16,17,28]. Importantly, the areas harboring the microreentrant sources were shown to be highly regular and spatiotemporally organized [15]. Fractionated activity and complex electrograms were identified mainly at boundaries separating different frequency domains [36]; for example, between the area of 1 : 1 activation by the microreentrant source and a neighboring lower frequency domain. We have also analyzed optical and electrogram recordings at the endocardial surface of the posterior LA of isolated sheep hearts to provide insight into the mechanisms that underlie the high frequency complex fractionated atrial electrograms (CFAEs) that have been used by some investigators as the target of radiofrequency ablation to terminate AF [37]. We tested the hypothesis that highly periodic electrical waves emerging from AF sources at or near the posterior LA give rise to the most fractionated activity in adjacent locations, which would explain the relatively high success of using CFAEs to guide AF ablation therapy.

For each signal, a regularity index (RI) was defined as the ratio of the power at the DF to the total power [36]. The power at the DF was calculated by summing the power values at the highest peak and its adjacent values (fixed band of about 0.75 Hz) and the total power was calculated as the sum over the range of 1 to 30 Hz. Average maps of the RI were constructed similar to the DF maps. Although the RI may not be a universal valid measure of irregularity [38], we verified that in our experimental setting this parameter correlates with the beat-by-beat variability in amplitude and the number of deflections in each beat.

Pixel-by-pixel quantification of the local RI enabled us to determine the spatial relation between DF and regularity. In Figure 5.3, panels (a) and (b) show, respectively, the DF and RI maps from one experiment [36]. The broken line outlining the outer boundaries of the DFmax (red) allows clear appreciation of the high RI inside the DFmax. The RI decreases very rapidly at the boundaries of the DFmax domain but then increases again toward the periphery of the field of view. This is confirmed by the single pixel recordings sampled from three different regions (points 1, 2, and 3). While the activation frequency decreases from 1 to 2 and then 3, the RI decreases from 1 to 2, but then increases at point 3, which corresponds to the lowest DF among all three points. Figure 5.3d depicts the relation between the DF and RI for all pixels in the same experiment. A clear biphasic relation is observed. The vertical dashed line corresponds to the DFmax boundary. It indicates that the minimum RI, i.e. the maximum fractionation, occurs at frequencies below the DFmax. At very low frequencies, the RI again increases.

To provide additional insight into the mechanisms underlying local fractionation during AF without the confounding effects of the complex atria, we utilized a numerical approach [36]. A stable reentry acted as the high frequency source of fibrillatory waves in a two-dimensional sheet that was divided in two areas set with markedly different IK_{ACh} conductances to simulate the conditions of heterogeneity in APD that prevail in the posterior LA. While the activity in the DFmax domain was highly organized, fragmentation (low RI) occurred at the boundary with the lower frequency domain. As in the optical mapping experiment of Figure 5.3, fragmentation was reduced (i.e. increased RI) at the low frequency domain, distal to the interface with the DFmax domain. Mechanistically, an analysis of sequential activations showed that the largest fractionation was found where the lowest consistency in direction of propagation and highest variability in beat-by-beat conduction velocity occurred.

Spatial distribution of dominant frequencies during atrial fibrillation in patients

Several recent studies have characterized the spatial distribution of DFs during AF in patients [12,39,40]. Using the CARTO electroanatomic mapping system, Sanders et al. sequentially acquired 5 s long bipolar recordings from about 120 points throughout both atria and the coronary sinus in 32 patients during sustained AF [12]. The recorded signals were rectified [41] and 3–15 Hz band-pass filtered. Then FFT was used to determine the DF of

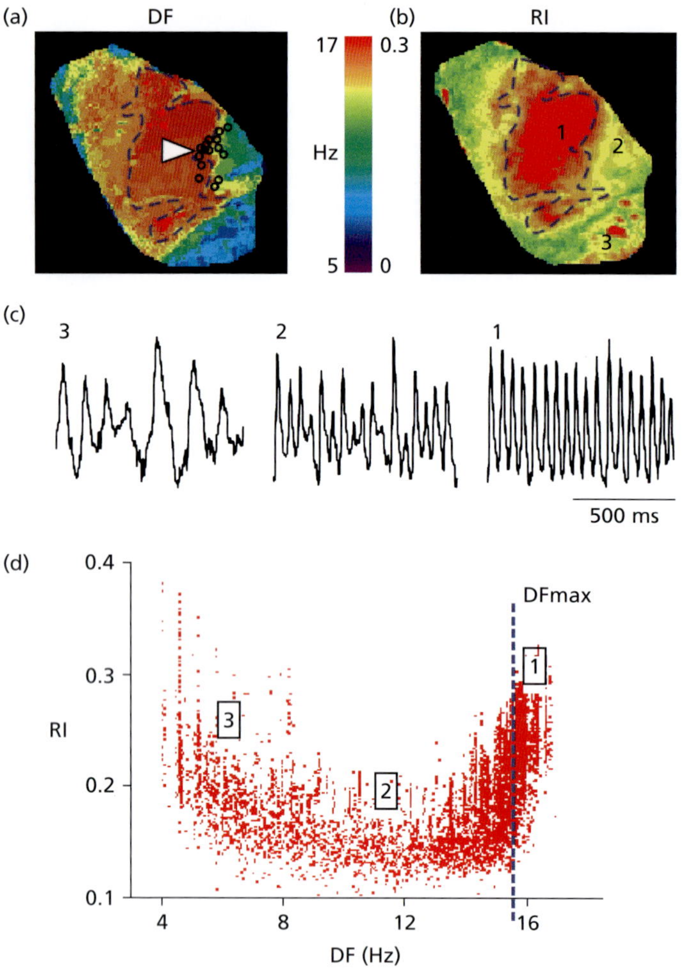

Figure 5.3 Spatial relationships between dominant frequency (DF) and fractionation. Average DF (a) and regulatory index (RI) (b) maps calculated from five movies recorded at the posterior LA for each of five isolated sheep hearts during AF. The dashed line shows the limit of the DFmax domain, the white arrowhead indicates the predominant direction of propagation, and the circles are the sites of wave break at the periphery of the DFmax domain. (c) Sample pixel signals from locations 1–3. (d) The biphasic relationship between the DF and RI. (Reproduced from [36] with permission.)

each of the 120 electrogram segments lasting 4.096 s at a resolution of 0.24 Hz [38]. Patients with both paroxysmal and permanent AF had DF gradients from the LA to RA to coronary sinus. However, compared to patients with paroxysmal AF, patients with permanent AF demonstrated significantly higher average frequencies of activation [12,13,40,42].

Figure 5.4 shows four sample bipolar electrograms with their respective power spectra acquired from endocardial sites in the LA and RA of a patient with paroxysmal AF of spontaneous onset [12]. On the left are typical AF recordings with variable amplitudes and interbeat intervals, precluding a robust cycle length analysis, particularly of the top recording. However, the spectra on the right show relatively narrow bands in the 3–15 Hz range with distinct peaks of DF corresponding to the inverse of the dominant cycle length in the electrograms.

In all patients, electrograms were collected from multiple sites (typically 120 in both atria) and their corresponding DFs were superimposed on the atrial geometry to generate color DF maps [12], as illustrated in Figure 5.5. On the DF map, those sites that demonstrated high frequency activity with a gradient of 20% or more relative to the surrounding atrial tissue were defined as high DF (HDF) sites. In this study most HDF sites involved a single point, but in some the HDF site extended over two or three adjacent points. Figure 5.5a reproduces left anterior oblique and posteroanterior views [12]

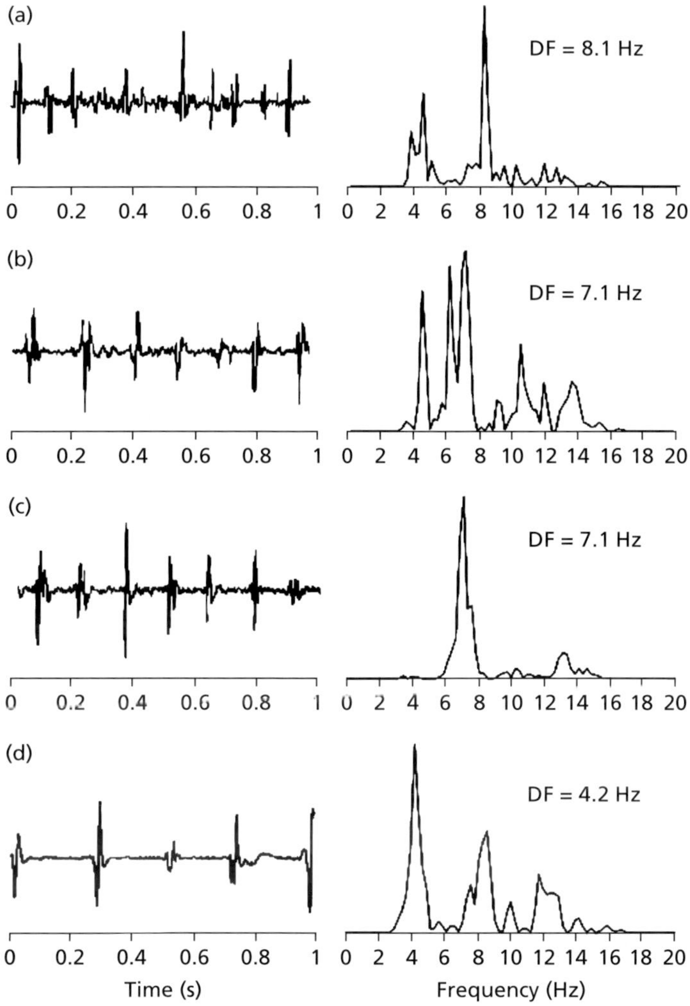

Figure 5.4 Bipolar electrograms and corresponding power spectra obtained from four points in a patient with spontaneous paroxysmal AF. Each site shows a distinct dominant frequency (DF). While the bipolar recording shows low amplitude complex signals that make accurate determination of frequency of activation difficult, the power spectrum clearly demonstrates the DF at 8.1 Hz (a). The DF map of this patient is shown in Figure 5.5a. Data from (a) the site of maximal DF at the right inferior PV; (b, c) other HDF sites in the right superior PV and left superior PV, respectively; and (d) the posterior RA. (Reproduced from [12] with permission.)

of the same map showing fibrillatory activity at a mean DF of ~4.8 Hz in the patient whose electrograms are shown in Figure 5.4. While frequency in the majority of the atria and coronary sinus was relatively low (≤ 5 Hz), the posterior wall of the LA was activated at faster rates (7–8 Hz), with notable HDF sites at each of the PVs. In this patient, focal radiofrequency ablation applied to the HDF site near the right inferior PV effectively terminated AF. Figure 5.5b shows a DF map from a patient with permanent AF. Compared with the previous case, this patient not only had a higher frequency at the maximal HDF site (13.7 Hz), but also both atria demonstrated higher global frequency of activity. In addition, many of the HDF sites were located in the atria rather in the PV region [12,13]. We concluded that in the cohort of patients studied, paroxysmal AF was characterized by the hierarchical spatial distribution of DFs where the LA and PVs are always the fastest regions. By contrast, in

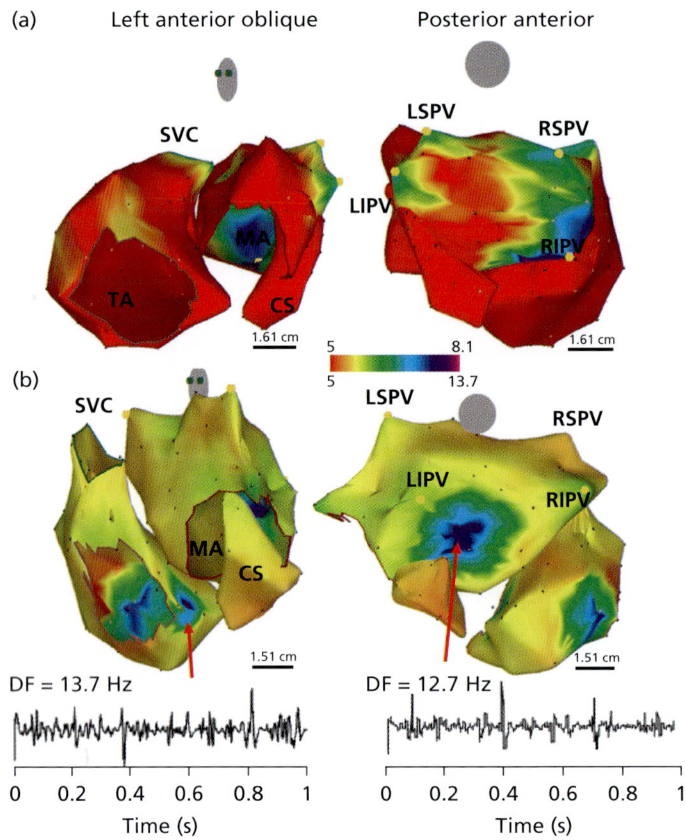

Figure 5.5 Dominant frequency (DF) maps of human AF. (a) A DF map in a patient with paroxysmal AF (6 h). Note HDF sites in each of the PVs. The ablation sequence in this patient was the left superior PV (LSPV), left inferior PV (LIPV), right superior PV (RSPV), and right inferior PV (RIPV; site of the AF termination). The AF cycle length increased by 10, 25, 9, and 75 ms, respectively, before termination. (b) A DF map in a patient with permanent AF (24 months). The maximal DF and atrial frequency are higher than in the patient in (a). In addition, many of the HDF sites are located outside the PVs. The ablation sequence in this patient was the RIPV, RSPV, LSPV, and LIPV. The AF cycle length increased by 5, 2, 0, and 5 ms, respectively. The electrograms of the site of maximal DF in the LA and RA are presented showing significant fractionation. CS, coronary sinus; MA, mitral annulus; SVC, superior vena cava; TA, tricuspid annulus. The color bar scale is in Hertz. (Reproduced from [12] with permission.)

persistent AF, a more uniform distribution of higher DF values was observed, where the highest DFs could not be found in the PV region [12,13].

High dominant frequency sites and maintenance of atrial fibrillation

Atrial fibrillation mapping studies have recognized the presence of temporally and spatially periodic activity [15,43–45] emanating from the PV region with regularity [14], suggesting that these structures may have a role in maintaining AF [15], by their ability to harbor either localized short cycle length reentrant sources and/or focal automatic activity [46,47]. A recent study utilizing a morphologically accurate computer model of the atria has demonstrated that the PV region is a preferential site for anchoring rotors [48]. In the clinic, paroxysms of short cycle length activity have been observed in the PVs of patients undergoing AF ablation [49–51]. In addition, sequential ablation of sites showing the shortest cycle lengths has been associated with a progressive slowing of AF frequency, culminating in termination in 75% of patients with paroxysmal AF [11].

Using a blind correlation between atrial DF distribution and ablation, without any attempt at identifying potentially arrhythmogenic sites at the time of the procedure, Sanders et al. [12] found that ablation at PVs harboring HDF sites resulted in an increase in the AF cycle length (> 5 ms) within the coronary sinus in 89% of cases. The latter was true in patients with either paroxysmal or permanent AF. However, eventual arrhythmia termination occurred during ablation in 15 (88%) out of 17 patients with paroxysmal AF, but in none with permanent AF ($P < 0.0001$). In 13 (87%) of the 15 paroxysmal AF patients, arrhythmia termination was associated with ablation at a HDF site; 11 localized to a PV and two to the LA roof and fossa ovalis.

The aforementioned data, together with those of Atienza et al. [13] and Lazar et al. [52], clearly indicate that the HDF sites play a role in the maintenance of AF in a significant number of patients. So, the following question arises: to what extent should one expect to be able to determine the role of the HDF sites in arrhythmia maintenance in the AF patient population at large? To address that question, consideration should be given to the relatively low resolution of currently available mapping systems and the substantial temporal limitation imposed by the need to sequentially acquire the electrograms needed to generate the DF maps. For example, in the study of Sanders et al. [12], a double-blinded analysis showed that the percentage of HDF sites ablated that resulted in AF termination was similar to the percentage of sites that did not result in termination in either group of patients. On the other hand, following ablation performed without knowledge of the HDF site offline analysis revealed significantly shorter RF duration (21.9 ± 18.6 min) per HDF site ablated in patients with AF termination compared with those in whom AF persisted (42.4 ± 26.4 min; $P = 0.008$). Such data suggested that due to the sequential nature of data acquisition, the distribution of HDF sites may have changed by the time the ablation was performed.

In this regard, studies on temporal stability of DFs at or near the PVs [39] and the entire atria [12] have found no significant change over periods of between 10 and 20 s. However, an assessment of the stability in the coronary sinus over a period of 50 min, which is more relevant to the time that is needed for mapping and ablation, demonstrated that while there was no trend of acceleration or slowing of the activation rate, the instantaneous rate fluctuated by about ± 1 Hz [12]. The presence of such fluctuations possibly reflected spatial shifts in the locations of the discrete drivers responsible for HDF sites, with concomitant transient alterations in the local rate of activation. Indeed, Schuessler et al. used intraoperatively bipolar electrograms from epicardial sites during AF and reported that in half of the patients the location of the HDF changed during the recording period [42]. Nevertheless, the study of Schuessler et al. [42] differs from others in that the location of the HDF was independent of the type of AF, which raises the possibility that the sites where DFs were measured may not have corresponded to the actual HDF site. The obvious conclusion here is that efficient use of DF mapping as a clinical electrophysiological tool to localize and terminate AF drivers by RF ablation in many patients will require higher resolution mapping, with multiple simultaneous electrograms and online power spectral analysis.

Activation frequency and driver mechanisms

Overall, it seems that the dynamic nature of AF keeps the spatiotemporal variability of the DF within a limit that allows consistent identification of HDF sites as discrete AF drivers despite the mapping limitations. The notion that a localized source of reentrant activity could maintain AF was first postulated by Lewis [53] in the early part of the twentieth century and subsequently by Scherf [54]. Many years later, Morillo et al. targeted ablation sites of short cycle length activity in the posterior LA and observed the termination of arrhythmia in a canine model of AF [8]. Using a sterile pericarditis model, Kumagai et al. identified in the septum dominant unstable reentrant circuits of very short cycle length that maintained AF and could be successfully terminated by focal ablation [55,56]. Others have reported that in some patients sustained focal activity at the PVs, coronary sinus, or superior vena cava initiated and maintained AF, and could be eliminated by discrete ablation [57]. However, to this date, whether such sites are either automatic, triggered, or reentrant and whether changes in the driver activity would alter spatial frequency gradients, remains unresolved.

Mapping an isolated canine atrial preparation, Schuessler et al. [58] found that with increasing concentrations of ACh, activation patterns

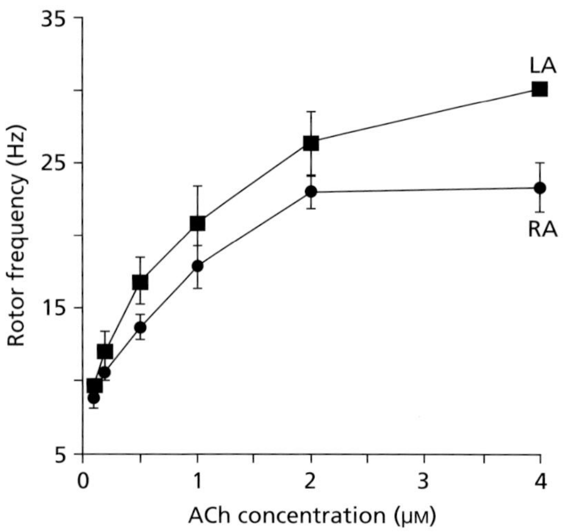

Figure 5.6 Relationship between acetylcholine (ACh) concentration and rotor frequency (l/cycle length). The ACh concentration–response curves are given for the left atrium (LA) and right atrium (RA) for the five longest living rotors for each of the six experiments. The rotor frequency is greater in the LA than the RA at all concentrations ($P = 2 \times 10^{-4}$). (Reproduced from [59] with permission.)

characterized by multiple reentrant circuits converted to a single, relatively stable, high frequency reentrant circuit that resulted in fibrillatory conduction. More recently, a systematic evaluation of the effect of ACh on the frequency of rotation in isolated sheep hearts was performed [59]. Figure 5.6 demonstrates the direct ACh concentration dependence of rotor frequency in both atria of six hearts, with frequency being significantly higher in the LA than the RA at all ACh concentrations. Moreover, the LA–RA rotor frequency gradient also increased with ACh concentration from 1.0 Hz at 0.1 μM ACh to 6.2 Hz at 4.0 μM ACh.

Identifying rotors as drivers of AF directly in patients is not feasible with the existing mapping techniques. Yet, the dose-dependent effects of ACh discussed above for Figure 5.6 offered an idea that led to the translation from animal experiments to the patient and gave us the opportunity to obtain evidence, though indirect, for the presence of rotors as drivers through pharmacological means. Translation was made possible also by the fact that adenosine, which is widely used in the clinic, is known to activate the same Kir3.x subfamily of inward rectifier potassium channels as ACh, albeit through a different signaling pathway [60–62]. By increasing K^+ conductance in the atrium, both ACh and adenosine hyperpolarize the cell membrane, abbreviate the action potential duration and the refractory period, and inhibit spontaneous pacemaker discharge as well as early and delayed depolarizations [60,61]. On the other hand, they both accelerate reentrant activity [59].

Thus, in a recent study we used adenosine to test the hypothesis that localized reentry maintains AF also in humans [13]. We determined the effects of adenosine infusion on DF at varying locations of both atria to test the idea that adenosine-induced acceleration of HDF sites reveals reentry as the mechanism of AF maintenance and therefore rules out an automatic or triggered mechanism. We generated baseline DF maps of the LA using novel real-time spectral analysis software that allowed determination of the specific HDF site locations likely to harbor the AF drivers [12] in paroxysmal AF patients. Then the adenosine effect was measured at the primary and secondary HDF sites in the LA. Figure 5.7a shows a representative example where the AF frequency at baseline was relatively slow (< 5 Hz) and three HDF sites were identified with the primary HDF site being located near the right inferior PV (red arrow). Figure 5.7b and c show that while the adenosine infusion practically abolished the ventricular activity as detected by V_5, the DF at the primary HDF site accelerated from 4.64 Hz at baseline to 6.35 Hz at the peak of the adenosine effect. An additional adenosine infusion performed while measuring activity at a secondary HDF site also showed an increase in DF, but to a lesser extent. Interestingly, in this patient the arrhythmia terminated during post-mapping ablation at the primary HDF site, supporting again the critical role of such sites as AF drivers [12]. Compared to baseline, adenosine significantly accelerated the primary and secondary HDF sites in these patients from about 5 to 6.7 Hz [13], demonstrating that the sites involved in the maintenance of AF are clearly affected by adenosine.

In a larger cohort of paroxysmal and persistent AF patients, Atienza et al. analyzed the effect of adenosine on the activation rate at specific regions at the junction of the PV and LA, the roof of the RA, and the coronary sinus [13]. In general, patients with persistent AF demonstrated significantly higher maximal baseline DFs than paroxysmal AF

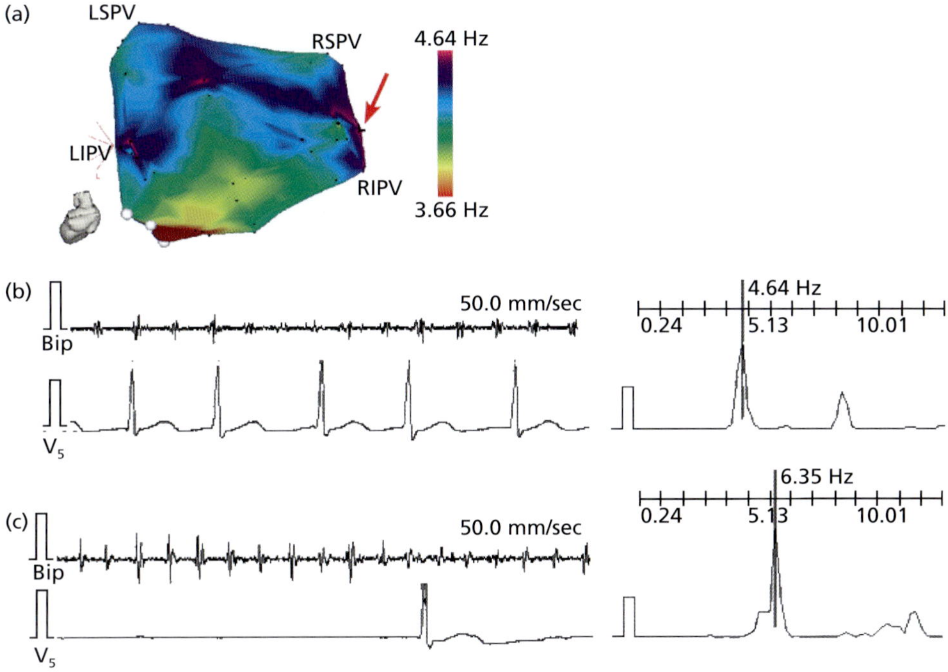

Figure 5.7 Accelerating effect of adenosine on HDF sites. (a) Left atrium posterior view DF map from a paroxysmal AF patient. The DF map was produced by the real-time frequency mapping CARTO system before the infusion of adenosine. The red arrow indicates the primary HDF site near the right inferior PV (RIPV). (b) Baseline recording at the primary HDF site with its power spectrum and simultaneous V_5 reference. (c) Recording at the primary HDF site with its power spectrum and simultaneous V_5 reference during the peak adenosine effect showing an increase of DF. Bip, bipolar catheter; LIPV, left inferior pulmonary vein; RSPV, right superior pulmonary vein; LSPV, left superior pulmonary vein. (Reproduced from [13] with permission.)

patients ($P < 0.001$). However, adenosine infusion in persistent AF patients increased local DFs only in the roof of the RA. The increase in the PV–LA junction was not statistically significant and there was no change in the coronary sinus DF. In sum, adenosine infusion increased frequency primarily at sites that activated at the highest rate at baseline. In paroxysmal AF patients, adenosine increased activation frequency in the PV–LA junction. In persistent AF patients, the highest frequency sources accelerated by adenosine were located in either atria but not at PV sites. Thus, the response to adenosine is consistent with reentrant drivers maintaining AF that have different locations in paroxysmal AF compared with persistent AF patients [13].

Conclusion

Experimental studies of cholinergic AF in the isolated sheep heart [63] demonstrated that high frequency sources in the posterior wall of the LA drive the fibrillatory activity throughout both atria. Motivated by these results and by a growing body of work investigating how measurements of the cycle length of activity in patients during AF can contribute to its treatment [10–13], we focused our analysis on the organization of DF activity during AF in animals and humans. In animal studies we have shown that the highest DF site harbors a driver of AF and is surrounded by a region of increased fractionated activity, while areas remote from the source are rather regular. Using electroanatomic mapping and Fourier spectral methods we generated three-dimensional, whole-atrial DF maps in patients undergoing AF ablation procedures and identified relatively small HDF sites. In patients with paroxysmal AF, the HDF sites are often localized to the posterior LA near the ostia of the PVs. In contrast, patients with permanent AF demonstrate HDF sites that are more often localized to either atrium than to the posterior LA–PV junction. In our study, ablation at HDF sites resulted in significant slowing of the arrhythmia and the termination of sustained AF in 87% of patients with paroxysmal AF [12]. The response of the arrhythmia to adenosine is consistent with the mechanistic hypothesis that reentry in those HDF sites maintains AF in humans, and that reentrant drivers have different locations in paroxysmal AF compared with persistent AF patients.

The ability to find whether AF depends on activity at discrete sites and identify their location promises to improve efficacy of ablation procedures in certain groups of patients. Overall, DF analysis on bipolar recordings obtained during AF ablation is found to be strongly suggestive of the local activation rate at specific sites and in particular at the HDF sites. Identification of these HDF sites and characterization of their stability may provide an efficient means of developing more patient-specific ablation procedures whereby targeting those sites, either directly or circumferentially, may reduce the burden of the ablation to terminate AF [52,64,65]. For that to occur, a better understanding of mechanisms of wave propagation dynamics in AF will be needed for each individual patient. The combination of time and frequency domain measures, such as fractionation [37] or the DF, as presented here, should help the clinician gain such a valuable insight.

Acknowledgements

Supported in part by grants PO1 HL039707 (JJ, OB), RO1 HL060843 (JJ) and RO1 HL087055 (JK) from the National Institutes of Health; Scientist Development Grant 0230311N from the American Heart Association (OB) and ACCF/GE Healthcare Career Development Award (JK).

References

1 Haissaguerre M, Jais P, Shah DC, et al. Spontaneous initiation of atrial fibrillation by ectopic beats originating in the pulmonary veins. *N Engl J Med* 1998;**339**:659–66.

2 Haissaguerre M, Shah DC, Jais P, et al. Mapping-guided ablation of pulmonary veins to cure atrial fibrillation. *Am J Cardiol* 2000;**86**:9K–19K.

3 Moe GK, Abildskov JA. Atrial fibrillation as a self-sustaining arrhythmia independent of focal discharges. *Am Heart J* 1959;**58**:59–70.

4 Haissaguerre M, Jais P, Shah DC, et al. Catheter ablation of chronic atrial fibrillation targeting the reinitiating triggers. *J Cardiovasc Electrophysiol* 2000;**11**:2–10.

5 Benussi S, Pappone C, Nascimbene S, et al. A simple way to treat chronic atrial fibrillation during mitral valve surgery: the epicardial radiofrequency approach. *Eur J Cardio-Thoracic Surg* 2000;**17**:524–9.

6 Knight BP, Weiss R, Bahu M, et al. Cost comparison of radiofrequency modification and ablation of the atrioventricular junction in patients with chronic atrial fibrillation. *Circulation* 1997;**96**:1532–6.

7 Oral H, Pappone C, Chugh A, et al. Circumferential pulmonary-vein ablation for chronic atrial fibrillation. *N Engl J Med.* 2006;**354**:934–41.

8 Morillo CA, Klein GJ, Jones DL, Guiraudon CM. Chronic rapid atrial pacing: structural, functional, and electrophysiological characteristics of a new model of sustained atrial fibrillation. *Circulation* 1995;**91**:1588–95.

9 Harada A, Sasaki K, Fukushima T, Ikeshita M, Asano T, Yamauchi S, Shoji T. Atrial activation during chronic atrial fibrillation in patients with isolated mitral valve disease. *Ann Thoracic Surg* 1996;**61**:104–12.

10 Pappone C, Rosanio S. Pulmonary vein isolation for atrial fibrillation. In: Zipes DP, Jalife J, eds. *Cardiac Electrophysiology – From Cell to Bedside.* Saunders, Philadelphia, 2004:1039–52.

11 Haissaguerre M, Sanders P, Hocini M, et al. Changes in atrial fibrillation cycle length and inducibility during catheter ablation and their relation to outcome. *Circulation* 2004;**109**:3007–13.

12 Sanders P, Berenfeld O, Hocini M, et al. Spectral analysis identifies sites of high-frequency activity maintaining atrial fibrillation in humans. *Circulation* 2005;**112**:789–97.

13 Atienza F, Almendral J, Moreno J, et al. Activation of inward rectifier potassium channels accelerates atrial fibrillation in humans: evidence for a reentrant mechanism. *Circulation* 2006;**114**:2434–42.

14 Skanes AC, Mandapati R, Berenfeld O, Davidenko JM, Jalife J. Spatiotemporal periodicity during atrial fibrillation in the isolated sheep heart. *Circulation* 1998;**98**:1236–48.

15 Mandapati R, Skanes A, Chen J, Berenfeld O, Jalife J. Stable microreentrant sources as a mechanism of atrial fibrillation in the isolated sheep heart. *Circulation* 2000;**101**:194–9.

16 Berenfeld O, Mandapati R, Dixit S, Skanes AC, Chen J, Mansour M, Jalife J. Spatially distributed dominant excitation frequencies reveal hidden organization in atrial fibrillation in the Langendorff-perfused sheep heart. *J Cardiovasc Electrophysiol* 2000;**11**:869–79.

17 Mansour M, Mandapati R, Berenfeld O, Chen J, Samie FH, Jalife J. Left-to-right gradient of atrial frequencies during acute atrial fibrillation in the isolated sheep heart. *Circulation* 2001;**103**:2631–6.

18 Skanes AC, Gray RA, Zuur CL, Jalife J. Spatio-temporal patterns of atrial fibrillation: role of the subendocardial structure. *Semin Interv Cardiol* 1997;**2**:185–93.

19 Gray RA, Pertsov AM, Jalife J. Incomplete reentry and epicardial breakthrough patterns during atrial fibrillation in the sheep heart. *Circulation* 1996;**94**:2649–61.

20 Cabo C, Pertsov AM, Baxter WT, Davidenko JM, Gray RA, Jalife J. Wave-front curvature as a cause of slow conduction and block in isolated cardiac muscle. *Circ Res* 1994;**75**:1014–28.

21 Spach MS, Josephson ME. Initiating reentry: the role of nonuniform anisotropy in small circuits. *J Cardiovasc Electrophysiol* 1994;**5**:182–209.

22 Rohr S, Kucera JP, Fast VG, Kleber AG. Paradoxical improvement of impulse conduction in cardiac tissue by partial cellular uncoupling. *Science* 1997;**275**:841–4.

23 Gray RA, Pertsov AM, Jalife J. Spatial and temporal organization during cardiac fibrillation. *Nature* 1998;**392**: 75–8.

24 Wellner M, Berenfeld O, Jalife J, Pertsov AM. Minimal principle for rotor filaments. *Proc Natl Acad Sci USA* 2002;**99**:8015–18.

25 Jalife J, Berenfeld O, Skanes A, Mandapati R. Mechanisms of atrial fibrillation: mother rotors or multiple daughter wavelets, or both? *J Cardiovasc Electrophysiol* 1998;**9**:S2–S12.

26 Fast VG, Kleber AG. Cardiac tissue geometry as a determinant of unidirectional conduction block: assessment of microscopic excitation spread by optical mapping in patterned cell cultured and in a computer model. *Cardiovasc Res* 1995;**29**:697–707.

27 Fast VG, Kleber AG. Block of impulse propagation at an abrupt tissue expansion: evaluation of the critical strand diameter in 2- and 3-dimensional computer models. *Cardiovasc Res* 1995;**30**:449–59.

28 Berenfeld O, Zaitsev AV, Mironov SF, Pertsov AM, Jalife J. Frequency-dependent breakdown of wave propagation into fibrillatory conduction across the pectinate muscle network in the isolated sheep right atrium. *Circ Res* 2002;**90**:1173–80.

29 Kim KB, Rodefeld MD, Schuessler RB, Cox JL, Boineau JP. Relationship between local atrial fibrillation interval and refractory period in the isolated canine atrium. *Circulation* 1996;**94**:2961–7.

30 Wang Z, Feng J, Nattel S. Idiopathic atrial fibrillation in dogs: electrophysiologic determinants and mechanisms of antiarrhythmic action of flecainide. *J Am Coll Cardiol* 1995;**26**:277–86.

31 Satoh T, Zipes DP. Unequal atrial stretch in dogs increases dispersion of refractoriness conductive to developing atrial fibrillation. *J Cardiovasc Electrophysiol* 1996;**7**:833–42.

32 Efimov IR, Huang DT, Rendt JM, Salama G. Optical mapping of repolarization and refractoriness from intact hearts. *Circulation* 1994;**90**:1469–80.

33 Feng J, Yue L, Wang Z, Nattel S. Ionic mechanisms of regional action potential heterogeneity in the canine right atrium. *Circ Res* 1998;**83**:541–51.

34 Spach MS, Dolber PC, Anderson PAW. Multiple regional differences in cellular properties that regulate repolarization and contraction in the right atrium of adult and newborn dogs. *Circ Res* 1989;**65**:1594–611.

35 Yamashita T, Nakajima T, Hazama H, Hamada E, Murakawa Y, Sawada K, Omata M. Regional differences in transient outward current density and inhomogeneities of repolarization in rabbit right atrium. *Circulation* 1995;**92**:3061–9.

36 Kalifa J, Tanaka K, Zaitsev AV, et al. Mechanisms of wave fractionation at boundaries of high-frequency excitation in the posterior left atrium of the isolated sheep heart during atrial fibrillation. *Circulation* 2006;**113**:626–33.

37 Nademanee K, McKenzie J, Kosar E, et al. A new approach for catheter ablation of atrial fibrillation: mapping of the electrophysiologic substrate. *J Am Coll Cardiol* 2004;**43**:2044–53.

38 Fischer G, Stuhlinger MC, Nowak CN, Wieser L, Tilg B, Hintringer F. On computing dominant frequency from bipolar intracardiac electrograms. *IEEE Trans Biomed Eng* 2007;**54**:165–9.

39 Lazar S, Dixit S, Marchlinski FE, Callans DJ, Gerstenfeld EP. Presence of left-to-right atrial frequency gradient in paroxysmal but not persistent atrial fibrillation in humans. *Circulation* 2004;**110**:3181–6.

40 Sahadevan J, Ryu K, Peltz L, Khrestian CM, Stewart RW, Markowitz AH, Waldo AL. Epicardial mapping of chronic atrial fibrillation in patients: preliminary observations. *Circulation* 2004;**110**:3293–9.

41 Botteron GW, Smith JM. Quantitative assessment of the spatial organization of atrial fibrillation in the intact human heart. *Circulation* 1996;**93**:513–18.

42 Schuessler RB, Kay MW, Melby SJ, Branham BH, Boineau JP, Damiano RJ, Jr. Spatial and temporal stability of the dominant frequency of activation in human atrial fibrillation. *J Electrocardiol* 2006;**39**(4 Suppl): S7–S12.

43 Wu TJ, Doshi RN, Huang HLA, et al. Simultaneous biatrial computerized mapping during permanent atrial fibrillation in patients with organic heart disease. *J Cardiovasc Electrophysiol* 2002;**13**:571–7.

44 Sih HJ, Zipes DP, Berbari EJ, Adams DE, Olgin JE. Differences in organization between acute and chronic atrial fibrillation in dogs. *J Am Coll Cardiol* 2000;**36**: 924–31.

45 Wu TJ, Ong JJC, Chang CM, et al. Pulmonary veins and ligament of Marshall as sources of rapid activations in a canine model of sustained atrial fibrillation. *Circulation* 2001;**103**:1157–63.

46 Arora R, Verheule S, Scott L, et al. Arrhythmogenic substrate of the pulmonary veins assessed by high-resolution optical mapping. *Circulation* 2003;**107**:1816–21.

47 Kalifa J, Jalife J, Zaitsev AV, et al. Intra-atrial pressure increases rate and organization of waves emanating from the superior pulmonary veins during atrial fibrillation. *Circulation* 2003;**108**:668–71.

48 Vigmond EJ, Tsoi V, Kuo S, Arevalo H, Kneller J, Nattel S, Trayanova N. The effect of vagally induced dispersion of action potential duration on atrial arrhythmogenesis. *Heart Rhythm* 2004;**1**:334–44.

49 Kumagai K, Yasuda T, Tojo H, et al. Role of rapid focal activation in the maintenance of atrial fibrillation originating from the pulmonary veins. *Pacing Clin Electrophysiol* 2000;**23**:1823–7.

50 O'Donnell D, Furniss SS, Bourke JP. Paroxysmal cycle length shortening in the pulmonary veins during atrial fibrillation correlates with arrhythmogenic triggering foci in sinus rhythm. *J Cardiovasc Electrophysiol* 2002;**13**: 124–8.

51 Oral H, Ozaydin M, Tada H, et al. Mechanistic significance of intermittent pulmonary vein tachycardia in patients with atrial fibrillation. *J Cardiovasc Electrophysiol* 2002;**13**:645–50.

52 Lazar S, Dixit S, Callans DJ, Lin D, Marchlinski FE, Gerstenfeld EP. Effect of pulmonary vein isolation on the left-to-right atrial dominant frequency gradient in human atrial fibrillation. *Heart Rhythm* 2006;**3**:889–95.

53 Lewis T. *The Mechanism and Graphic Registration of the Heart Beat.* Shaw & Sons, London, 1925.

54 Scherf D. Studies on auricular tachycardia caused by aconitine administration. *Proc Soc Exp Biol Med* 1947;**64**:233–9.

55 Kumagai K, Khrestian C, Waldo AL. Simultaneous multisite mapping studies during induced atrial fibrillation in the sterile pericarditis model. Insights into the mechanisms of its maintenance. *Circulation* 1997;**95**:511–21.

56 Kumagai K, Uno K, Khrestian C, Waldo AL. Single site radiofrequency catheter ablation of atrial fibrillation: studies guided by simultaneous multisite mapping in the canine sterile pericarditis model. *J Am Coll Cardiol* 2000;**36**:917–23.

57 Jais P, Haissaguerre M, Shah DC, Chouairi S, Gencel L, Hocini M, Clementy J. A focal source of atrial fibrillation treated by discrete radiofrequency ablation. *Circulation* 1997;**95**:572–6.

58 Schuessler RB, Grayson TM, Bromberg BI, Cox JL, Boineau JP. Cholinergically mediated tachyarrhythmias induced by a single extrastimulus in the isolated canine right atrium. *Circ Res* 1992;**71**:1254–67.

59 Sarmast F, Kolli A, Zaitsev A, et al. Cholinergic atrial fibrillation: I-K,I-ACh gradients determine unequal left/right atrial frequencies and rotor dynamics. *Cardiovas Res* 2003;**59**:863–73.

60 Kabell G, Buchanan LV, Gibson JK, Belardinelli L. Effects of adenosine on atrial refractoriness and arrhythmias. *Cardiovasc Res* 1994;**28**:1385–9.

61 Belardinelli L, Shryock JC, Song Y, Wang D, Srinivas M. Ionic basis of the electrophysiological actions of adenosine on cardiomyocytes. *FASEB J* 1995;**9**:359–65.

62 Khositseth A, Clapham DE, Ackerman MJ. Intracellular signaling and regulation of cardiac ion channels. In: Zipes DP, Jalife J, eds. *Cardiac Electrophysiology – From Cell to Bedside.* WB Saunders, Philadelphia, 2004:33–41.

63 Jalife J, Berenfeld O, Mansour M. Mother rotors and fibrillatory conduction: a mechanism of atrial fibrillation. *Cardiovasc Res* 2002;**54**:204–16.

64 Oral H, Chugh A, Good E, et al. A tailored approach to catheter ablation of paroxysmal atrial fibrillation. *Circulation* 2006;**113**:1824–31.

65 Lemola K, Ting M, Gupta P, et al. Effects of two different catheter ablation techniques on spectral characteristics of atrial fibrillation. *J Am Coll Cardiol* 2006;**48**:340–8.

6

CHAPTER 6

Three-dimensional images in catheter ablation of atrial fibrillation

Hsuan-Ming Tsao, Mei-Han Wu, & Shih-Ann Chen

Introduction

Atrial fibrillation (AF) remains a major clinical disease, not only because it is the most common arrhythmia that contributes to significant cardiovascular mortality and morbidity, but also due to its socioeconomic impact [1,2]. Abundant human and experimental studies have provided mechanistic insight into the initiation and perpetuation of AF in recent years, with great progress made in the elucidation of the pathophysiology and catheter-based therapy of AF [3–8]. The pulmonary veins (PVs) play an important role in both ectopy generation and substrate maintenance in AF. It has been well documented that elimination or isolation of these ectopic triggers can cure a subset of AF. Therefore, the interventional therapy of paroxysmal AF has been focused initially on the interruption of electric conduction by isolating the AF initiators of the PVs from left atrial tissues. Recently, modification of the substrate within the left atrium (LA) has been shown to improve the long-term success rate of AF ablation. Furthermore, more extensive ablation strategies, including multiple linear and point ablations within the LA and ablation of the continuous fractionated atrial electrogram [9–11], have become popular in catheter ablation of persistent AF. From a practical point of view, understanding the morphological characteristics of the LA and PVs in detail can achieve a more efficient and successful ablation and prevent potential procedure-related complications. Non-invasive imaging modalities, including magnetic resonance angiography (MRA) and multidetector computed tomography (MDCT), are useful and powerful enough to depict the PVs and LA. They can provide a valuable road map before the catheter ablation of AF [12–20].

Catheter Ablation of Atrial Fibrillation Edited by Etienne Aliot, Michel Haïssaguerre and Warren M. Jackman

Anatomic characteristics of the pulmonary veins and left atrium

Evolving techniques in catheter ablation of AF have led to an expansion in knowledge of the anatomy of the LA. Detailed information of PV anatomy and the relationship between the PVs and the LA is mandatory for mapping and ablation procedures.

Basic anatomy and morphological patterns of the pulmonary veins

Structural information regarding PV size and shape, and the angle between the PV and LA have been obtained in AF patients using MRA and computed tomography (CT) scans. PV ostia are ellipsoid with a longer superioinferior dimension.

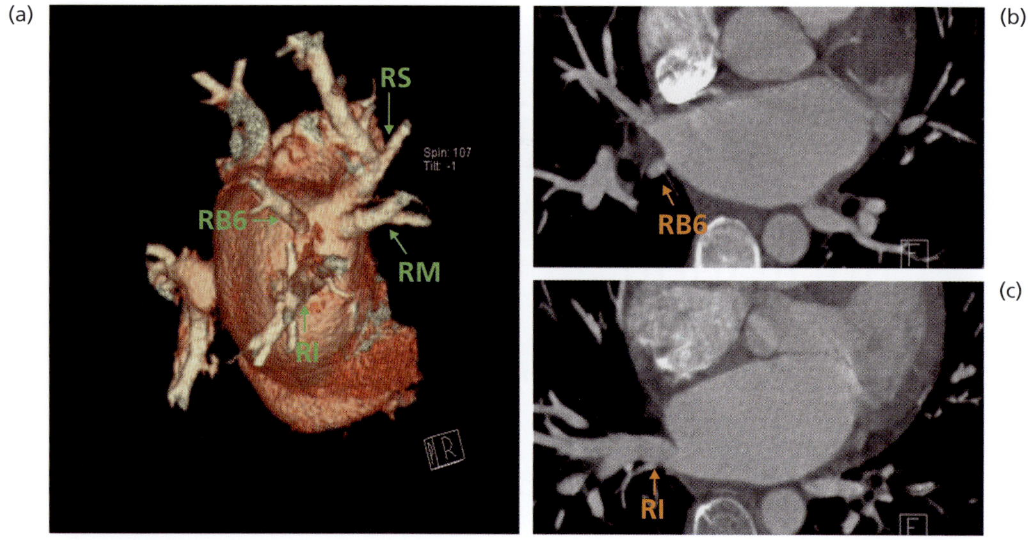

Figure 6.1 Supernumerary right pulmonary veins (PVs). (a) Three-dimensional image showing four discrete PVs, including a right superior PV (RS), a right middle PV (RM), an additional PV of the RB6 segment, and a right inferior PV (RI) in the right lateral projection. (b, c) Axial views showing different orientations of the RB6 PV (b) and RI PV (c).

Funnel-shaped ostia are frequently noted in AF patients. Although the PVs have a certain basic pattern, they are more variable than we predicted. The anatomic variations of PVs can be readily demonstrated by cardiac CT/MRA. The variability can substantially influence the success rate of catheter ablation if the variant veins are inadequately treated.

Tsao et al. [15] utilized MRA to demonstrate a variant of a discrete right middle PV that had an independent orifice other than the typical two PV ostia in the right side. Several investigators have reported the existence of supernumerary right PVs (Figure 6.1), with the incidence ranging from 18% to 29% [12,15,17–20]. Lickfett et al. recognized a right top PV in 3% of AF patients using MRA [21]. Awareness of this variant can avoid inadvertent catheter manipulation. Perez-Lugones et al. showed that multiple ramifications and early branching of the right inferior PV can be observed and this might explain the low incidence of firing of the right inferior PV [22]. A common trunk of left or right PVs can be occasionally identified using cardiac CT/MRA images. The common ostium is more frequently found on the left-sided PVs (6–35%) and results in a broad PV–atrial junction (Figure 6.2). In addition, the common left PV has been reported to be a common source of arrhythmogenic ectopy [23]. Thus, it is critical to understand these anatomic variations before catheter ablation of AF. A more accurate localization of the true PV–atrial junction in these patients can be made with the assistance of three-dimensional imaging prior to mapping and ablation procedures [24].

Anatomic landmarks within the left atrium

Linear lesions delivered within the LA were reported to improve the long-term success rate of catheter ablation of AF. Various strategies have been advocated recently to gain a good outcome of AF ablation. From the experience of typical atrial flutter ablation, the anatomic variation of the cavotricuspid isthmus can influence significantly the procedure time and results. Therefore, a knowledge of the topographic anatomy of the mitral isthmus, LA roof, and left atrial appendage (LAA) is important for deploying linear lesions over these areas.

By using virtual endoscopic views, the endocardial configurations of the LA and PV can be delineated and the ablation strategy can be modified if

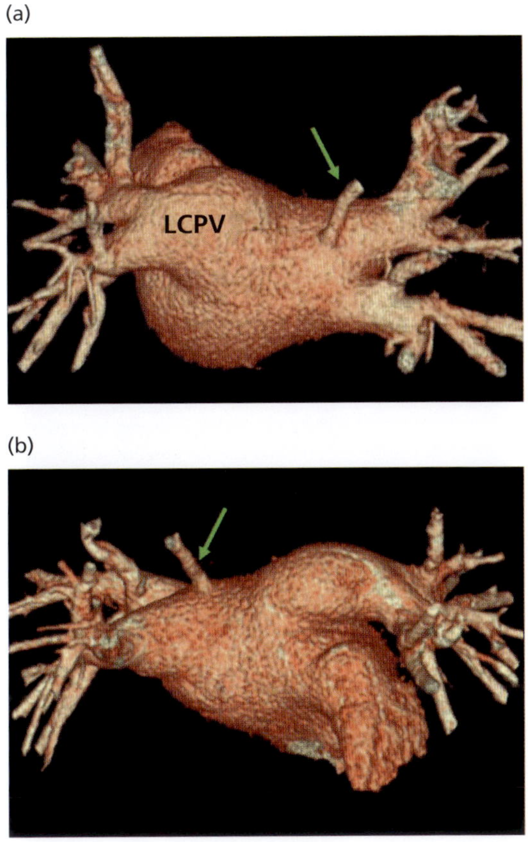

Figure 6.2 Volume-rendering technique of MDCT showing three-dimensional images of an unusual case of a coexisting large left common pulmonary vein (LCPV) and right top PV (green arrows) in different projections (a, b).

any variant morphology exists. We have reported that the configuration and length of the LA roof and isthmuses were variable in controls and AF patients [25,26] (Table 6.1). Three types of roof shape, including concave, straight, and convex, were noted. In some cases with a convex roof, the pulmonary artery was very close to the LA roof near the right superior PV antrum. In addition, pouches were recognized in the LA roof and isthmuses in about 5–15% of AF cases, which might develop into a gap formation after linear ablation (Figure 6.3a). The endocardial configurations of the LA isthmus included concave, straight, and pouch-like shapes. In addition, a prominent ridge was found to course between the right inferior PV and medial mitral annulus in 13% of AF patients (Figure 6.3b), which might cause difficulty in making a complete block in this area.

We also investigated the structure of the LAA and classified the location of the LAA into three types according to the relationship between the LAA and left superior PV (LSPV) orifice: (i) type I – the LAA orifice was superior to the LSPV orifice (ii) type II – the LAA orifice was horizontal to the LSPV orifice; (iii) type III – the LAA orifice was inferior to the LSPV orifice (Figure 6.4). There were higher incidences of the LAA type I and type III in the AF group as compared to the control subjects. In addition, a prominent ridge interposed between the LAA and LSPV orifice was demonstrated by CT imaging. Two types of LAA ridges, long and short,

Table 6.1 Morphological characteristics of left atrium structures in atrial fibrillation patients

	Roof	*Lateral isthmus*	*Medial isthmus*
Length (cm)	3.8 ± 1.0	3.3 ± 0.7	5.1 ± 0.9
Distance (cm)	3.6 ± 0.9	2.7 ± 0.5	4.7 ± 0.8
Depth (cm)	0.2 ± 0.2	0.6 ± 0.3	0.6 ± 0.3
Configuration (%)			
Concave	18	82	73
Straight	50	13	9
Convex	17	0	0
Pouch	15	5	5
Ridge	0	0	13

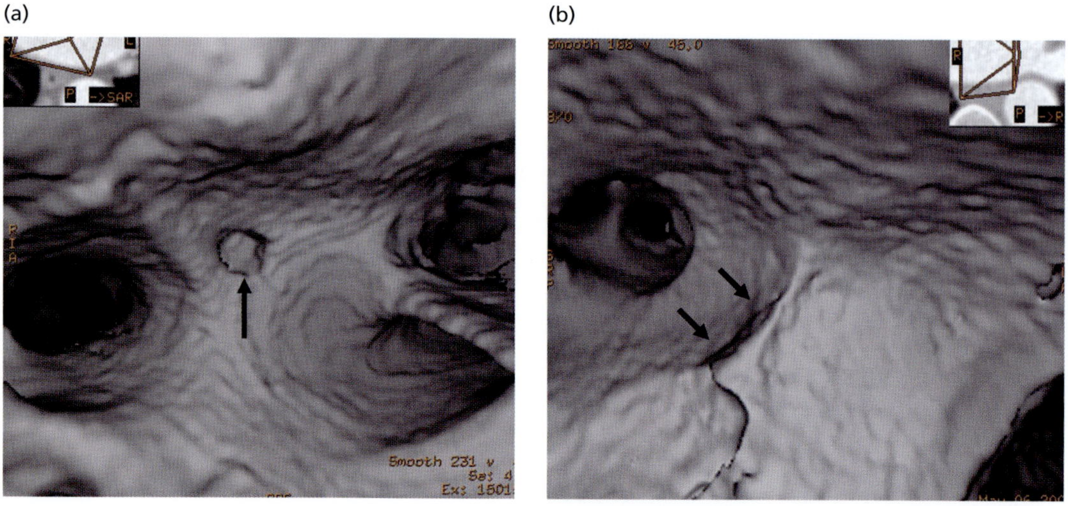

Figure 6.3 Virtual endoscopic views showing peculiar structures within the LA. (a) Roof pouch (arrow) between the left and right superior PVs. (b) A prominent ridge (arrows) coursing between the right inferior PV orifice and septal mitral annulus. (Reproduced with permission from [25,26].)

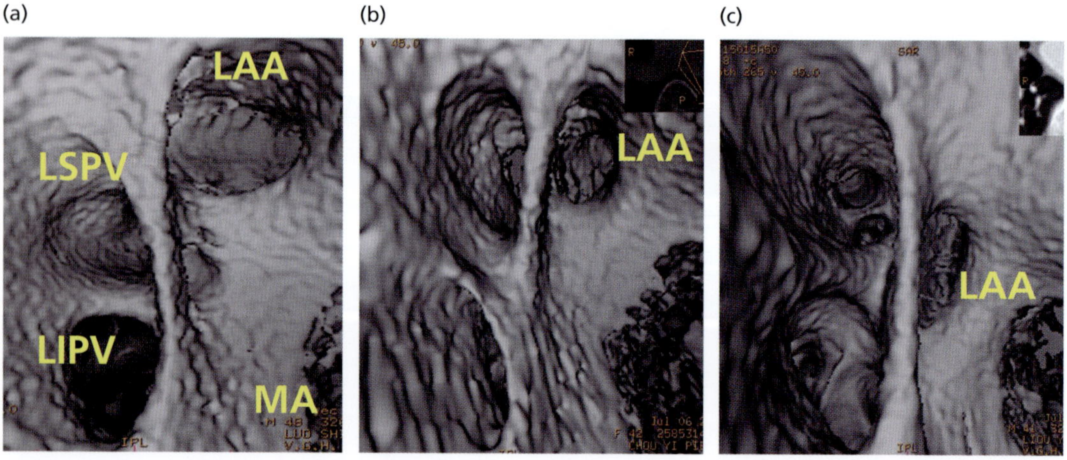

Figure 6.4 Virtual endoscopic views showing the three types of location of the left atrial appendage (LAA) and the length of ridge between the LAA and left pulmonary veins (PVs). (a) Superior type and long ridge. (b) Horizontal type and short ridge. (c) Inferior type and long ridge. LIPV, left inferior pulmonary vein; LSPV, left superior pulmonary vein; MA, mitral annulus. (Reproduced with permission from [25].)

were illustrated. Schmidt et al. also found narrow ridges between the ipsilateral PVs and between the left PVs and appendage using an endoluminal reconstruction of MRA [27]. The extension of the myocardial ridges may influence the stability of catheter placement and increase the difficulty in creating a complete block of mitral isthmus ablation at the inferior border of the left inferior PV ostium.

Anatomic structures surrounding the left atrium (Table 6.2)

Esophagus

Atrioesophageal fistulae have been reported during intraoperative radiofrequency ablation of AF using the endocardial approach, or after percutaneous catheter ablation of the PV and LA [28–30]. An atrioesophageal fistula is a lethal complication

Table 6.2 Potential complications related to anatomic proximity between the adjacent structures and left atrium (LA)

Complications	*Possible danger area*
Atrioesophageal fistula	Posterior LA wall and PV ostia
Atriobronchial fistula	Superior PV ostia
Coronary artery injury	Distal coronary sinus and LA appendage orifice
Phrenic nerve injury	Superior vena cava, right superior PV, and LA appendage

PV, pulmonary vein.

and is associated with a high mortality rate. Thus, understanding the anatomic relationship between the esophagus and PV/LA may be the first step to avoid esophageal injury during the catheter ablation procedure. Several studies have demonstrated the close relationship between the posterior LA, PVs, coronary sinus, and esophagus by CT scan [31–34] (Figure 6.5). In addition, the contact between the upper portion of the lateral LA isthmus and esophagus was noted in about half of our AF patients [26]. In these patients, delivering energies over the junction of the left inferior PV and lateral isthmus should be carried out with caution. It might be a good policy to avoid repeated ablations and overheating this area. The esophagus was separated from the lateral isthmus gradually as it went down. Thus, it was less likely that the esophagus would be injured during ablation of the lower portion of the lateral isthmus.

Although peristalsis and dynamic movement of the esophagus can influence the exact location of the esophagus, the anatomic parameters gained from static CT images are still of value for modification of ablation lesions in the posterior LA. However, real-time demonstration of the esophageal route by swallowing barium contrast may be a simple and reliable method to guide ablation lesions.

Coronary arteries

Takahashi et al. reported that the left circumflex coronary artery (LCX) was occluded acutely during ablation within the coronary sinus for achievement of mitral isthmus block [35]. Autopsy results from Maselli et al. have shown that the LCX coursed between the coronary sinus and mitral isthmus in 63.9% of the studied cases [36]. The CT images can also illustrate the close relation between the distal coronary sinus and LCX (Figure 6.6). Therefore, the LCX may be vulnerable to thermal injury from radiofrequency ablation deep within the coronary sinus in these patients. In addition, the very close vicinity between the LAA orifice and proximal LCX was also demonstrated by the CT images. Because energy applications around the LAA have recently

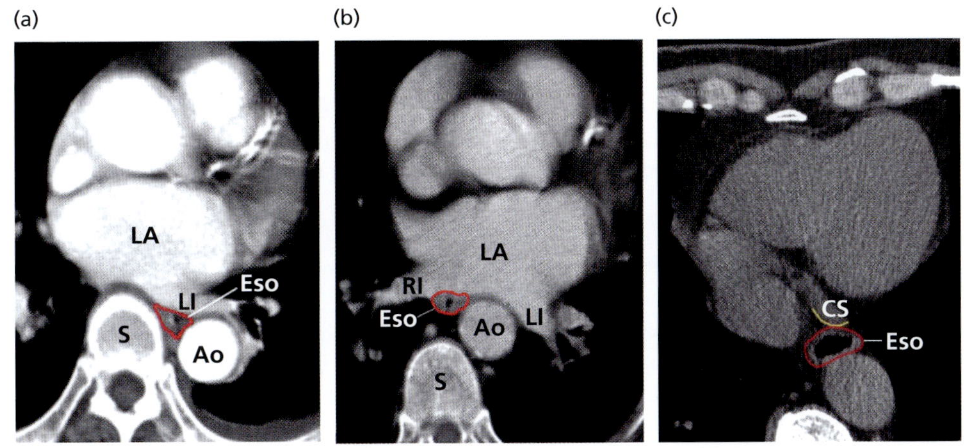

Figure 6.5 Close relationship between the esophagus (Eso) and (a) PVs, (b) posterior left atrium (LA), and (c) coronary sinus (CS). Ao, aorta; LI, left inferior pulmonary vein; RI, right inferior pulmonary vein; S, spine. (Reproduced with permission from [33,34].)

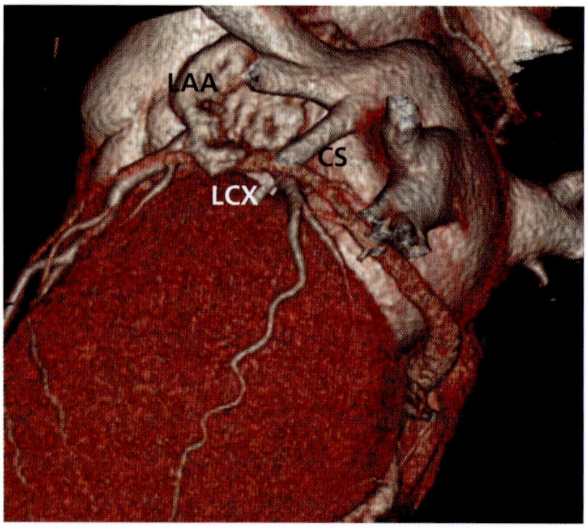

Figure 6.6 Three-dimensional images demonstrating the close anatomic relationship between the left atrial appendage (LAA), left circumflex coronary artery (LCX), and coronary sinus (CS).

been proposed to increase the success rate in treating persistent AF, ablation near the anterior base of the LAA orifice must be performed carefully in order to prevent any potential risk of proximal LCX injury.

Bronchial tree

Atriobronchial fistula is a very rare but devastating complication after catheter ablation of AF. Because of its high mortality rate, atriobronchial fistulae should be suspected with high priority in any patient who presents with hemoptysis and/or stroke after AF ablation. Doshi et al. reported a case that suffered from recurrent hemoptysis after a second ablation procedure for AF [37]. A fistula between the LSPV and bronchus was demonstrated during surgical exploration. This complication raises concern about the anatomic proximity between the LA/PVs and the bronchial trees. Our experience has shown that the right main bronchus can be in proximity to the posterior wall of the RSPV ostium and the left main bronchus can be in proximity to the posterior wall of the LSPV ostium. PV isolation procedures may carry a potential hazard of injury to the main bronchi. However, the cartilage of the main bronchi and the fat plane between the bronchi and PVs are protective, which may account for the very low incidence of bronchial injury during AF ablation.

Morphological remodeling of the pulmonary veins and left atrium in atrial fibrillation patients

The ostial geometries of the PVs have been comprehensively evaluated by CT and MRA. We first reported that different sizes of PVs were noted in control, paroxysmal AF (PAF), and chronic AF (CAF) groups using MRA images [38]. Significant dilation of both superior PVs with simultaneous LA enlargement was demonstrated among patients with PAF and CAF. After successful ablation of arrhythmogenic PV, the dilated (non-ablated) PVs could regress during a long-term follow-up [39]. Our later study showed that the morphological remodeling and reverse remodeling of LAA appendage in AF patients were also demonstrated by the MRA images [40] (Figure 6.7). Jayam et al. investigated the changes of PV and LA size after segmental isolation of the PV by MRA [41]. They found that the LA volume decreased significantly after successful ablation. Further, significant reductions of LA volume and PV ostial size were revealed by CT scan in patients with maintenance of sinus rhythm after left atrial circumferential ablation [42]. In addition, MDCT was effective in demonstrating the anatomic remodeling process manifested as recession of the pectinate muscle and a thinning and dilated LA in patients with chronic AF [43].

Detection of complications after catheter ablation

The feasibility and safety of catheter ablation within the LA have been well documented. However, procedure-related complications, including PV stenosis, thrombosis and dissection, pericarditis, cardiac perforation, pulmonary hypertension, and systemic embolism, are encountered occasionally. MRA and CT scans play an important role in disclosing the complications [44]. Acquired PV stenosis after PV ablation is a major concern when radiofrequency energy is applied around or inside the PV ostia (Figure 6.8a, b). Although a single PV stenosis can be asymptomatic, the severity of clinical symptoms may be related to the number, stenostic degree, and chronicity of the involved veins. MDCT and MRA can effectively delineate the lesions and provide the information needed to

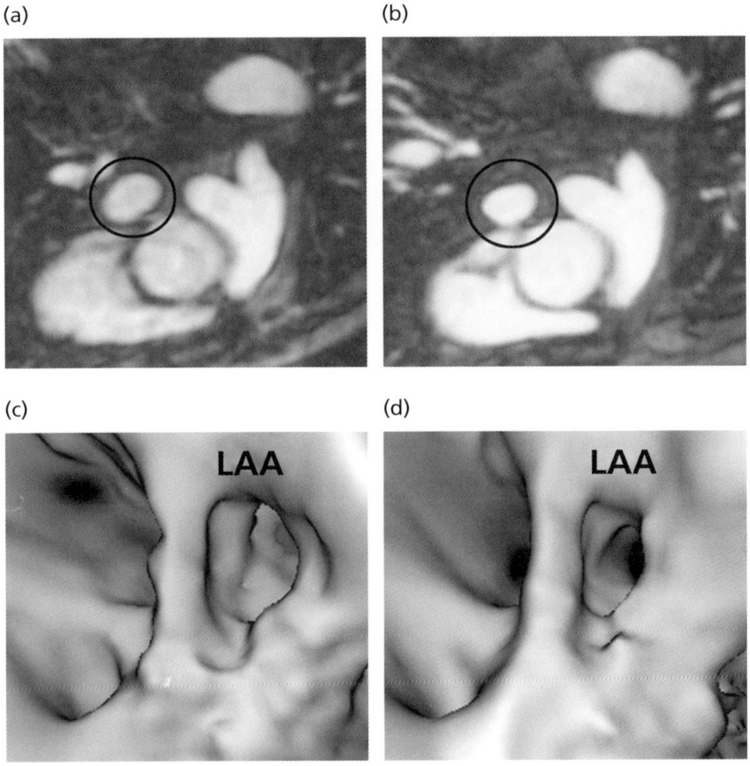

Figure 6.7 MRA images showing the morphological changes of the PVs and left atrial appendage (LAA) after successful ablation of AF. (a, b) Regression of ostial size of the right superior PV. (c, d) Decrease of the size of the LAA orifice. (Reproduced with permission from [39,40].)

plan further management [45–48]. However, we would like to emphasize the necessity of pre-procedural CT scans for the detection of pre-existing PV stenosis [49] (Figure 6.8c, d). Finally, the images can facilitate the diagnosis of mediastinitis, pericardial effusion, and cardiac tamponade post-procedurally.

Delineation of the right atrial structure and superior vena cava

Our laboratory has demonstrated the morphological alterations of the superior vena cava (SVC) in patients with AF initiated from the SVC using cardiac MRA [50]. A dilated SVC and increased eccentricity of the middle part of the SVC were revealed in these patients. Another interesting issue is the left SVC. The left SVC is the embryological precursor of the ligament of Marshall. It is an important arrhythmogenic structure for non-PV AF. CT scans are useful to demonstrate the left SVC and an integration of CT images with a three-dimensional mapping system can assist ablation of the left SVC [51]. Understanding of the SVC structures can also prevent potential complications related to the ablation procedure, including sinus node injury, SVC stenosis, and phrenic nerve palsy. Furthermore, Komatsu et al. have used MDCT to evaluate the cavotricuspid isthmus and right atrium in patients with common atrial flutter [52]. Cardiac MRA images with three-dimensional reconstruction of the right atrium can reveal the details of the right atrium structures and can be integrated with biplane fluoroscopic images to facilitate the mapping and ablation procedure in treating right atrial arrhythmias [53]. These reports suggest that CT and MRA are also valuable in characterizing the anatomic structures of the right atrium.

Conclusion

Advances in imaging technology have improved the quality of cardiac CT and MRA. Three-dimensional

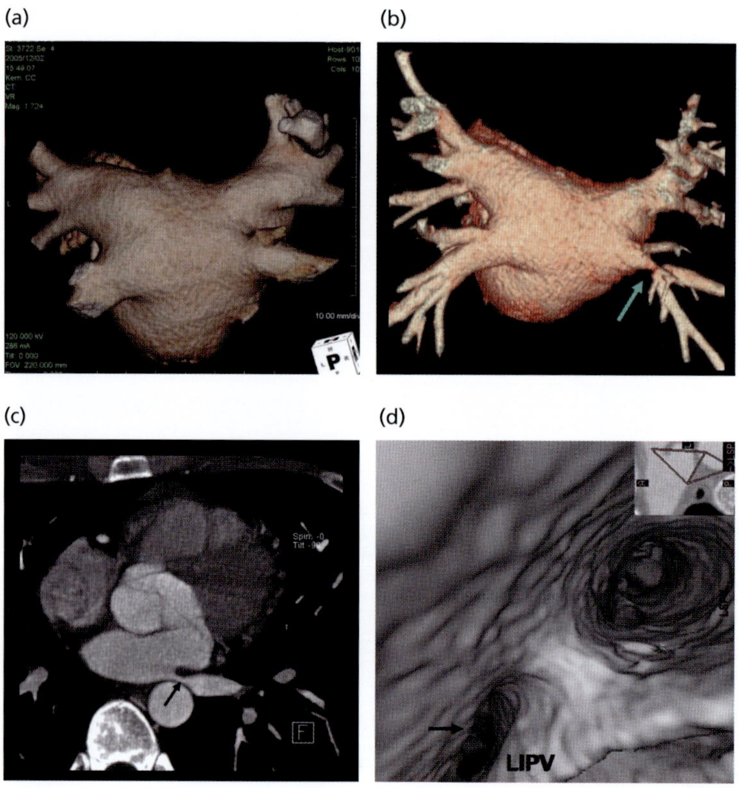

Figure 6.8 MDCT images of acquired PV stenosis (a, b) and pre-existing PV stenosis (c, d). (a) Three-dimensional images before ablation. (b) Right inferior PV stenosis (arrow) after ablation. (c) Axial view showing a left inferior pulmonary vein (LIPV) stenosis (arrow) before ablation. (d) Virtual endoscopic view showing a pre-existing stenosis (arrow) caused by compression of the descending aorta. (Adapted with permission from [49].)

image, multiplanar images, and endoscopic views can provide crucial information for electrophysiologists to perform ablations within the LA with more efficiency and safety. We should be familiar with normal and variant patterns of PVs, important landmarks within the LA, and the topographic relationship between the LA, esophagus, bronchial tree, and surrounding vascular structures before the ablation procedure is started. In addition, we can understand the morphological changes of the PV and LA and procedure-related complications after ablation by utilizing CT and MRA images. In the near future, the integration of three-dimensional CT/MRA with three-dimensional mapping systems will become more popular and make AF ablation an easier and safer treatment.

References

1 Go AS, Hylek EM, Phillips KA, Chang Y, Henault LE, Selby JV, Singer DE. Prevalence of diagnosed atrial fibrillation in adults: national implications for rhythm management and stroke prevention: the AnTicoagulation and Risk Factors in Atrial Fibrillation (ATRIA) Study. *J Am Med Assoc* 2001;**285**:2370–5.

2 Wattigney WA, Mensah GA, Croft JB. Increasing trends in hospitalization for atrial fibrillation in the United States, 1985 through 1999: implications for primary prevention. *Circulation* 2003;**108**:711–16.

3 Nattel S. New ideas about atrial fibrillation 50 years on. *Nature* 2002;**415**:219–26.

4 Wyse DG, Gersh BJ. Atrial fibrillation: a perspective: thinking inside and outside the box. *Circulation* 2004; **109**:3089–95.

5 Haissaguerre M, Jais P, Shah DC, et al. Spontaneous initiation of atrial fibrillation by ectopic beats originating from pulmonary veins. *N Engl J Med* 1998;**339**: 659–66.

6 Chen SA, Hsieh MH, Tai CT, et al. Initiation of atrial fibrillation by ectopic beats originating from the pulmonary veins: electrophysiologic characteristics, pharmacologic response and effects of radiofrequency ablation. *Circulation* 1999;**100**:1879–86.

7 Pappone C, Rosanio S, Oreto G, et al. Circumferential radiofrequency ablation of pulmonary vein ostia: a new anatomic approach for curing atrial fibrillation. *Circulation* 2000;**102**:2619–28.

8 Oral H, Scharf C, Chugh A, et al. Catheter ablation for paroxysmal atrial fibrillation: segmental pulmonary vein ostial ablation versus left atrial ablation. *Circulation* 2003; **108**:2355–60.

9 Haissaguerre M, Hocini M, Sanders P, et al. Catheter ablation of long-lasting persistent atrial fibrillation: clinical outcome and mechanisms of subsequent arrhythmias. *J Cardiovasc Electrophysiol* 2005;**16**:1138–47.

10 Nademanee K, McKenzie J, Kosar E, et al. A new approach for catheter ablation of atrial fibrillation: mapping of the electrophysiological substrate. *J Am Coll Cardiol* 2004;**43**: 2044–53.

11 Chen SA, Tai CT. Catheter ablation of atrial fibrillation originating from the non-pulmonary vein foci. *J Cardiovasc Electrophysiol* 2005;**16**:229–32.

12 Kato R, Lickfett L, Meininger G, et al. Pulmonary vein anatomy in patients undergoing catheter ablation of atrial fibrillation: lessons learned by use of magnetic resonance imaging. *Circulation* 2003;**107**:2004–10.

13 Dill T, Neumann T, Ekinci O, et al. Pulmonary vein diameter reduction after radiofrequency catheter ablation for paroxysmal atrial fibrillation evaluated by contrast-enhanced three-dimensional magnetic resonance imaging. *Circulation* 2003;**107**:845–50.

14 Wittkampf FH, Vonken EJ, Derksen R, et al. Pulmonary vein ostium geometry: analysis by magnetic resonance angiography. *Circulation* 2003;**107**:21–3.

15 Tsao HM, Wu MH, Yu WC, et al. Role of right middle pulmonary vein in patients with paroxysmal atrial fibrillation. *J Cardiovasc Electrophysiol* 2001;**12**:1353–7.

16 Scharf C, Sneider M, Case I, et al. Anatomy of the pulmonary veins in patients with atrial fibrillation and effects of segmental ostial ablation analyzed by computed tomography. *J Cardiovasc Electrophysiol* 2003;**14**:150–5.

17 Schwartzman D, Lacomis J, Wigginton WG. Characterization of left atrium and distal pulmonary vein morphology using multidimensional computed tomography. *J Am Coll Cardiol* 2003;**41**:1349–57.

18 Mansour M, Holmvang G, Sosnovik D, Migrino R, Abbara S, Ruskin J, Keane D. Assessment of pulmonary vein anatomic variability by magnetic resonance imaging: implications for catheter ablation techniques for atrial fibrillation. *J Cardiovasc Electrophysiol* 2004:**15**: 387–93.

19 Cirillo S, Bonamini R, Gaita F, et al. Magnetic resonance angiography virtual endoscopy in the assessment of pulmonary veins before radiofrequency ablation procedures for atrial fibrillation. *Eur Radiol* 2004;**14**:2053–60.

20 Marom EM, Herndon JE, Kim YH, McAdams HP. Variations in pulmonary venous drainage to the left atrium: implications for radiofrequency ablation. *Radiology* 2004;**230**:824–9.

21 Lickfett L, Kato R, Tandri H, et al. Characterization of a new pulmonary vein variant using magnetic resonance angiography: incidence, imaging, and interventional implications of the "right top pulmonary vein". *J Cardiovasc Electrophysiol* 2004;**15**:538–43.

22 Perez-Lugones A, Schvartzman PR, Schweikert R, et al. Three-dimensional reconstruction of pulmonary veins in patients with atrial fibrillation and controls: morphological characteristics of different veins. *Pacing Clin Electrophysiol* 2003;**26**:8–15.

23 Schwartzman D, Bazaz R, Nosbisch J. Common left pulmonary vein: a consistent source of arrhythmogenic atrial ectopy. *J Cardiovasc Electrophysiol* 2004;**15**:560–6.

24 Ahmed J, Sohal S, Malchano ZJ, Holmvang G, Ruskin JN, Reddy VY. Three-dimensional analysis of pulmonary venous ostial and antral anatomy: implications for balloon catheter-based pulmonary vein isolation. *J Cardiovasc Electrophysiol* 2006;**17**:251–5.

25 Wongcharoen W, Tsao HM, Wu MH, et al. Morphologic characteristics of left atrial appendage, roof and septum. Implication for the ablation of atrial fibrillation. *J Cardiovasc Electrophysiol* 2006;**17**:951–6.

26 Chiang SJ, Tsao HM, Wu MH, et al. Anatomic characteristics of left atrial isthmus in patients with atrial fibrillation. Lessons from computed tomographic images. *J Cardiovasc Electrophysiol* 2006;**17**:1274–8.

27 Schmidt B, Ernst S, Ouyang F, et al. External and endoluminal analysis of left atrial anatomy and the pulmonary veins in three-dimensional reconstructions of magnetic resonance angiography: the full insight from inside. *J Cardiovasc Electrophysiol* 2006;**17**:957–64.

28 Doll N, Borger MA, Fabricius A, et al. Esophageal perforation during left atrial radiofrequency ablation: is the risk too high? *J Thoracic Cardiovasc Surg* 2003;**125**: 836–42.

29 Pappone C, Oral H, Santinelli V, et al. Atrio-esophageal fistula as a complication of percutaneous transcatheter ablation of atrial fibrillation. *Circulation* 2004;**109**:2724–6.

30 Scanavacca MI, Davila A, Parga J, Sosa E. Left atrial-esophageal fistula following radiofrequency catheter ablation of atrial fibrillation. *J Cardiovasc Electrophysiol* 2004:**15**:960–2.

31 Lemola K, Sneider M, Desjardins B, et al. Computed tomographic analysis of the anatomy of the left atrium and the esophagus: implications for left atrial catheter ablation. *Circulation* 2004;**110**:3655–60.

32 Kottkamp H, Piorkowski C, Tanner H, et al. Topographic variability of the esophageal left atrial relation influencing ablation lines in patients with atrial fibrillation. *J Cardiovasc Electrophysiol* 2005;**16**:146–50.

33 Tsao HM, Wu MH, Higa S, et al. Anatomic relationship of the esophagus and left atrium: implication for

catheter ablation of atrial fibrillation. *Chest* 2005;**128**: 2581–7.

34 Tsao HM, Wu MH, Chern MS, et al. Anatomic proximity of the esophagus to the coronary sinus: implication for catheter ablation within the coronary sinus. *J Cardiovasc Electrophysiol* 2006;**17**:266–9.

35 Takahashi Y, Jais P, Hocini M, et al. Acute occlusion of the left circumflex coronary artery during mitral isthmus linear ablation. *J Cardiovasc Electrophysiol* 2005;**16**: 1104–7.

36 Maselli D, Guarracino F, Chiaramonti F, Mangia F, Borelli G, Minzioni G. Percutaneous mitral annuloplasty: an anatomic study of human coronary sinus and its relation with mitral valve annulus and coronary arteries. *Circulation* 2006;**114**:377–80.

37 Doshi RN, Kaushal R, Cesario DA, Shivkumar K. Atrio-bronchial fistula formation as a devastating complication of left atrial catheter ablation for atrial fibrillation. *Heart Rhythm* 2006;**3**:S59 (abstract).

38 Tsao HM, Yu WC, Cheng HC, et al. Pulmonary vein dilation in patients with atrial fibrillation: detection by magnetic resonance imaging. *J Cardiovasc Electrophysiol* 2001;**12**:809–13.

39 Tsao HM, Wu MH, Huang BH, et al. Morphologic remodeling of pulmonary veins and left atrium after catheter ablation of atrial fibrillation: insight from long-term follow-up of three-dimensional magnetic resonance imaging. *J Cardiovasc Electrophysiol* 2005;**16**:7–12.

40 Chang SH, Tsao HM, Wu MH, et al. Morphological changes of left atrial appendage after catheter ablation of atrial fibrillation. *J Cardiovasc Electrophysiol* 2007;**18**: 47–52.

41 Jayam VK, Dong J, Vasamreddy CR, et al. Atrial volume reduction following catheter ablation of atrial fibrillation and relation to reduction in pulmonary vein size: an evaluation using magnetic resonance angiography. *J Interv Cardiac Electrophysiol* 2005;**13**:107–14.

42 Lemola K, Sneider M, Desjardins B, et al. Effects of left atrial ablation of atrial fibrillation on size of the left atrium and pulmonary veins. *Heart Rhythm* 2004;**1**: 576–81.

43 Imada M, Funabashi N, Asano M, Uehara M, Ueda M, Komuro I. Anatomical remodeling of left atria in subjects with chronic and paroxysmal atrial fibrillation evaluated by multislice computed tomography. *Int J Cardiol* 2006; **7**:164.

44 Tsao HM, Chen SA. Evaluation of pulmonary vein stenosis after catheter ablation of atrial fibrillation. *Cardiac Electrophysiol Rev* 2002;**6**:397–400.

45 Saad EB, Rossillo A, Saad CP, et al. Pulmonary vein stenosis after radiofrequency ablation of atrial fibrillation: functional characterization, evolution, and influence of the ablation strategy. *Circulation* 2003;**108**:3102–7.

46 Packer DL, Keelan P, Munger TM, et al. Clinical presentation, investigation, and management of pulmonary vein stenosis complicating ablation for atrial fibrillation. *Circulation* 2005;**111**:546–54.

47 Arentz T, Jander N, von Rosenthal J, et al. Incidence of pulmonary vein stenosis 2 years after radiofrequency catheter ablation of refractory atrial fibrillation. *Eur Heart J* 2003;**24**:963–9.

48 Dong J, Vasamreddy CR, Jayam V, et al. Incidence and predictors of pulmonary vein stenosis following catheter ablation of atrial fibrillation using the anatomic pulmonary vein ablation approach: results from paired magnetic resonance imaging. *J Cardiovasc Electrophysiol* 2005;**16**:845–52.

49 Wongcharoen W, Tsao HM, Wu MH, et al. Preexisting pulmonary vein stenosis in patients undergoing atrial fibrillation ablation: a report of five cases. *J Cardiovasc Electrophysiol* 2006;**17**:423–5.

50 Huang BH, Wu MH, Tsao HM, et al. Morphology of the thoracic veins and left atrium in paroxysmal atrial fibrillation initiated by superior caval vein ectopy. *J Cardiovasc Electrophysiol* 2005;**16**:411–17.

51 Elayi CS, Fahmy TS, Wazni OM, Patel D, Saliba W, Natale A. Left superior vena cava isolation in patients undergoing pulmonary vein antrum isolation: impact on atrial fibrillation recurrence. *Heart Rhythm* 2006;**3**:1019–23.

52 Komatsu S, Okuyama Y, Omori Y, et al. Evaluation of the cavotricuspid isthmus and right atrium by multidetector-row computed tomography in patients with common atrial flutter. *Heart Vessels* 2005;**20**:264–70.

53 Ector J, De Buck S, Adams J, Dymarkowski S, Bogaert J, Maes F, Heidbuchel H. Cardiac three-dimensional magnetic resonance imaging and fluoroscopy merging: a new approach for electroanatomic mapping to assist catheter ablation. *Circulation* 2005;**112**:3769–76.

CHAPTER 7

Signal processing of fibrillatory electrograms

Thomas H. Everett, IV & Jeffrey E. Olgin

Introduction

Signal processing has been used in the medical arena for speech therapy, analyzing electroencephalographs (EEGs) and electromyographs (EMGs) for several years [1]. While signal processing has been used to analyze cardiac signals, it has not been until the last 10 years that it has become a popular tool for analyzing fibrillatory electrograms. Signal processing is used to analyze fibrillatory electrograms as a research tool to characterize atrial fibrillation (AF) and has the potential to be a useful clinical tool to identify sites for possible target ablation. As scientists, researches, and clinicians continue to use signal processing, an increased understanding of fibrillation and improved ablation therapies will continue to develop.

The basics of signal processing

Signal processing is a broad term used whenever any filtering or analysis is performed on a signal. However, many of these processes are very technical, difficult to understand, and can cause unwanted changes to the recorded signal. In general, filtering of signals is employed to eliminate or reduce any signal components that would interfere with the analysis such as 50 or 60 Hz noise, any unwanted cardiac activation such as QRS complexes, and any farfield artifacts. Filtering is also used to enhance the signal generated by cardiac activation. Specific signal processing aimed at signal analyses can be employed to uncover fundamental characteristics of the recorded signal and to aid in understanding the characteristics of the fibrillatory signals.

When filtering and analyzing fibrillatory electrograms there are two types of frequency components within the signal that we need to be concerned with (Figure 7.1). One is the frequency of the fibrillation, which can vary from 3 to 15 Hz; the other is the frequency that composes each individual activation spike. These frequencies can be greater than 20 Hz.

Filtering

When filtering the signals, there are several different types of filters that can be used. Ideal filters are shown in Figure 7.2. A high-pass filter is one that passes high frequencies and attenuates low frequencies. A low-pass filter is one that passes frequencies below a specified frequency and attenuates higher frequencies. A band-pass filter has a range of frequencies that pass unfiltered while frequencies below and above the specified frequencies of the filter are attenuated. Finally, a notch filter or a bandstop filter is one that rejects a narrow band of frequencies and passes all others. This filter is often used to eliminate specific frequencies such as 60 Hz noise.

As mentioned earlier when filtering and analyzing fibrillatory electrograms, there are two different types of frequencies that compose the signal – the actual frequency of the fibrillation, and the frequency components that compose each individual

Catheter Ablation of Atrial Fibrillation Edited by Etienne Aliot, Michel Haïssaguerre and Warren M. Jackman
© 2008 Blackwell Publishing, ISBN: 978-1-4501-6349-1.

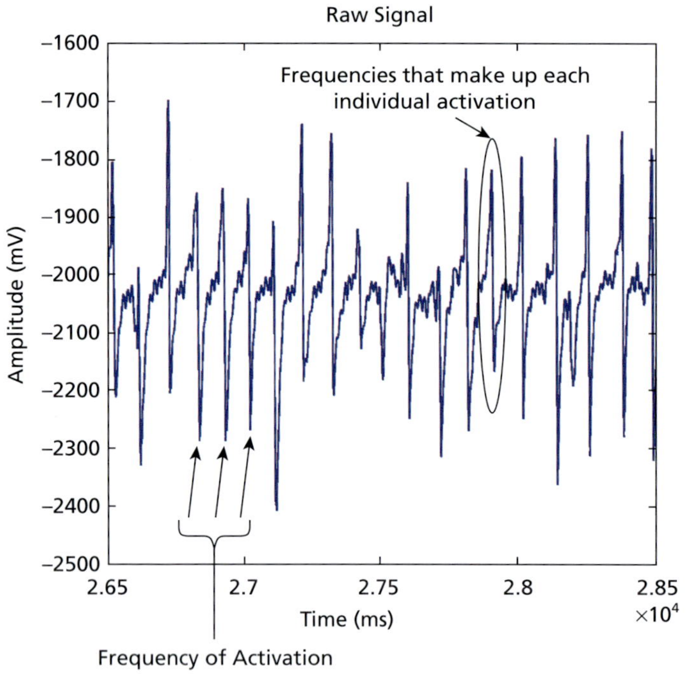

Figure 7.1 An example of a raw unipolar atrial fibrillation signal. The frequencies that compose the cycle length of the fibrillation are different from the frequencies that compose the unipolar deflection that indicates an atrial activation.

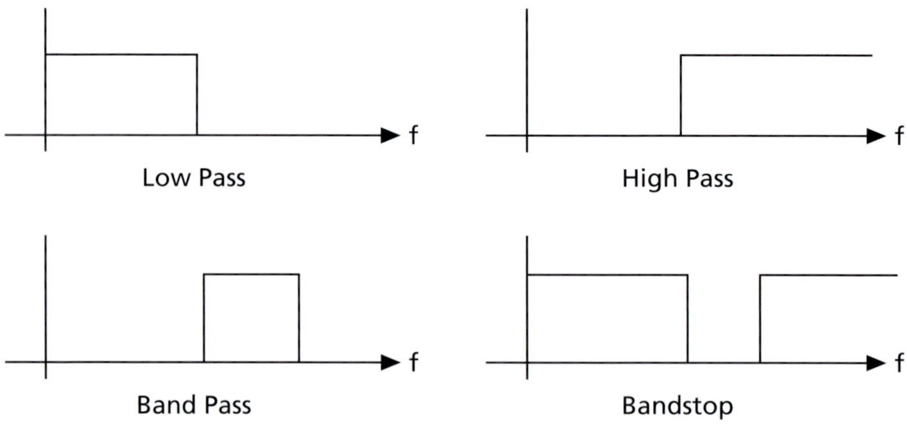

Figure 7.2 Ideal filters for signal processing.

activation. This becomes important when performing signal analysis. One type of signal analysis is frequency domain analysis using a fast Fourier transform (FFT), the results of which indicate the frequencies that compose the signal. The high frequency content that composes each atrial activation can dominate the FFT, masking the frequency of the fibrillation [2]. Filtering the electrograms can bring the frequency of the actual atrial activation frequency to the foreground [3,4]. Filtering can also increase the probability that an atrial activation occurred at that point in time, and reduce the influence of low frequency farfield artifacts such as farfield QRS complexes or low frequency respiration that can create unwanted noise in the recording [3].

Signal analysis

Regardless of the type of filtering that is performed on the signal, there are several different tools that are then used to analyze the resulting waveform. These tools include cross-correlation [3], wavelet analysis [5], entropy [6,7], chaos theory [8,9], signal linearity [10], and frequency domain analysis using the FFT [4,11,12]. These tools of signal analysis have been used to research the characteristics of fibrillation and are currently being explored for use clinically. The FFT can be used to study the dominant frequency of the signal, organization [4], and conduction block [13]. All of these analyses are being used to help find organization within a seemingly chaotic rhythm, identifying and study mechanism which could possibly be used to identify ablation sites [14,15], and to time defibrillation and pacing for AF termination [16,17].

Frequency domain analysis

In order to generate a signal, Jean Baptiste Fourier, a French mathematician, first claimed that any repetitive signal could be composed of sums of sinusoids. Figure 7.3 shows two examples, one of a square wave (Figure 7.3a) and the corresponding sinusoids that are added together to generate this signal, and one of a triangle wave (Figure 7.3b) and its corresponding sinusoids. This same theory can also be applied to cardiac signals.

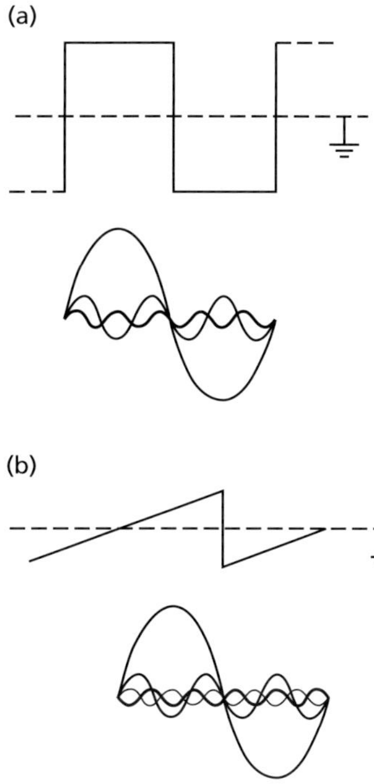

Figure 7.3 Every repetitive signal can be represented by adding sine waves of different frequencies together. An example of (a) a square wave and (b) a triangle wave are shown with their corresponding sine waves that added together compose that particular signal.

Fourier also developed what is known as the Fourier transform, which is based on the concept that signals can be approximated by a sum of sinusoids, each at a different frequency. The Fourier transform is a description of what frequencies are present and how much of each frequency composes the signal. The results of a FFT are either given as a magnitude spectrum or a power spectrum, which is a graph of peaks at the frequencies that are present within the signal. The more a certain frequency is influencing a signal, the higher the peak. The highest peak of a magnitude spectrum is considered the dominant frequency (DF). The DF indicates the main frequency that composes the signal. The magnitude spectrum also composes peaks at frequencies that are integer multiples of the dominant peak. These peaks are called the harmonic peaks. Figure 7.4 shows an example of a raw fibrillatory signal, the signal after digital filtering, and its corresponding FFT which shows a dominant peak at 9.7 Hz.

One example of using frequency domain analysis to aid in characterizing and understanding AF is by analyzing a global AF signal as shown in Figure 7.5. Figure 7.5 shows an example of a global AF signal with a high amount of organization, or more flutter-like characteristics. The part of the signal to be analyzed is the atrial component of the waveform, so the ventricular components of the electrogram were averaged and digitally subtracted. The resulting waveform is shown in Figure 7.5b. Figure 7.5c shows the results of the signal after digital filtering and Figure 7.5d shows the result of the FFT performed on the processed AF signal. In this particular example, there is a main peak with discrete harmonic peaks. Also, there is little frequency content at other frequencies.

Figure 7.6 shows another example of a global AF signal. This signal was recorded from the same AF episode at a different time from the same animal as in Figure 7.5, and it shows an example of more

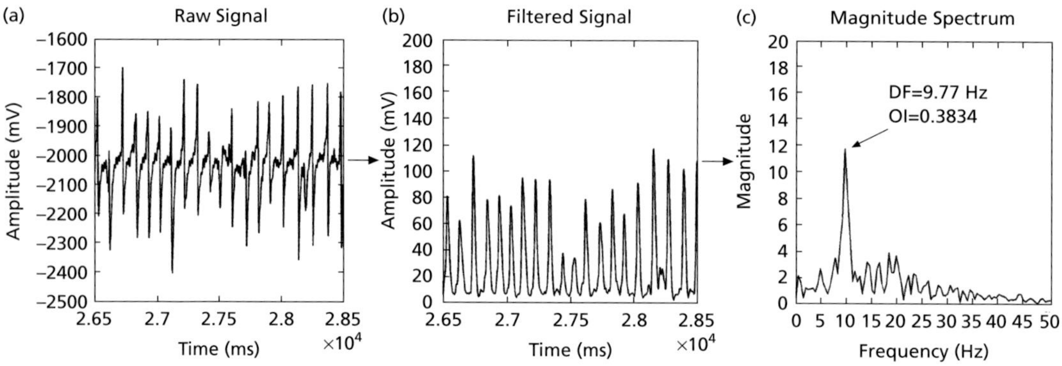

Figure 7.4 A 2 s window of AF is shown (a) along with the signal after digital filtering (b). Also shown is the corresponding FFT of the digitally filtered waveform (c). DF, dominant frequency; OI, organization index. (Reproduced from [23] with permission)

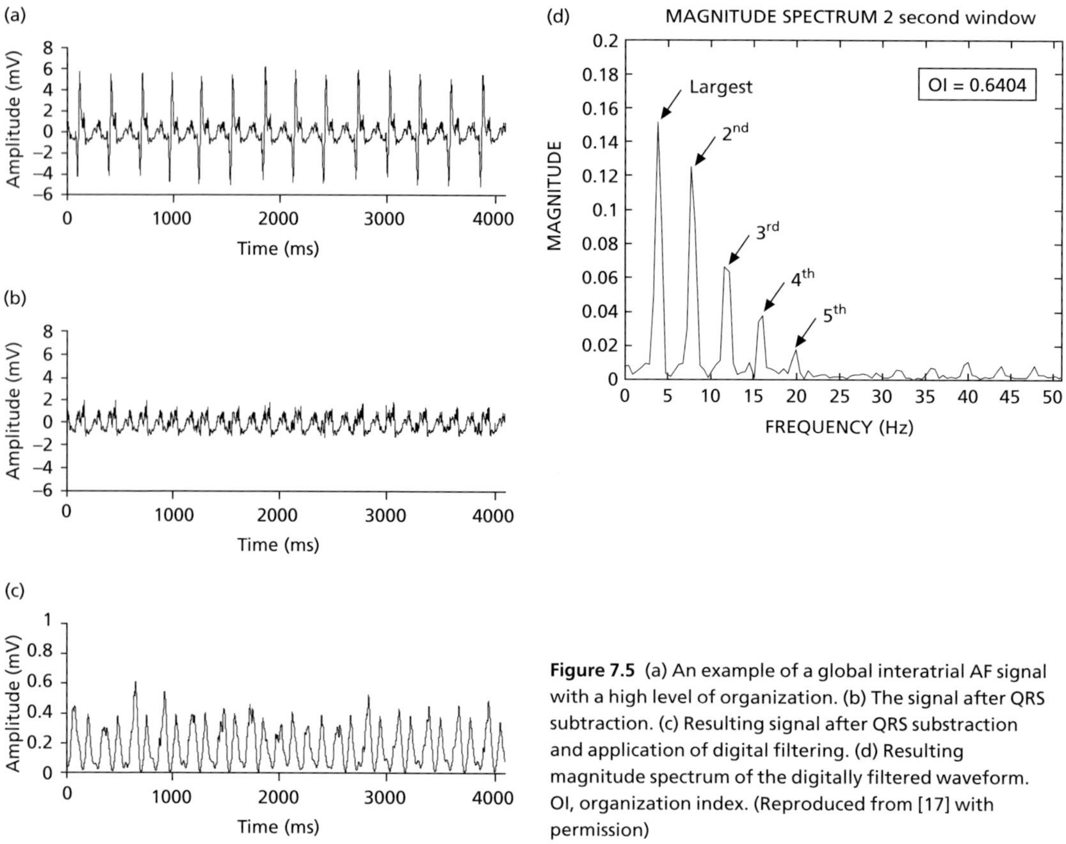

Figure 7.5 (a) An example of a global interatrial AF signal with a high level of organization. (b) The signal after QRS subtraction. (c) Resulting signal after QRS substraction and application of digital filtering. (d) Resulting magnitude spectrum of the digitally filtered waveform. OI, organization index. (Reproduced from [17] with permission)

disorganized activity. The same ventricular component subtraction and filtering process was applied. Figure 7.6a shows the raw signal. Figure 7.6b is the signal after QRS subtraction, and Figure 7.6c shows the resulting signal after filtering. Figure 7.6d shows the result of a FFT calculated on the more disorganized AF signal. In contrast to the previous example (Figure 7.5), this magnitude spectrum has a main peak, but there is a large amount of frequency content between the harmonics. The resulting

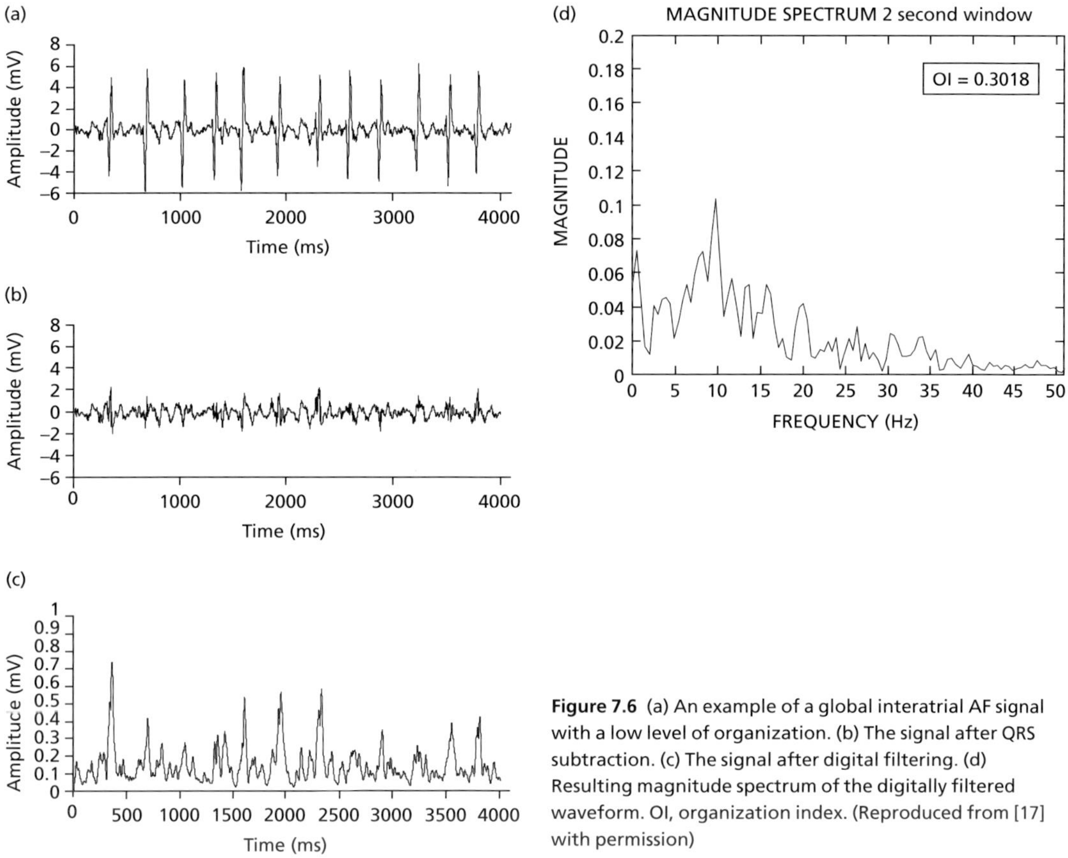

Figure 7.6 (a) An example of a global interatrial AF signal with a low level of organization. (b) The signal after QRS subtraction. (c) The signal after digital filtering. (d) Resulting magnitude spectrum of the digitally filtered waveform. OI, organization index. (Reproduced from [17] with permission)

magnitude spectra from the FFTs of the two signals are obviously quite different, and these signals show how the AF can transition between periods of higher and lower organization. A simple method to quantitate this difference has been devised. This method is called the organization index or the OI number [4]. To calculate the OI from the frequency domain results, the largest peak and its harmonics were identified. The areas under the maximum peak and three of its harmonics were calculated over a 1 Hz window. The total area of the spectrum was calculated up to the fifth harmonic peak. The OI was the ratio of the area under the harmonic peaks to the total area [4].

In addition to measuring the organization of a signal, FFT analysis can also be used to detect areas of conduction block. Areas of block alter the frequency of the fibrillation at that site. The recording electrodes then record a signal that is influenced by other frequencies. These other frequencies then appear in the resulting FFT as peaks that are not associated with the dominant one as a harmonic. When compared to an isochronal map of activation during AF, the signals that result in FFTs that have secondary peaks within their magnitude spectrum are located in and around areas of conduction block [13]. These extra peaks within the magnitude spectrum also decrease the organization of the signal as measured from the resulting FFT by the OI.

Results from experimental data

Signal processing has been used as a tool to aid in the analysis of fibrillatory electrograms in experimental data. From this analysis, a better understanding of the characteristics, mechanisms, and treatment of fibrillation has been achieved.

Defibrillation thresholds

Frequency domain analysis has shown that global AF has periods of both high and low organization

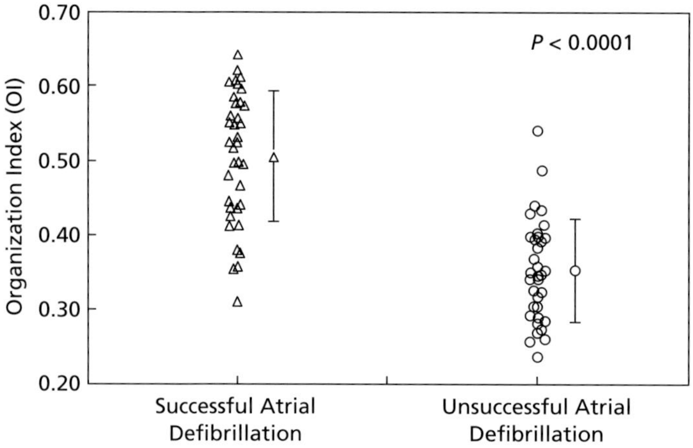

Figure 7.7 Organization index numbers calculated from 4 s of the electrogram just prior to energy delivery. Triangles represent the OI calculated before a successful shock and circles represent the OI calculated before an unsuccessful shock. The mean ± SD is also displayed. A Student's *t*-test was used to compare OI values from successful and unsuccessful shocks. (Reproduced from [4] with permission)

[17]. It was theorized that the efficacy of AF defibrillation would increase if the energy delivery occurred during the periods of higher organization. Using an up-down-up defibrillation protocol to determine the atrial defibrillation threshold ($ADFT_{50}$) as previously described [18], multiple shocks were then delivered at the $ADFT_{50}$ and the signal just prior to each shock was analyzed. This study showed that the period of AF before a successful shock is more organized than the period of AF before an unsuccessful shock [4]. Figure 7.7 shows data showing the measured OI prior to $ADFT_{50}$ energy delivery in 10 dogs. The OI before unsuccessful shocks is significantly lower than the OI before successful shocks. Based on these data, an OI of 0.5 or greater was thought to be associated with improved defibrillation efficacy [4]. Defibrillation shocks were then timed to periods of increased global AF organization. Figure 7.8a shows the results of the 50% defibrillation success voltage determined with QRS synchronized shocks delivered randomly or when the OI was > 0.5, in 15 dogs. The 50% defibrillation success voltage was reduced from a mean of 183 V to 142 V [17]. Figure 7.8b shows the distribution function curves for both random shocks and shocks delivered when the OI was > 0.5 for 15 dogs that were conditioned with 48 h of rapid atrial pacing. In each of the dogs,

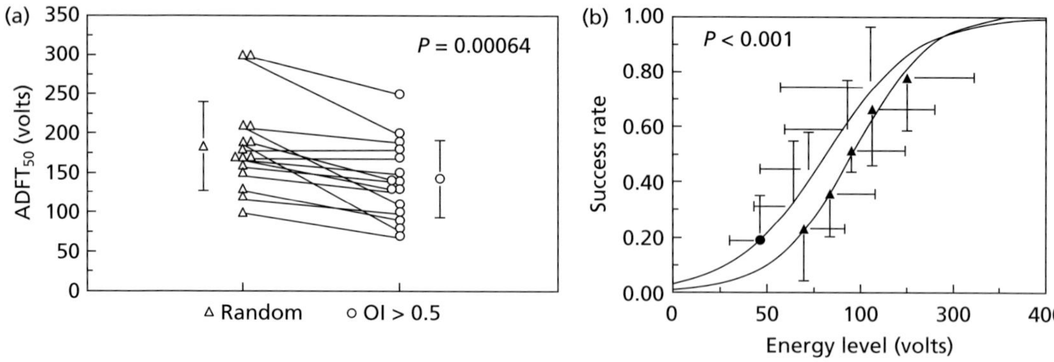

Figure 7.8 (a) Energy level for atrial defibrillation threshold ($ADFT_{50}$) shocks delivered either randomly, or when the OI > 0.5. Triangles represent the $ADFT_{50}$ when QRS-synchronized shocks were delivered randomly. Circles represent the $ADFT_{50}$ when QRS-synchronized shocks were delivered with an OI > 0.5. Using the OI to guide timing of shock delivery, the $ADFT_{50}$ in these paired comparisons was decreased by 23%. (b) Distribution function curves for both random shocks (black triangles) and shocks delivered during OI > 0.5 (black circles). The *x*-axis gives the defibrillation voltage and the *y*-axis the success rate. The five data points for each curve represent the $ADFT_{50}$, $ADFT_{50}$ ± 10%, and $ADFT_{50}$ ± 20% for both conditions for all dogs. A leftward shift of the distribution function was seen when shocks were delivered with OI values > 0.5. (Reproduced from [17] with permission)

shocks were randomly delivered at fixed energy levels above and below the 50% defibrillation success level while randomly alternating between random shocks and when the OI was > 0.5. The data are fit with a Boltzman equation. Even though there is a large amount of variability in the data, shocks synchronized to high OI values were more successful at any energy level producing a significant leftward shift in the curve [17]. Following a similar protocol, burst pace termination attempts were administered randomly and when the OI was > 0.5. It was shown that burst pace termination for AF is more efficacious when pacing is timed to periods of higher organization [16].

Optical mapping data

Over the last decade, optical mapping has been a powerful tool in helping to understand the mechanisms of fibrillation. During these studies, FFTs have been used to analyze optical mapping signals to help characterize AF. Skanes et al. showed that AF could be characterized by stable, high frequency sources [11]. Mandepati et al. then demonstrated that the high frequency sources were associated with spiral waves that were seen with optical mapping [19]. When a FFT was performed on the signals from the spiral wave and on the signals from the other areas of both the right atrium and left atrium, the signals from the spiral wave had the highest frequency found in both atria, which brought about the theory that this high frequency area could be responsible for driving the AF.

Frequency domain analysis of optical mapping signals has also shown that there exists a DF gradient between the left and right atria [20] (Figure 7.9), and, in AF characterized with stable, high frequency areas, these areas consist of a small area of an organized high frequency signal [21] (Figure 7.10). Figure 7.9 shows dominant frequencies from both the right and left atria, demonstrating that the left atrium has higher frequencies than the right atrium [20]. Figure 7.10 shows both the DF and organization maps from an episode of AF that was characterized by a stable, high frequency area. The signals and resulting FFTs from this area show that it consists of an organized high frequency signal. As you move away from the center of the high frequency area, the signals still result in an FFT with a high frequency dominant peak, however the signals are more disorganized [21]. All of these optical mapping studies were performed with an acetylcholine model of AF, and it was not clear whether these findings were unique to this model and AF substrate.

A study was performed by Everett et al. looking at the characteristics of AF in canine models of rapid atrial pacing, mitral regurgitation, and control. The characteristics of AF from these different canine models were analyzed with optical mapping, and signal processing was used to aid in this analysis [22]. The results from the signal analysis are shown in Figure 7.11 (left atrium) and Figure 7.12 (right atrium). The activation maps represent conduction during a paced rhythm at 250 ms from the same direction as the dominant AF activation. For the control left atrium as shown in Figure 7.11, homogenous conduction is seen throughout the field of view. The APD80 map shows action potential durations ranging from 76.2 to 117.8 ms. Homogeneous conduction was also seen with pacing at 250 ms, and varying APD80 levels in the control right atrium (Figure 7.12). Also similar to control, the rapid atrial pacing (RAP) model had homogeneous conduction with pacing at 250 ms.

Figure 7.11 also shows a representative DF map from a control left atrium and demonstrates two different frequencies with most of the field of view being composed of 5.86 Hz with a small area of 6.84 Hz. The variations that were seen in APD80 occurred even in the area that is mostly composed of a single DF. Statistical analysis showed that APD80 did not correlate with DF (correlation = 0.41, $R^2 = 0.16$). In the control right atrium, the DF map (Figure 7.12) has discreet regions of both high and low frequencies of 7.3 and 5.8 Hz. Similar to the left atrium, a majority of the field of view of the right atrium was composed of a single DF, which for this particular example was 7.3 Hz. Also, the DFs did not correlate with the APD80 (correlation = 0.56, $R^2 = 0.32$).

A representative example of a DF map for the RAP left atrium is shown in Figure 7.11 and demonstrates that most of the region consists of 7.8 Hz and a smaller region of 5.3 Hz. The DF map for the right atrium (Figure 7.12) shows the entire area having the same frequency of 5.86 Hz. These findings in the right and left atria, as demonstrated by these examples, were found in all episodes in all

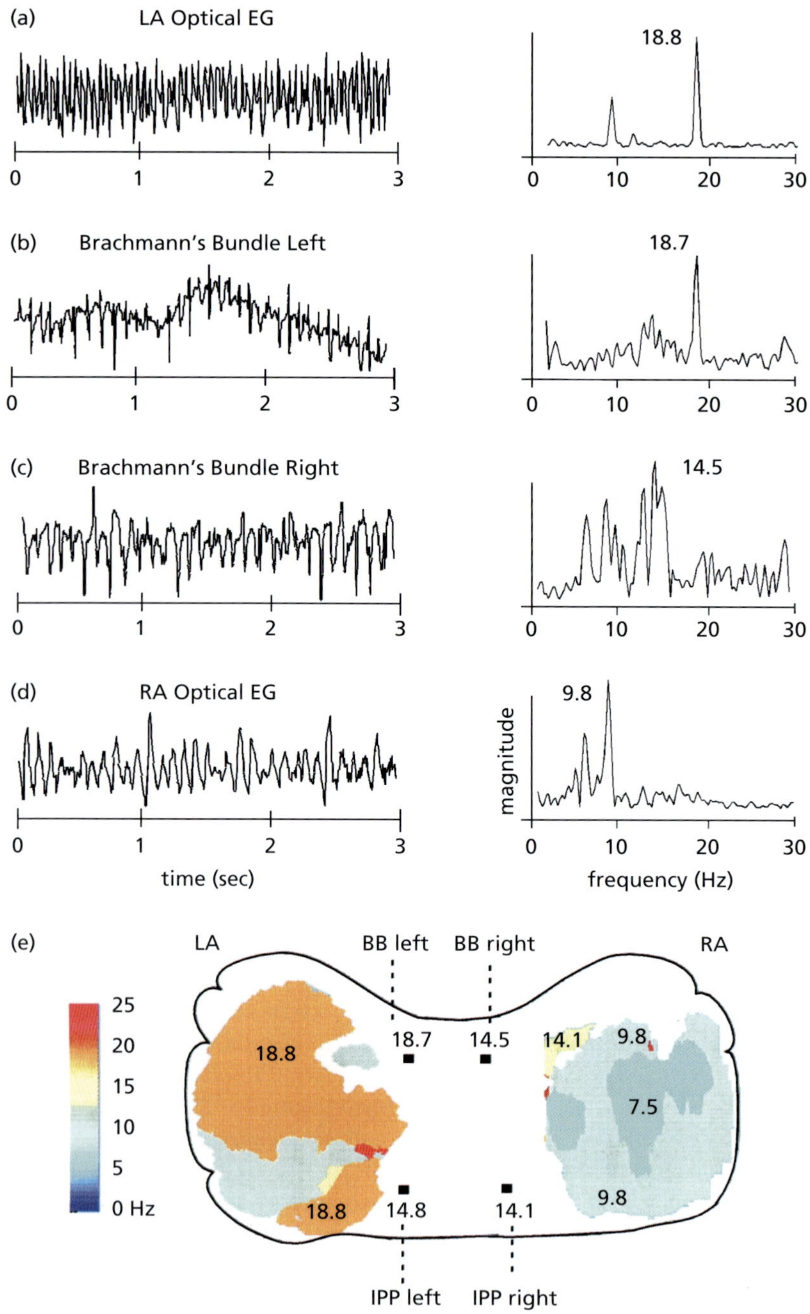

Figure 7.9 Left-to-right gradient of dominant frequencies. (a–d) Optical electrograms from different areas of the right atrium (RA) and left atrium (LA) and corresponding FFTs. (e) Dominant frequency map of the epicardial surface of the right and left atria. The highest frequencies are seen in the LA. BB, Brachmann's bundle; EG, electrogram; IPP, inferoposterior pathway. (Reproduced from [20] with permission)

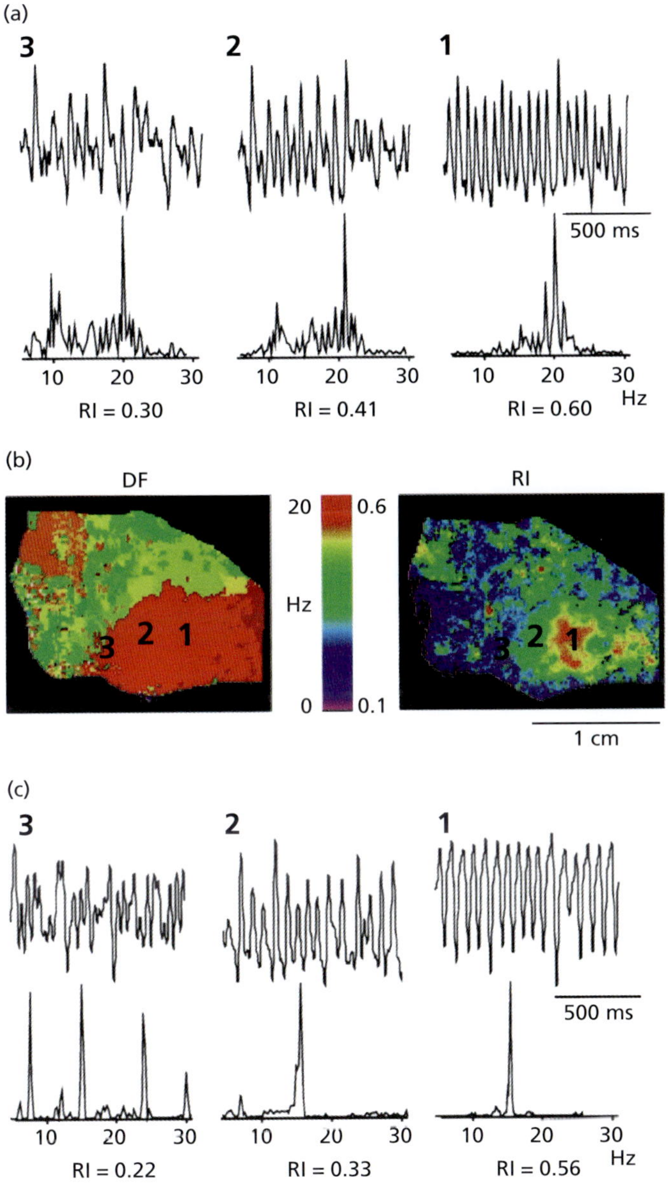

Figure 7.10 Dominant frequency (DF) and organization maps from optical signals of AF. A high frequency area is shown and within that area there is a high frequency, organized signal. Representative pixel recordings from locations 1, 2, and 3 are shown along with their corresponding FFTs in (a). As samples of signals are shown away from the high frequency, organized area, the frequency remains high but the organization decreases. Bipolar electrograms recorded from locations 1, 2, and 3 are shown along with their corresponding FFTs in (c). Similar results are seen when compared to the optical recordings. RI, regularity index. (Reproduced with permission from [21].)

animals in the RAP group. As with the controls, the dominant frequencies did not correlate with the APD80 in the left atrium (correlation = −0.69, R^2 = 0.48) or in the right atrium (correlation = −0.61, R^2 = 0.37). The highest dominant frequencies for all the models are shown in Figure 7.13. As the figure shows, the RAP group had similar frequencies to that of the control for both the left and right atria.

In contrast to the control and RAP left atrium, the DF maps in the mitral regurgitation (MR) left atrium show several distinct regions of widely disparate frequencies, as shown in the example in Figure 7.11. In this example, there is a small region with the highest DF of 14.16 Hz, and there is a small region with the lowest frequency of 3.9 Hz. This type of frequency map was seen in all of the MR left atrial preparations. Areas where slow conduction is indicated corresponded to areas of lower dominant frequencies in all episodes of AF. Similar to the control and RAP, the APD80 did not correlate with the DF (correlation = −0.30, R^2 = 0.09). The corresponding right atrial DF maps were also very similar

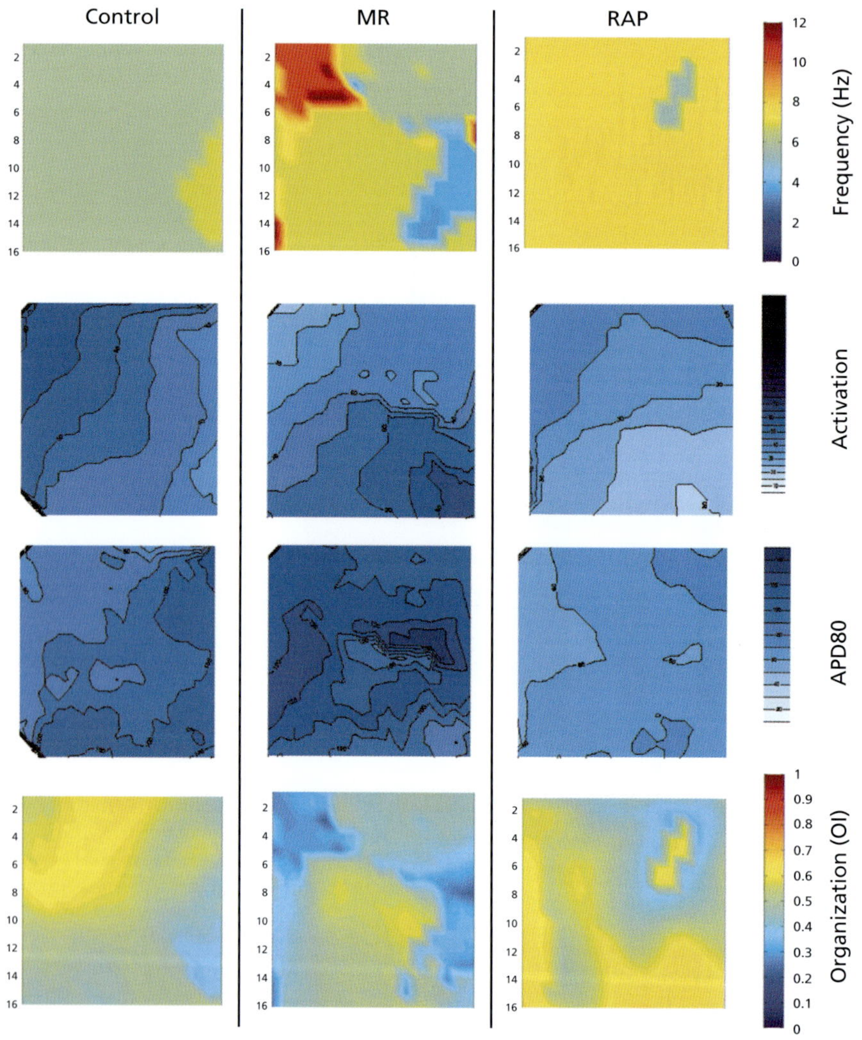

Figure 7.11 Dominant frequency (row 1), activation patterns (row 2), APD80 (row 3), and organization (row 4) maps in the left atrium for controls, mitral regurgitation (MR), and rapid atrial pacing (RAP) models. All scales are shown to the right for their corresponding panels. As these figures demonstrate, the AF in the left atrium of the MR model was significantly different from the AF in the other models. The MR DF map shows several discrete areas of different frequencies, including an area composed of the highest frequencies. This frequency pattern was not observed in the frequency maps from the other AF models. The MR organization map shows large areas of lower OI values than is shown in the organization maps for the other models. Also shown is that the dominant frequencies followed conduction patterns and not the distribution of APD80. (Reproduced with permission from [22].)

to those of the right atrium in the control and RAP groups.

Figure 7.13a shows the highest DF found in each preparation. The left atrium of the MR group had a small discrete area of higher frequencies, which was significantly different from that of the right atrium (10.8 ± 2.4 Hz vs 6.7 ± 2.9 Hz; $P < 0.04$). Figure 7.13b shows the results from measuring the largest frequency difference and dividing that by the distance over which it occurs. In the left atrium of the MR group, this ratio was more than double that of the control or RAP, and four times greater than the right atrium of the MR group. This data begins to show that through signal processing with frequency dominant analysis, AF has different characteristics within different atrial substrates.

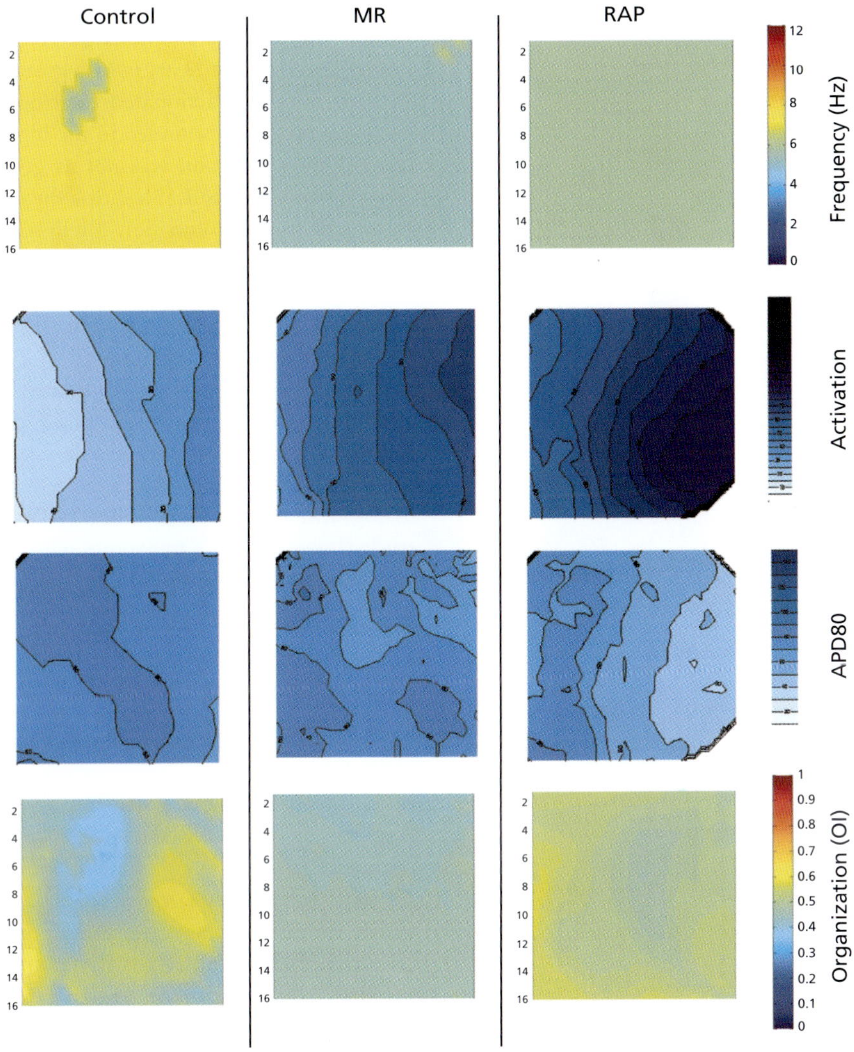

Figure 7.12 Dominant frequency (row 1), activation patterns (row 2), APD80 (row 3), and organization (row 4) maps in the right atrium for controls, mitral regurgitation (MR), and rapid atrial pacing (RAP) models. All scales are shown to the right for their corresponding panels. As these figures demonstrate, the AF in the right atrium was very similar for each of the models as the majority of each DF map is composed of a signal frequency, and the organization maps are composed of large areas of higher OI values. Also shown is that the dominant frequencies followed conduction patterns and not the distribution of APD80. (Reproduced with permission from [22].)

Whole animal data

To look at the characteristics of AF within different models in vivo, custom-built epicardial plaques with 240 unipoles were placed on the epicardial surface of the atria of canines conditioned with RAP, pacing-induced heart failure, MR, or methylcholine, or controls [23]. In each of the models, 30 s AF episodes were recorded. Figure 7.14 shows examples of static DF maps (top panels) and organization maps (bottom panels) for each of the canine models. Dominant frequencies and the organization index are shown from an FFT performed on a 2 s window of AF. Stable, discrete high DF areas were seen in the MR and heart failure dogs. For the methylcholine dogs, the representative DF map shows the stable, discrete high DF

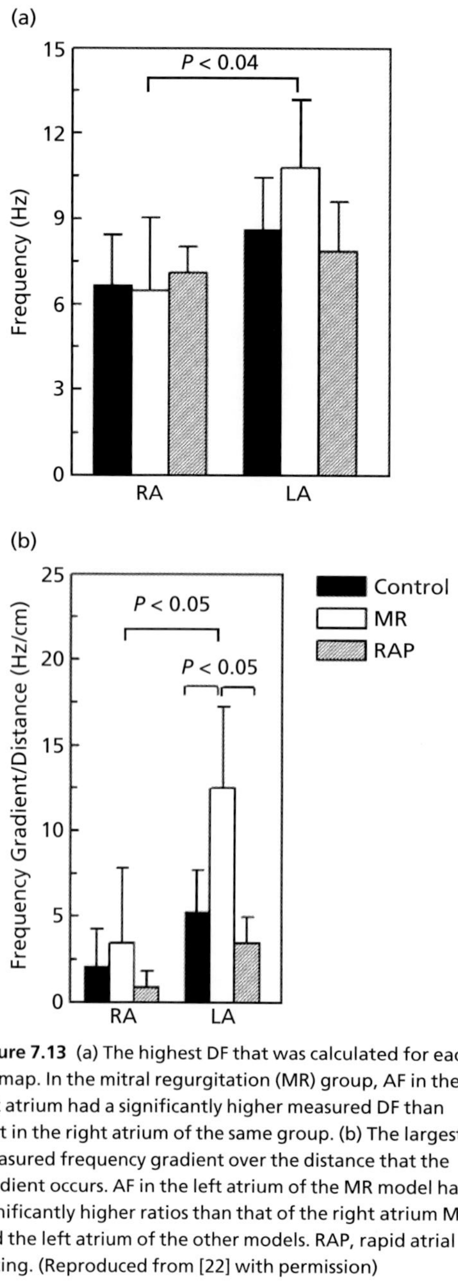

Figure 7.13 (a) The highest DF that was calculated for each DF map. In the mitral regurgitation (MR) group, AF in the left atrium had a significantly higher measured DF than that in the right atrium of the same group. (b) The largest measured frequency gradient over the distance that the gradient occurs. AF in the left atrium of the MR model had significantly higher ratios than that of the right atrium MR and the left atrium of the other models. RAP, rapid atrial pacing. (Reproduced from [22] with permission)

areas in both the right and left atria. The high frequency areas in the MR and heart failure dogs correlated with poorly organized fractionated electrograms. From all of the canine models, all of the signals recorded during each AF episode were observed for fractionation. Figure 7.15a shows the percent area of the total mapped atria that contained fractionated electrograms. As the graph shows, the area of fractionated electrograms is model-specific. The heart failure group shows the smallest area of fractionated electrograms; however, this area corresponded to the high frequency areas. This correlation was not as good with the other models. Figure 7.15b shows the organization of the fractionated and non-fractionated electrograms for each canine model. As expected, for most of the models, the fractionated electrograms had lower levels of organization than the unfractionated electrograms.

Ryu et al. also performed frequency domain analysis on in vivo recordings of AF signals in an attempt to provide insights into the mechanisms of the fibrillation. The authors analyzed AF recorded in dogs with pacing-induced heart failure [24]. This study showed that AF in canines with heart failure was characterized with stable, high frequency sources in both the right and left atria.

Signal analysis in clinical data

FFT analysis is now being applied to AF in the clinical setting both as a research tool and to aid in AF therapies. Figure 7.16 shows a DF map by Sanders et al. from a patient with paroxysmal AF in (a), and a DF map from a patient with permanent AF in (b) [15]. High frequency areas were seen within the pulmonary vein region in both patients. However, each of the points that composed these maps was a short duration of signal recorded on a point-by-point basis over time. Sahadevan et al. recorded simultaneous epicardial electrograms from both the right and left atria in nine patients with chronic AF. Seven of the nine patients had areas of higher dominant frequencies that may have been driving the AF [25]. However, in both of these studies, in the clinical setting, it is not known if these frequencies are stable. As was seen in the canine models of AF, stable, high frequency areas were model-specific; as shown in Figure 7.14, AF in a dog conditioned with pacing-induced heart failure, there is a stable, high frequency area in the left atrium. Throughout the rest of the atria there are transient high frequency areas that are not stable. In a dog conditioned with RAP, there is a left-to-right frequency gradient; however, there are no stable, high frequency areas [23]. This demonstrates that

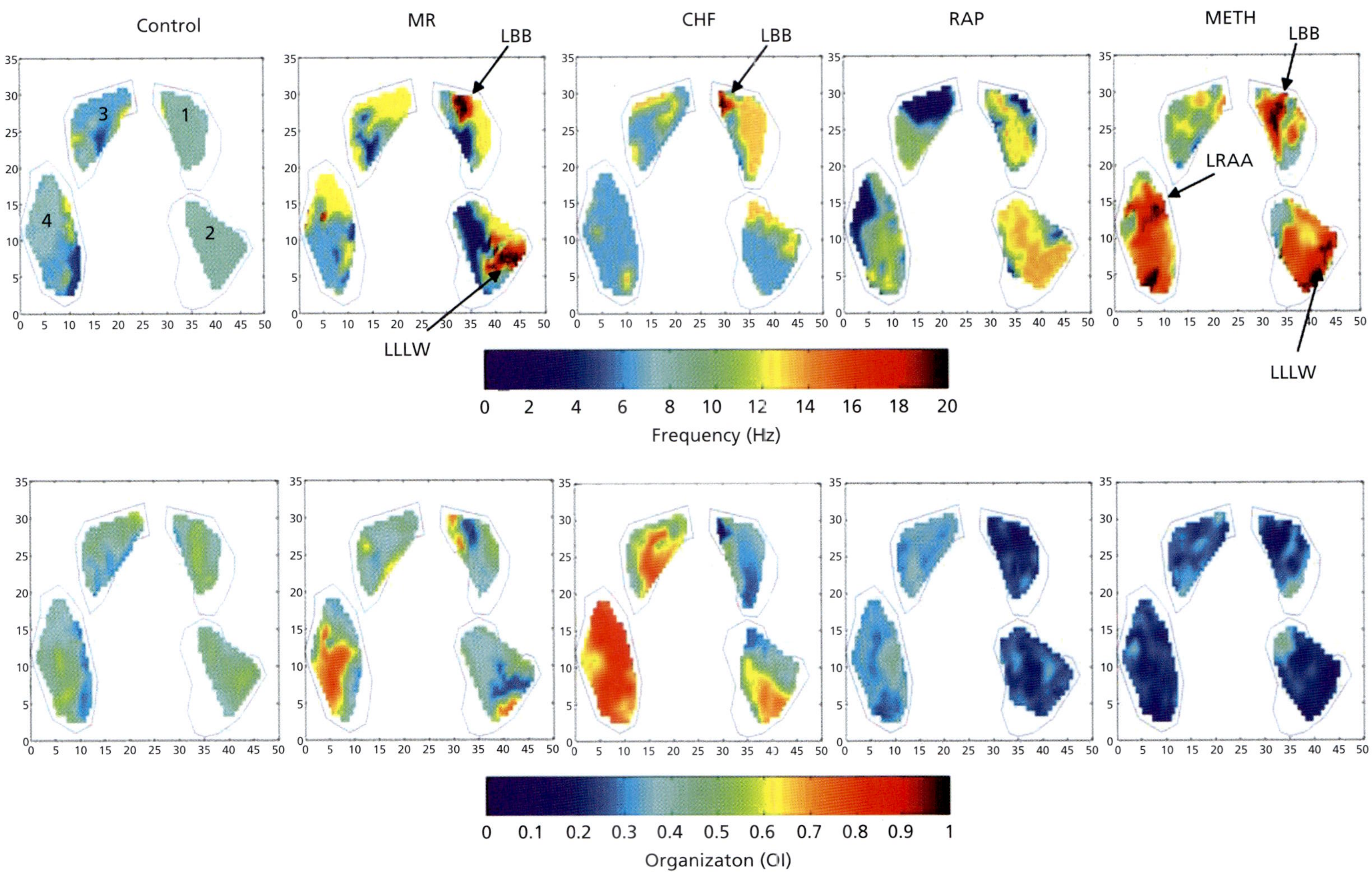

Figure 7.14 Examples of static DF maps (top panels), and organization maps (bottom panels) for each of the animal models used in the study. DFs and OIs are shown from an FFT performed on a 2 s window of AF. The stable, discrete high DF areas are identified in the mitral regurg tation (MR) and congestive heart failure (CHF) dogs, along with their atrial location. For the methylcholine (METH) dogs, the representative DF map shows the stable, discrete high DF areas in both the right and left atria. The arrows indicate the locations of discrete, stable, high frequency areas. LBB, left atrial Brachmann's bundle; LLLW, left atrial low lateral wall; RAP, rapid atrial pacing. (Reproduced from [23] with permission)

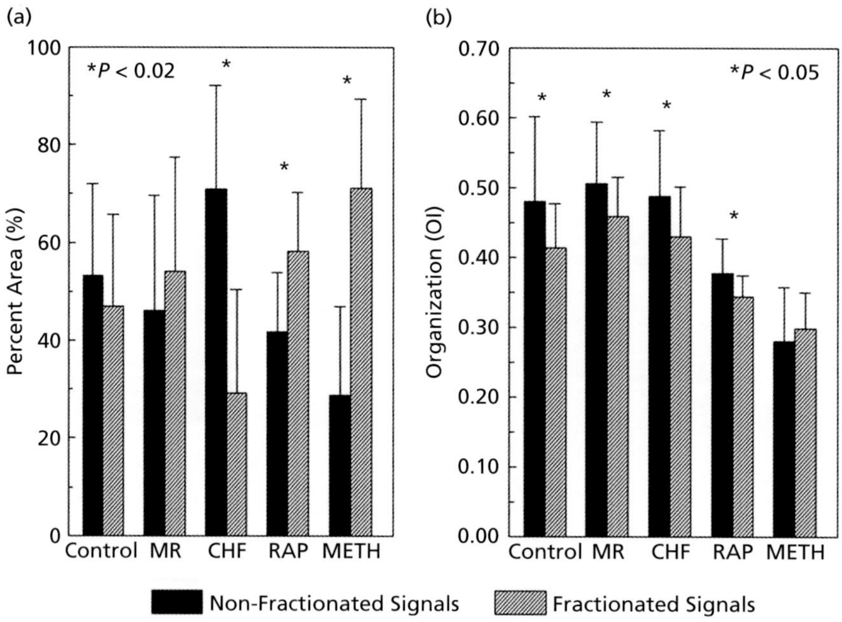

Figure 7.15 All of the signals recorded during each AF episode in every canine model were observed for fractionation. (a) The percent area of the total mapped atria that contained fractionated (hashed bars) or non-fractionated (solid bars) electrograms. (b) Organization index (OI) of the fractionated and non-fractionated electrograms for each canine model. (Reproduced from [23] with permission)

when searching for a high frequency area that could be driving the AF, it is more than just finding the highest DF, it is also finding a stable area with a steep frequency gradient.

To use signal processing as a research tool in clinical AF to help characterize the AF, dominant frequencies were determined in signals from patients with AF coming from either the pulmonary veins or from the superior vena cava (SVC) in a study from Lin et al. [26]. The area from which the AF originated had the highest DF. When the AF originated from the pulmonary veins, a left atrium to right atrium (LA–RA) frequency gradient existed. A gradient was not seen when the AF originated from the SVC. In a study by Lazar et al., recordings were made in both the right and left atria in patients with paroxysmal and persistant AF [27]. A LA–RA frequency gradient was observed, but this gradient was only seen in patients with paroxysmal AF and it was not present in patients with persistent AF. Sanders et al. also looked at the effects of pulmonary vein isolation on the AF frequencies. Figure 7.17 shows the dominant frequencies in patients with permanent and paroxysmal AF before and after pulmonary vein isolation [28]. When pulmonary vein isolation was performed in patients with permanent AF, the frequencies did not change. When this procedure was performed in patients with paroxysmal AF, there was a significant decrease in the dominant frequencies. In another study by Lazar et al., it was shown that a LA–RA frequency gradient disappears with pulmonary vein isolation [29]. Takahashi et al. used signal processing techniques to show that the organization of AF increases after catheter ablation of the pulmonary veins [30]. It was also shown that a high OI value was associated with AF termination. With all of these studies using signal processing to study fibrillation in the clinical setting, a limited number of points are collected and short recordings of AF are obtained and the stability of frequencies is unknown. Using dominant frequencies during AF as a clinical tool shows promise, but it is too early to tell if it will be useful for finding areas for target ablation as a possible therapy.

Pachon et al. are using FFT to locate fractionated electrograms or AF nests [14]. Any sort of

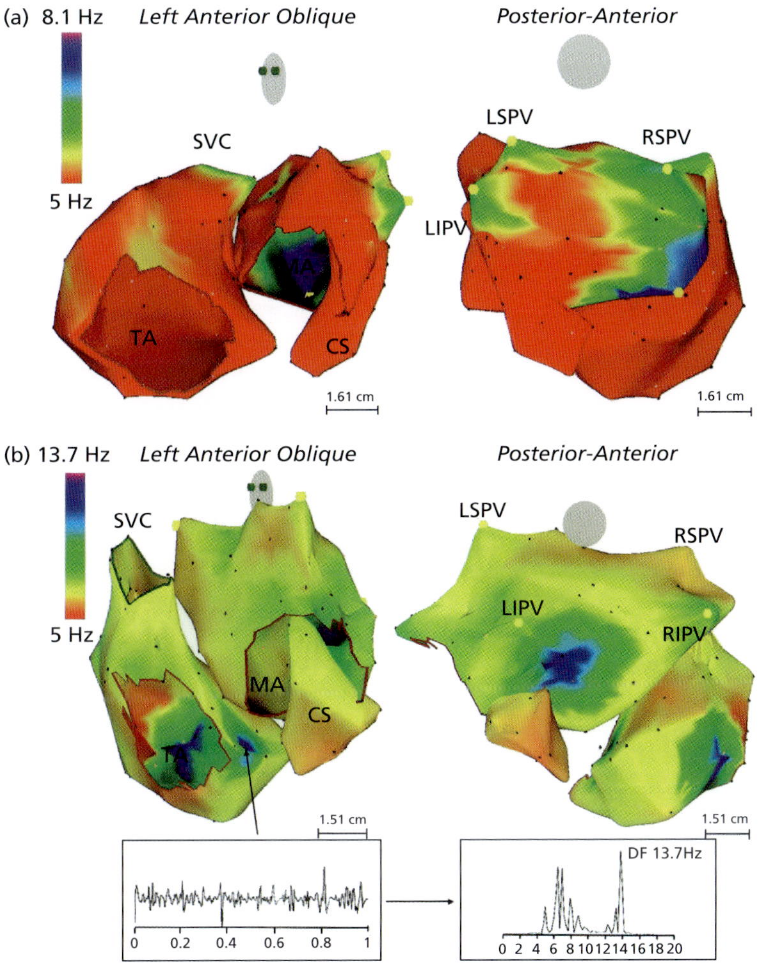

Figure 7.16 Dominant frequency maps in a patient with paroxysmal AF (a) and in a patient with permanent AF (b). Also shown is an electrogram and the corresponding power spectrum from a high frequency area. CS, coronary sinus; LIPV, left inferior pulmonary vein; LSPV, left superior pulmonary vein; RIPV, right inferior pulmonary vein; RSPV, right superior pulmonary vein; SVC, superior vena cava; TA, tricuspid annulus. (Reproduced from [15] with permission)

fractionation within the atrial activation sequence will add other peaks in the magnitude spectrum other than the dominant peak. Normal conduction produces an electrogram with no extra peaks within it. Heterogeneous depolarization produces extra peaks in the activation sequence, which then produces extra peaks in the magnitude spectrum. A recording electrode can exhibit a fractionated electrogram if the signal is subject to block, fibrillatory conduction, or multiple waves. Targeting the sites with fractionated electrograms for ablation has been shown to decrease the incidence of AF.

The future of signal processing

In summary, signal processing of fibrillatory electrograms is used to both filter the signal and then for analysis. Filtering is used to eliminate noise and farfield artifacts, and to enhance activation sequences. The FFT is used to analyze the characteristics of the recorded signal, which then aids in understanding the characteristics of the fibrillation that will ultimately aid in therapeutic measures. Using signal processing to aid in therapies for AF is still in its infancy of transitioning from a research

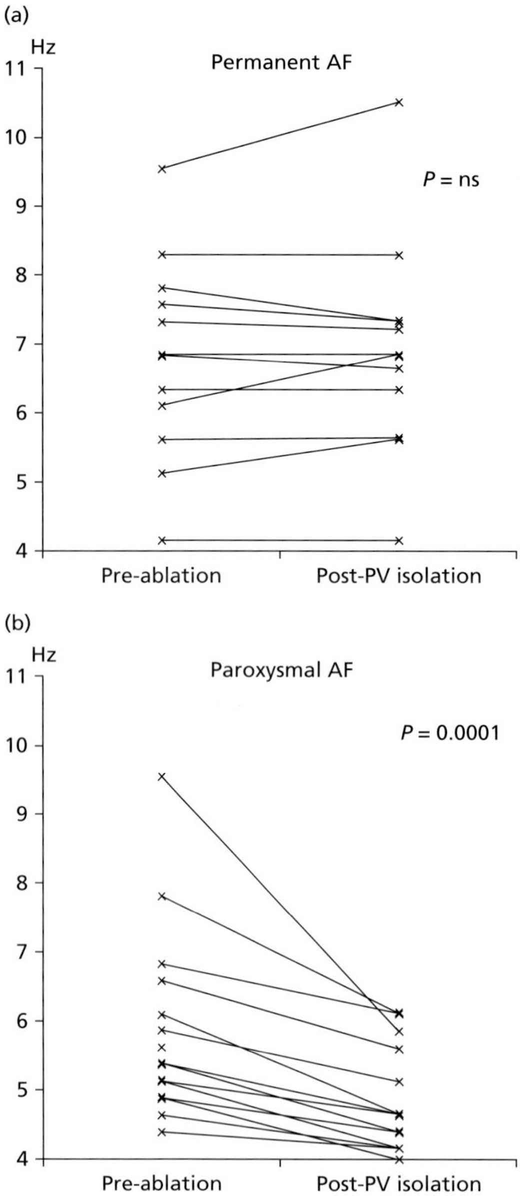

Figure 7.17 Dominant frequencies calculated in patients with both paroxysmal AF (a) and permanent AF (b) before and after pulmonary vein (PV) isolation. After PV isolation, there was no difference in the DFs in the patients with permanent AF. However, after PV isolation in patients with paroxysmal AF, there was a significant decrease in the DFs in the AF ns, not significant. (Reproduced from [28] with permission)

tool to a clinical tool. Until the technology advances such that several AF signals can be recorded simultaneously to help characterize clinical AF, this transition will continue.

References

1 Bronzino JD, ed. *The Biomedical Engineering Handbook*, 2nd edn. CRC Press/IEEE Press, Boca Raton, Florida, 2000.
2 Ng J, Kadish AH, Goldberger JJ. Effect of electrogram characteristics on the relationship of dominant frequency to atrial activation rate in atrial fibrillation. *Heart Rhythm* 2006;**3**(11):1295–305.
3 Botteron GW, Smith JM. A technique for measurement of the extent of spatial organization of atrial activation during atrial fibrillation in the intact human heart. *IEEE Trans Biomed Eng* 1995;**42**(6):579–86.
4 Everett TH, Kok LC, Vaughn RH, Moorman JR, Haines DE. Frequency domain algorithm for quantifying atrial fibrillation organization to increase defibrillation efficacy. *IEEE Trans Biomed Eng* 2001;**48**(9):969–78.
5 Lee KW, Everett TH, Ilhan HT, Linscott I, Olgin J. Feature extraction of the atrial fibrillation signal using the continuous wavelet transform. In: *Proceedings of the 26th Annual International Conference of the IEEE EMBS, 2004 September, San Francisco, CA*, 2004:275–8.
6 Akar JG, Everett TH, Kok LC, Moorman JR, Haines DE. Effect of electrical and structural remodeling on spatiotemporal organization in acute and persistent atrial fibrillation. *J Cardiovasc Electrophysiol* 2002;**13**(10):1027–34.
7 Richman JS, Moorman JR. Physiological time-series analysis using approximate entropy and sample entropy. *Am J Physiol Heart Circ Physiol* 2000;**278**(6):H2039–H2049.
8 Garfinkel A, Chen PS, Walter DO, et al. Quasiperiodicity and chaos in cardiac fibrillation. *J Clin Invest* 1997;**99**(2):305–14.
9 Gray RA, Jalife J. Ventricular fibrillation and atrial fibrillation are two different beasts. *Chaos* 1998;**8**(1):65–78.
10 Sih HJ, Zipes DP, Berbari EJ, Olgin JE. A high-temporal resolution algorithm for quantifying organization during atrial fibrillation. *IEEE Trans Biomed Eng* 1999;**46**(4):440–50.
11 Skanes AC, Mandapati R, Berenfeld O, Davidenko JM, Jalife J. Spatiotemporal periodicity during atrial fibrillation in the isolated sheep heart. *Circulation* 1998;**98**(12):1236–48.
12 Ryu K, Sahadevan J, Khrestian CM, Stambler BS, Waldo AL. Use of fast fourier transform analysis of atrial electrograms for rapid characterization of atrial activation-implications for delineating possible mechanisms of atrial tachyarrhythmias. *J Cardiovasc Electrophysiol* 2006;**17**(2):198–206.
13 Evans FG, Rogers JM, Smith WM, Ideker RE. Automatic detection of conduction block based on time-frequency analysis of unipolar electrograms. *IEEE Trans Biomed Eng* 1999;**46**(9):1090–7.

14 Pachon MJ, Pachon ME, Pachon MJ, et al. A new treatment for atrial fibrillation based on spectral analysis to guide the catheter RF-ablation. *Europace* 2004;**6**(6):590–601.

15 Sanders P, Berenfeld O, Hocini M, et al. Spectral analysis identifies sites of high-frequency activity maintaining atrial fibrillation in humans. *Circulation* 2005;**112**(6):789–97.

16 Everett TH, Akar JG, Kok LC, Moorman JR, Haines DE. Use of global atrial fibrillation organization to optimize the success of burst pace termination. *J Am Coll Cardiol* 2002;**40**(10):1831–40.

17 Everett TH, Moorman JR, Kok LC, Akar JG, Haines DE. Assessment of global atrial fibrillation organization to optimize timing of atrial defibrillation. *Circulation* 2001;**103**(23):2857–61.

18 Mangrum JM, Everett TH, Mitchell MA, McRury ID, Li H, Haines DE. The effects of reverse atrial electrical remodeling on atrial defibrillation thresholds. *Pacing Clin Electrophysiol* 2002;**25**(4 Pt 1):470–6.

19 Mandapati R, Skanes A, Chen J, Berenfeld O, Jalife J. Stable microreentrant sources as a mechanism of atrial fibrillation in the isolated sheep heart. *Circulation* 2000; **101**(2):194–9.

20 Mansour M, Mandapati R, Berenfeld O, Chen J, Samie FH, Jalife J. Left-to-right gradient of atrial frequencies during acute atrial fibrillation in the isolated sheep heart. *Circulation* 2001;**103**(21):2631–6.

21 Kalifa J, Tanaka K, Zaitsev AV, et al. Mechanisms of wave fractionation at boundaries of high-frequency excitation in the posterior left atrium of the isolated sheep heart during atrial fibrillation. *Circulation* 2006;**113**(5):626–33.

22 Everett TH, Verheule S, Wilson EE, Foreman S, Olgin JE. Left atrial dilatation resulting from chronic mitral regurgitation decreases spatiotemporal organization of atrial fibrillation in left atrium. *Am J Physiol Heart Circ Physiol* 2004;**286**(6):H2452–H2460.

23 Everett TH, Wilson EE, Verheule S, Guerra JM, Foreman S, Olgin J. Structural atrial remodeling alters the substrate and spatiotemporal organization of AF: a comparison in canine models of structural and electrical atrial remodeling. *Am J Physiol Heart Circ Physiol* 2006;**291**:H2911–H2923.

24 Ryu K, Shroff SC, Sahadevan J, Martovitz NL, Khrestian CM, Stambler BS. Mapping of atrial activation during sustained atrial fibrillation in dogs with rapid ventricular pacing induced heart failure: evidence for a role of driver regions. *J Cardiovasc Electrophysiol* 2005;**16**(12):1348–58.

25 Sahadevan J, Ryu K, Peltz L, et al. Epicardial mapping of chronic atrial fibrillation in patients: preliminary observations. *Circulation* 2004;**110**(21):3293–9.

26 Lin YJ, Tai CT, Kao T, et al. Frequency analysis in different types of paroxysmal atrial fibrillation. *J Am Coll Cardiol* 2006;**47**(7):1401–7.

27 Lazar S, Dixit S, Marchlinski FE, Callans DJ, Gerstenfeld EP. Presence of left-to-right atrial frequency gradient in paroxysmal but not persistent atrial fibrillation in humans. *Circulation* 2004;**110**(20):3181–6.

28 Sanders P, Nalliah CJ, Dubois R, et al. Frequency mapping of the pulmonary veins in paroxysmal versus permanent atrial fibrillation. *J Cardiovasc Electrophysiol* 2006;**17**(9):965–72.

29 Lazar S, Dixit S, Callans DJ, Lin D, Marchlinski FE, Gerstenfeld EP. Effect of pulmonary vein isolation on the left-to-right atrial dominant frequency gradient in human atrial fibrillation. *Heart Rhythm* 2006;**3**(8): 889–95.

30 Takahashi Y, Sanders P, Jais P, et al. Organization of frequency spectra of atrial fibrillation: relevance to radiofrequency catheter ablation. *J Cardiovasc Electrophysiol* 2006;**17**(4):382–8.

PART 2
Practical approaches in atrial fibrillation

CHAPTER 8

Emerging technologies in the treatment of atrial fibrillation

Matthew Wright, Christian de Chillou, Etienne Aliot & D. Wyn Davies

Introduction

Pulmonary vein isolation is an effective treatment for atrial fibrillation (AF), the commonest arrhythmia in man. Since the initial report [1] that ectopic triggers within the pulmonary veins (PVs) can lead to paroxysms of AF, our understanding of the mechanisms of initiation and perpetuation of atrial fibrillation have increased [2–12]. However, the success of radiofrequency ablation for paroxysmal atrial fibrillation (PAF) is not yet comparable to radiofrequency ablation of other common atrial arrhythmias such as atrial flutter or atrioventricular nodal reciprocating tachycardia. In addition, radiofrequency ablation of AF is relatively time-consuming and technically challenging, especially when treating recurrent persistent or permanent AF [7,8]. This combination of factors has served as an impetus for companies and individuals to design new tools for the electrophysiologist to improve the treatment of AF.

Current ablation techniques and results

Paroxysmal atrial fibrillation

Since the initial report that radiofrequency ablation of ectopic foci within the PVs resulted in freedom from AF for 62% of patients with a mean follow-up of 8 months [1], there have been two broad classes of ablation strategies for PAF. One strategy is targeted ablation of the muscular sleeves at the ostia of the PVs (PV isolation [1]), whilst another is an anatomic approach (wide anatomic circumferential ablation [2]) encircling the PVs within the left atrium. One of the potential problems of ablation within the PVs is PV stenosis [13]. The incidence of PV stenosis is variable and the reported incidence depends in part on the imaging modality used. In the initial studies, the reported incidence was between 4% and 42% [13,14]. However, the use of a circumferential multipolar catheter made the procedure safer. Using this mapping catheter within the PVs demonstrated that there are usually a number of muscular sleeves that electrically connect the PVs with the left atrium. Targeting these sleeves outside the veins' ostia to achieve PV isolation reduces unnecessary ablation of bystander tissue and reduces the risk of PV stenosis.

An alternative approach to PV isolation is an anatomically based approach, wide anatomic circumferential ablation [2]. With this technique, ablation is carried out more distally to the PV ostia within the left atrium, with many operators utilizing a non-fluoroscopic mapping system. The non-fluoroscopic mapping system, such as Carto™ or Ensite NavX® both guide the ablation catheter and confirm continuous lesions encircling either individual or ipsilateral PV ostia. The results from this anatomic approach seem similar to PV isolation for PAF.

Catheter Ablation of Atrial Fibrillation Edited by Etienne Aliot, Michel Haïssaguerre and Warren M. Jackman
© 2008 Blackwell Publishing, ISBN: 978-1-4501-6349-1.

Persistent and permanent atrial fibrillation

With both persistent and permanent AF, sometimes referred to as chronic AF, it has been demonstrated that PV isolation alone is not usually sufficient to achieve long-term freedom from AF. Over the last few years different groups have tried a number of strategies. These have ranged from making linear lesions of block, similar to the surgical maze procedure described by Cox [15], targeting complex fractionated atrial electrograms [5,16], ablation at areas of short cycle length activity [5,17], and ablation of focal sources in addition to PV foci [12,18]. In an elegant study from Bordeaux the relative importance of these mechanisms was studied [7,8].

In a prospective randomized study of 60 patients with persistent AF, patients underwent ablation within the left and right atrium in up to four steps, ending when sinus rhythm had been achieved or all four steps completed [7,8]. The ablation sites were PV isolation, isolation of other thoracic veins (coronary sinus, superior vena cava), and ablation of left atrial tissue at sites of fractionation or continuous activation. If sinus rhythm had not been restored then linear lines of block were created at the left atrial roof between the two superior PVs, a cavotriscuspid line, and a line from the mitral annulus to the left inferior PV. This procedure resulted in a very high procedural success rate, with 87% of patients being in sinus rhythm at the end of the procedure without the need for either antiarrhythmic medication or DC cardioversion. However, in the following 3 months, 40% of patients developed atrial tachycardias. Following further ablation, 95% were in sinus rhythm at 11 months, with only four of the 57 patients in sinus rhythm requiring antiarrhythmic medication.

Procedural times

Whilst with any procedure there is a learning curve, AF ablation is a lengthy procedure, even when non-fluoroscopic mapping systems are utilized [2,4,19]. Even in experienced hands PV isolation takes approximately 1 hour to perform [7,8], more than half of which is due to radiofrequency ablation. The increasing complexity of substrate modification for persistent and permanent AF increases procedural time even further [7,8]. Conventional catheters require multiple pulses of energy to be delivered around the ostia of the PVs to achieve electrical isolation. This necessarily demands that the catheter is manipulated several times for each individual vein and that at each position there has to be adequate catheter stability, prior to energy delivery. This limitation has served as one of the main drivers to develop catheters specifically for PV isolation.

Pulmonary vein anatomy

An understanding of PV anatomy is crucial both to the understanding of the technologies used in AF ablation and for the planning of the procedure for the individual patient. The majority of patients will have four PVs, two superior and two inferior with independent ostia [20]. A number of variations have been described in the literature [20–24]. In one series a common ostium for the left PVs was described in 83% of patients, however a common ostium for the right PVs was less frequent, occurring in 40% of patients [25]. Other reports confirm that a common ostium for the superior and inferior veins is more frequent on the left than the right but the overall frequency is much less at 15% and 10% of patients, respectively [22]. One of the reasons for the difference in the reported frequency of common PV ostia are the different imaging modalities used (magnetic resonance angiography (MRA) [23], computed tomography (CT) angiography [25], echocardiography [26], postmortem specimens [22]), and the definition used for the border between the left atrial wall and the PV.

The other common variant described in the literature is a separate origin for the right middle PV. The majority of the population will have the middle PV drain into the right superior PV. A separate origin has been described in 17–23%, with insertion into the right inferior PV the least frequent, at 3–8%, in surgical series [27,28]. More recently, a separate origin for the middle PV has been described in 22% in one study, using multidetector row CT [25], but only 10% in another study using MRA [23], and with none being seen in a postmortem study utilizing 20 hearts [22]. Additional left-sided PVs are far less frequent, but are described [25,29].

The diameter of the PVs is also important, both for risk of PV stenosis, which is greater in smaller veins [23], and the sizing of catheters. A study compared PV diameters in patients with AF as measured by intracardiac echocardiography (ICE) and multislice CT [26]. The majority of patients were in PAF and there was a statistically significant difference in the measured size of the PVs between the two imaging modalities. The diameter of the veins tended to be undersized when using ICE compared to CT. The mean diameters of the PVs in patients vary between 11 and 19 mm for left-sided veins and 15 and 19 mm for right-sided veins. The average diameter for common ostia is between 18 and 27 mm for common left-sided ostia and between 26 and 34 mm for right-sided common ostia. These results encompass a number of imaging modalities and patient populations [20–24,26,29,30].

Although size is important, a number of new ablation catheters are balloon-based and are circular in the axial plane. However, several studies have shown that the PVs themselves are not circular [23,25,26]. All studies that have reported upon the geometry of the PVs have shown that the left-sided veins are oval, with a greater superior–inferior diameter compared to anterior–posterior diameter. The right-sided veins tend to be more circular, but they still tend to have a larger superior–inferior diameter. In a study utilizing MRA, the ratio of the superior–inferior diameter to the anterior–posterior diameter was 1.5 for the left-sided PVs and 1.2 for the right-sided veins [23]. When using projection imaging, such as fluoroscopy, the oval nature of the left-sided PVs is not as easily appreciated as when using CT or MRA reconstructions. This means that PV stenosis could easily be missed if fluoroscopy is the only imaging modality used.

Emerging ablation technologies

Over the last few years AF ablation has become more widespread and there has been a tendency to move towards an anatomically driven approach for isolation of the PVs. Upon this basis a number of companies have designed catheters that can deliver a circumferential lesion around the PVs, with minimal applications of energy. The potential benefit of all such systems is that procedure times should be shorter, the learning curve should be quicker, and lesions could be contiguous around the ostium of the PVs. Three of the most promising technologies are the High Intensity Focused Ultrasound (HIFU)™ balloon (ProRhythm, Inc.), the Arctic Front™ balloon (CryoCath), and the High Density Mesh™ (C.R. Bard).

Pro Rhythm High Intensity Focused Ultrasound™ balloon

The HIFU® balloon (Figures 8.1 and 8.2) is designed to create circumferential lesions at the antrum of the PVs. The ablation catheter consists of an inner non-compliant balloon, which is filled with sterile water and contrast. This balloon tapers distally to allow placement within the PV. Within the balloon is an ultrasound crystal, which when excited emits ultrasound waves at 9 MHz. An outer, non-compliant balloon is filled with carbon dioxide (CO_2), and this creates an impedance mismatch at the interface of the two balloons between the fluid and the gas that allows it to act as a reflector. The parabolic shape of the balloon focuses the ultrasound waves in a ring, distal to the balloon catheter. The depth of the lesion is controlled by the duration of the application, with the circumference of the lesion dependent upon the size of the balloon. An inner steerable shaft allows placement of the

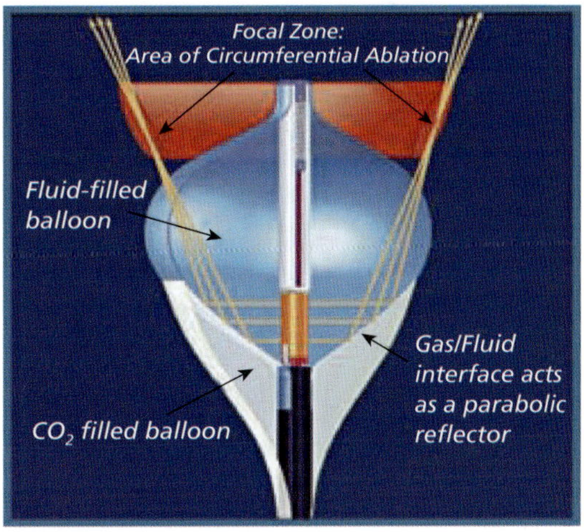

Figure 8.1 The HIFU™ balloon is an over-the-wire design balloon. Ultrasound waves are generated in the distal fluid-filled balloon (50 : 50 contrast : sterile water). The proximal balloon is filled with CO_2 and acts as a parabolic reflector focusing the ultrasound waves distal to the balloon. In this way a circumferential lesion can be formed at the ostium of the PV to be treated.

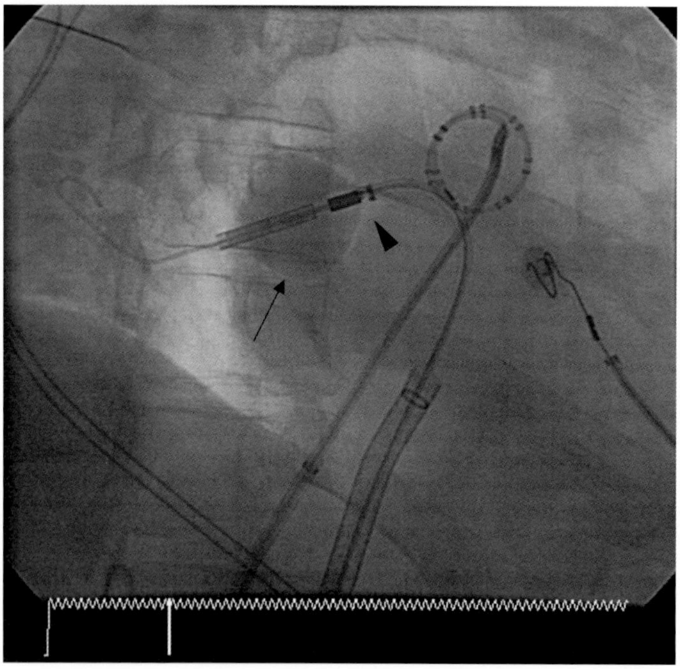

Figure 8.2 HIFU™ balloon ablation of the right inferior PV. The HIFU™ balloon is seen here in the right inferior PV. The distal balloon (arrowed) is filled with a 50 : 50 mix of contrast and water and is placed at the ostium of the vein to be treated. The proximal balloon (arrowhead) is filled with CO_2, acting as a parabolic mirror. The ultrasound transducer is seen within the distal balloon. In this patient a double transseptal puncture was used and the 8 Fr sheath and Lasso™ catheter can be seen. Note that the HIFU™ balloon catheter needs the large 14 Fr transseptal sheath.

catheter within the PVs over a guidewire and is the delivery system for the fluid and CO_2. The whole system is quite bulky and the investigational catheters have required 14 and 16 Fr transseptal sheaths. The latest versions of the catheter allow the passage of a specifically designed circumferential mapping catheter to be placed distal to the balloon to check for electrical isolation of the vein during energy delivery.

The initial studies in dogs with the HIFU™ balloon were very encouraging [31]. Transmural, circumferential lesions were created in four of 14 veins treated, and a further five had near-circumferential lesions. In the veins that had been inadequately treated the HIFU™ balloon had either not been located ideally within the vein or the transducer was not aligned with the balloon optimally. A redesign of the catheter rectified this problem. There was no obvious PV stenosis identified at postmortem, nor was there any damage to extracardiac tissue, including the esophagus and phrenic nerve. Further work in dogs tested for electrical isolation of the PVs following application of energy using the HIFU™ balloon [32]. A single application resulted in block in 88% of veins, with the remaining 12% requiring a second application. In addition they were able to demonstrate isolation of the veins at up to 3 months post ablation. However, it was noted that PV stenosis occurred in early branching vessels in two of the 32 veins treated [32].

The first clinical experience, presented in 2004 at the American Heart Association, was on a group of eight patients with both paroxysmal and persistent AF [33]. Whilst the investigators were unable to position the HIFU™ catheter into the right inferior PV, they were able to target the rest of the PVs successfully. With a median of three applications they were able to successfully isolate the veins treated, with six of the patients being free from AF at a median of 6 months. A similar study, presented at the Heart Rhythm Society meeting, confirmed these initial results in a further group of five patients [34]. An improvement to the catheter was the addition of steerability [35], and this allowed the right inferior PV to be reached. Although procedure and fluoroscopy times were reduced with this catheter, the mean procedure time was still over 4 h. In part this is due to the experimental nature of the catheter, as the actual duration of energy delivery to achieve isolation of all four PVs can be as short as 5 min [36].

Recently there have been reports of serious complications with the use of the HIFU™ balloon catheter [35,37]. Phrenic nerve injury has been reported in a canine model when delivering energy to the right superior vein [35]. This was using one of the smaller 20 mm balloon, (compared to the 25 and 30 mm balloons), which has a depth of focus that is approximately 3 mm outside the distal balloon. Unfortunately there have also been reports of phrenic nerve injury in humans [37]. The published case report was about a case utilizing the 20 mm balloon for application of energy to the right superior PV. The diameter of the PV was 16 mm fluroscopically, and the diameter of the balloon that causes the 20 mm circumferential lesion is actually 24 mm, and thus was not deeply intubated within the PV. However after 19 s of energy delivery, the right hemidiaphragm was seen to stop contracting. Despite immediate cessation of energy delivery, the phrenic nerve did not recover at the time of the procedure. Up to 20% of phrenic nerve injury have since been experienced with this system. Although phrenic nerve injury is a well-recognized complication, especially of balloon ablation procedures, typically when treating the right superior PV, it usually seems to cause remarkably few symptoms [38].

A far more grave complication is an atrioesophageal fistula [39]. In a canine study this complication was specifically studied. The left inferior PV is the closest to the esophagus, so this vein was targeted to try and see if a lesion could be created within the esophagus. To get close to the esophagus, as assessed by ICE and also by opacification of the esophagus with barium, the HIFU™ balloon had to be pushed towards the esophagus. However, by doing this, a lesion was seen within the esophagus in one of five dogs [40]. Although there was no reported left atrioesophageal fistula the dogs were sacrificed within 2 h (two dogs) and 7–8 days, whilst reported cases of left atrioesophageal fistula in humans, using conventional radiofrequency ablation, have been reported at later time points. In clinical practice, one fatal atrioesophageal fistula and one non-communicating esophageal injury have been seen with this system [41].

In summary, the HIFU™ balloon with the steerable shaft is able to deliver circumferential lesions to the antrum of all four PVs, causing electrical isolation. The lesions persist histologically in dogs for at least 6 months, and electrical isolation and freedom from AF is seen in small case series in clinical trials. At the present time there appears to be no benefit in terms of procedural time or safety when compared to conventional procedures; however, it is one of the more promising technologies that has undergone a lot of developmental work.

CryoCath Arctic Front™ balloon

The CryoCath Arctic Front™ balloon (Figures 8.3 and 8.4) is designed to create circumferential PV isolation. This catheter again consists of two balloons; the inner balloon containing the refrigerant when inflated, with an outer balloon under constant vacuum to prevent any refrigerant from

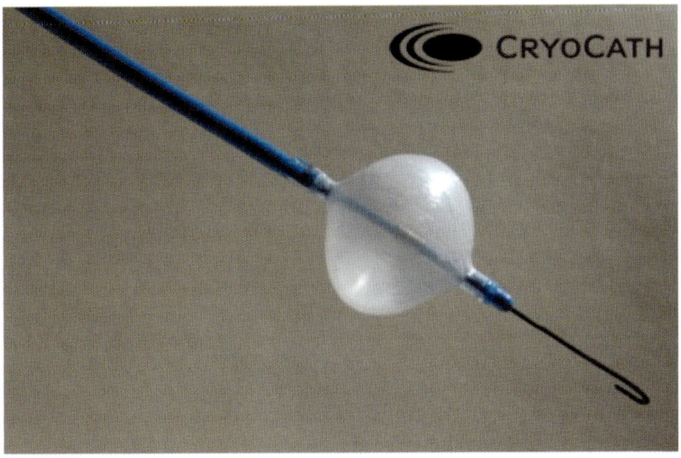

Figure 8.3 The Arctic Front™ balloon is mounted on a steerable catheter, and is an over-the-wire design. The balloon itself consists of two separate balloons, both of which are under vacuum. The inner balloon contains refrigerant, whilst the outer balloon is designed to collect any inadvertant leak.

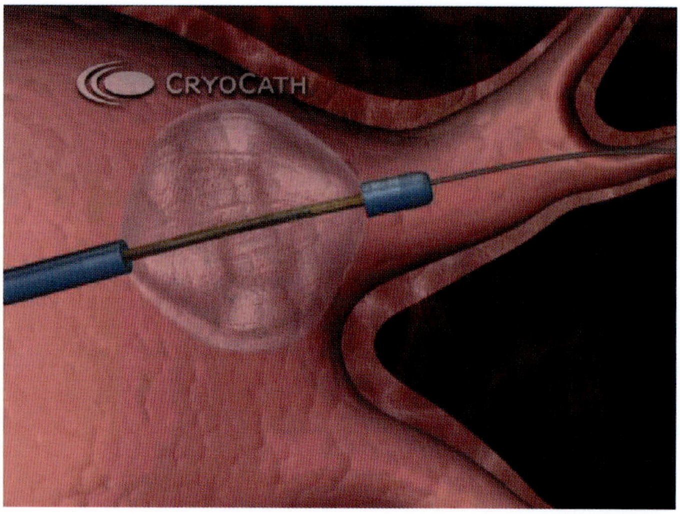

Figure 8.4 Placement of the Arctic Front™ balloon within a PV. The Arctic Front™ balloon is designed to be placed at the ostium of the PV. Ideally when engaged and cooled to –80°C there should be no leak of blood around the balloon.

entering into the patient in the event of a leak from the inner balloon. The balloon is mounted on a steerable catheter, which delivers the refrigerant, using an over-the-wire system, and is designed to be used with a steerable sheath. With cryothermy endothelial integrity is maintained, and the lesions created are well demarcated, transmural, and free of inflammation. This has potential benefits compared to both radiofrequency ablation and focused ultrasound, in that lesions should be less thrombogenic – hence with a lower risk of thromboembolic complications and with significantly reduced chance of perforation.

The balloon catheter was developed following the use of an earlier technology, the Arctic Circler™, which demonstrated that PV isolation was feasible with cryothermy [42]. In a trial, 52 patients – with the majority of patients having PAF – underwent PV isolation using the curvilinear cryoablation catheter marketed as the Arctic Circler™. The acute procedural success, as determined by electrical isolation of the vein targeted, was high, with 97% of veins successfully treated. Follow-up data was encouraging with 62% of patients free from AF, as determined by event recorder analysis. This may give a falsely high success rate, as other studies using more rigorous monitoring protocols have shown that there is an increase in asymptomatic AF following AF ablation on ambulatory monitoring [43]. In a further study of 31 patients with both PAF and permanent AF, the results were less favourable, with 43% of patients unchanged with an average of 18 months' follow-up [44]. One of the benefits of using cryothermy was the low complication rate in this study, with no evidence of significant PV stenosis [42]. Despite this relative success there were a number of important drawbacks to this catheter; the main problem was the very long procedural time, with a range of 3.5 to 13 h and a mean procedural time of 7.5 ± 2 h.

The evolution of the Arctic Circler™ was the Arctic Front™, with the aims of improving cryolesions and shortening procedural time. As the Arctic Front™ is balloon-based and the entire balloon is cooled to –80°C, a circumferential lesion can be formed. A feasibility and safety study in canines was promising. In each dog the right and left superior PVs were targeted. Acute procedure success, as measured by PV isolation using a Lasso™ catheter, was promising with 14 of the 16 veins treated isolated. When the animals were sacrificed at 1 week post ablation, the Lasso™ catheter was placed within the PVs and 10 of 12 veins remained isolated. There was no difference with the duration of energy delivery, or number of ablations performed. The mean duration of energy delivery was 8 min per vein, which compares favorably to an earlier study with the curvilinear catheter, in humans, where it took approximately 65 min to isolate each vein [44].

It was demonstrated that successful isolation was dependent upon occlusive engagement of the balloon within the PV ostium. Non-occlusive engagement, measured by ICE, was seen in three veins, only one of which was isolated. The temperature that was achieved with these non-occlusive applications was significantly lower. Whilst only one balloon size (23 mm) was used in this study, a 28 mm balloon is also produced. None of the dogs had common ostia to the PVs. A further problem identified in this canine study was a high incidence of phrenic nerve injury, which occurred in 50% of the dogs and was still present at 1 week. This complication occurred when two applications of 4 min duration had to be applied to the right superior PV to achieve isolation. At 16 weeks, six animals were assessed for PV stenosis by CT; there were no significant changes seen. Occasional right phrenic nerve injuries have been seen whilst treating the right upper and right lower PVs. Close monitoring of right phrenic nerve function by pacing the nerve or by monitoring diaphragmatic movement during inspiration allows immediate cessation of freezing when diaphragmatic movement attenuates or stops. This is followed by phrenic nerve recovery within minutes.

At the present time there are no published efficacy studies of the Arctic Front™ in patients.

Bard High Density Mesh Ablator™

The Bard High Density (HD) Mesh Ablator™ (Figure 8.5) is another new technology for PV isolation. In comparison to the two previous technologies, this is not balloon-based. Instead, the HD Mesh Ablator™ is based upon two helices of 18 individual wires. Each of the 36 wires is isolated and can also deliver conventional radiofrequency energy, up to 100 W. There are four temperature sensors mounted around the equator of the mesh. The HD Mesh Ablator™ comes in two sizes, 25 and 30 mm when fully expanded, and the manufacturers advise that it should not be used for PVs greater than 20 mm in diameter. A further difference compared to the two balloon-based products

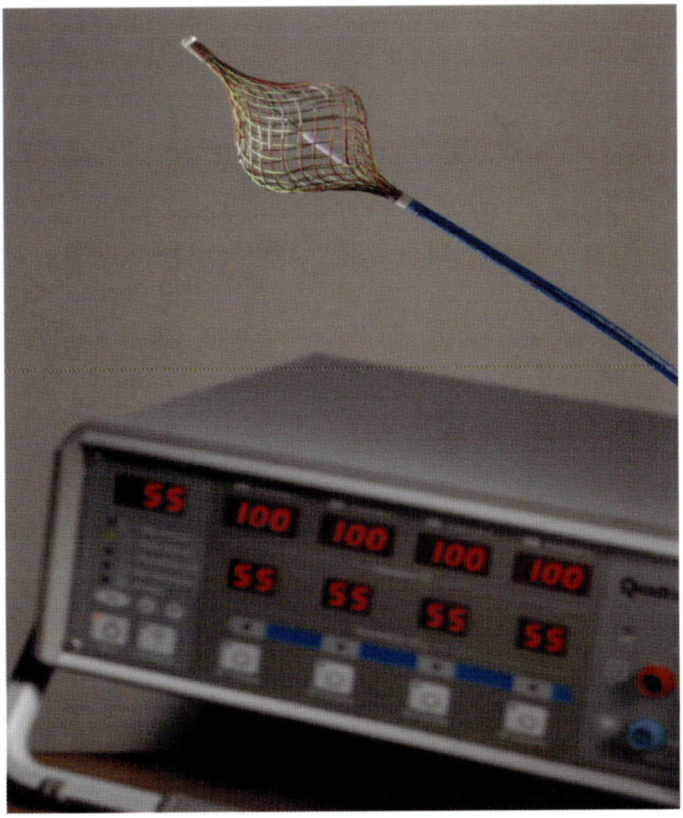

Figure 8.5 The Bard HD Mesh Ablator™ consists of two interlinked helices of 18 individually isolated wires. Power is delivered at the equator of the mesh, which can be seen as a silver band.

is that the HD Mesh Ablator™ is able to record electrograms whilst also ablating, without the need for a separate catheter.

As the HD Mesh Ablator™ is a new product there are less clinical data regarding its use and efficacy compared to the HIFU™ balloon and the Arctic Front™ balloon. However, there are some data that have been presented at major conferences. In a small study in dogs, the 8 Fr HD Mesh Ablator™ was able to electrically isolate nine of the 10 PVs targeted [45]. The energy is delivered in a pulsed fashion, up to 300 s at a maximum power output of 100 W. In the canine study there were no procedural complications reported, although only six dogs were used. In a study presented at the Heart Rhythm Society last year, a further study was reported using the HD Mesh Ablator™ [46]. The current catheter is non-steerable, and in this study the Daig™ transseptal sheath was used. This only allowed the superior PVs to be targeted. However, 21 of the 22 superior veins were treated. Each application of energy lasted for a total of 300 s, but this was delivered in pulses of 5 ms, followed by a 5 ms pause, with a fixed output of 100 W. The average number of deliveries per vein was 2.8, and isolation at the end of the procedure was seen in most of the PVs treated. There were no long-term follow-up data presented. There was only one complication reported, late pericardial tamponade, and no reports of esophageal fistula or pulmonary vein stenosis in this small sample. The very first paper reporting on the use of the Mesh Ablator™ in a canine model has been published recently [47]. This study showed that PV disconnection could be obtained in 13 of 19 treated right superior PVs after one to four radiofrequency applications. No significant PV stenosis was observed but a left atrial mural thrombus was present in three of 19 animals.

Emerging navigation and mapping technologies

All of the new technologies discussed above in this chapter have focused on energy delivery and catheter-based systems. Navigation and mapping technologies that have been developed since the mid 1990s are now widely used by most teams performing AF ablation. Such systems are aimed to improve the linearity of the deployed ablation lesions and to decrease fluoroscopy time. One of the most recent and remarkable engineering feats has been the development of robotic systems to actually control the catheters that we use.

Carto™ and NavX™/Ensite™

The use of the Carto™ system (Biosense Webster, Johnson & Johnson) has been promoted by Pappone et al. [2] to perform an anatomic approach that consists of deploying continuous radiofrequency lesions within the left atrium to encircle either individual or ipsilateral PV ostia. The most recent version of the CARTO™ system (CartoMerge™, Figure 8.6) allows the fusion of an electroanatomic three-dimensional reconstruction of the left atrium (virtual anatomy) with a three-dimensional shell of the same heart chamber, obtained by a CT scan or MRA performed prior to the electrophysiological study. The first paper reporting on the use of CartoMerge™ in patients undergoing AF ablation was published in 2005 [48]. This paper showed that the CT scan images could be successfully fused with the electroanatomic mapping with an average mean distance of 2.1 ± 0.2 mm between the mapping points and the CT scan surface. Similar results have been published [49] with the use of integrated electroanatomic mapping (CartoMerge™) with three-dimensional MRA images to guide catheter ablation of AF. In the near future, the next version of the Carto™ system will provide real-time anatomic images with simultaneous use of ICE, which will be incorporated into the Carto™ platform.

The use of another non-fluoroscopic navigation system (NavX™, St. Jude Medical, Figure 8.7) has been evaluated recently in 44 patients undergoing left atrial linear ablation to modify the substrate of AF [50]. Use of this navigation system was associated with a significant 35% shorter fluoroscopic exposure when creating the ablations lines and was also associated with a trend toward shorter procedure times. Using a multielectrode array catheter (non-contact Ensite™ mapping technology), the NavX™ system also offers the possibility to map spontaneous atrial premature beats that trigger atrial fibrillation episodes [51]. In the near future, the next version of the NavX™ system will permit the fusion of virtual anatomy images with images obtained from CT scans or MRA.

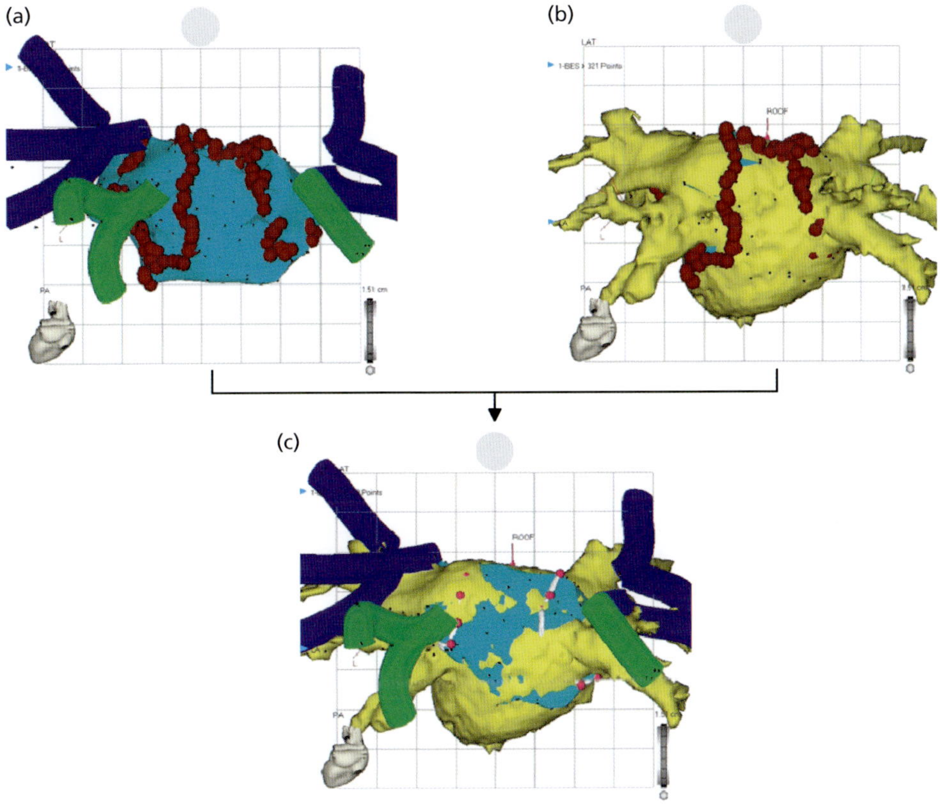

Figure 8.6 The CartoMerge™ system. Posteroanterior views of a three-dimensional left atrium reconstructed with Carto™ in a patient undergoing an ablation procedure for PAF. (a) Three-dimensional shell of a Carto™ reconstructed left atrium with the blue and green tubes representing the PVs. (b) CT scan shell of the left atrium in the same patient. (c) Image showing the fusion between the two three-dimensional shells. The brown dots (a, b) represent sites where radiofrequency energy was delivered to isolate the PVs.

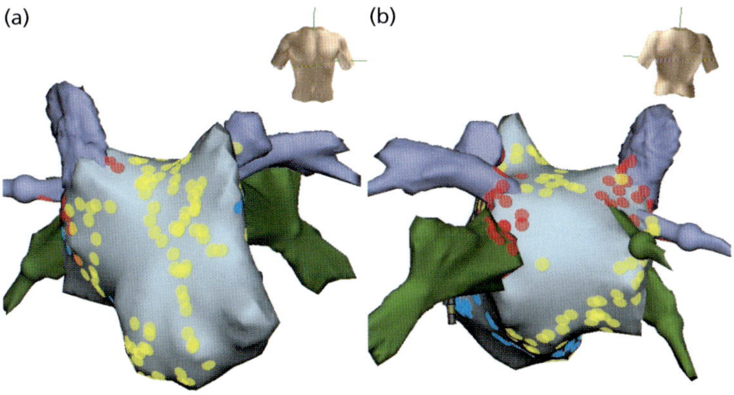

Figure 8.7 The NavX™ system. Anteroposterior (a) and posteroanterior (b) views of a three-dimensional left atrium reconstructed with NavX™ in a patient undergoing an ablation procedure for chronic AF. The red dots are the sites of radiofrequency energy application to isolate the PVs. The yellow dots represent the sites where radiofrequency energy was delivered to create ablation lines in the left atrium.

Hansen Medical Sensei™ robotic catheter remote control system

The theoretical benefits of such robotic systems are that there should be greater catheter stability, and catheters should be able to be placed within areas that are typically difficult to reach. Another benefit of the robotic system is that the operator does not need to be next to the patient, so the radiation dose to the operator can be radically cut down. The Sensei™ robotic system uses a proprietary control catheter, Artisan™, which has 6° of movement. Currently this system is undergoing clinical evaluation in a number of centers, but in our hands we have found the Sensei™ system very easy to use. Saliba et al. recently showed the feasibility and safety of this system to facilitate navigation, precise positioning, and control of percutaneous catheters to specific and discrete regions of all four chambers of the heart in an experimental canine model [52]. This study also first reported on remote endocardial transeptal puncture.

Stereotaxis Niobe™ robotic magnetic navigation system

The magnetic navigation system (Niobe™, Stereotaxis, Inc.) consists of two permanent magnets (neodymium–iron–boron compound), the positions of which, relative to each other, are computer controlled inside a fixed housing and positioned on either side of the fluoroscopy table. While positioned in "navigate" position, they create a relatively uniform and spherical (~20 cm diameter) magnetic field (0.08 T) inside the patient's chest. The combination of rotation, translation, and tilt movements of the magnets adjusts the magnetic field to any desired orientation in the spherical 20 cm diameter navigation volume. The mapping and ablation catheter is equipped with a small permanent magnet positioned at the tip that aligns itself with the direction of the externally controlled magnetic field to enable it to be steered effectively. Changing the orientation of the magnetic field thereby leads to a deflection of the catheter. The position of the magnetic catheter within the heart is also controlled by a mechanical catheter advancer system (Cardiodrive™, Stereotaxis, Inc.). Indeed, after the extracorporeal portion of the catheter is secured into the catheter advancer system, remote advancement and retraction of the catheter through a standard intravascular sheath is accomplished via changes in the externally controlled magnetic field. The system is controlled by joystick and allows remote control of the ablation catheter from inside the control room.

The magnetic navigation system has been integrated in a newly developed electroanatomic platform using Carto™ technology: the Carto RMT™ mapping system (Biosense Webster, Johnson & Johnson). The Carto RMT™ system sends real-time catheter tip location and orientation data to the magnetic navigation system. It also sends target locations, groups of points, and anatomic surface information from the electroanatomic map to the magnetic navigation system. The real-time catheter location information can be displayed on the reference X-ray images, enabling continuous real-time monitoring of the catheter tip position even without acquiring a fresh X-ray image.

The first human study of AF ablation with the use of this technology has been published recently [53]. This study showed that remote control navigation for AF ablation is safe and feasible with a short learning curve (~12 patients).

Conclusion

In the short space of time since radiofrequency ablation for PAF was demonstrated to be possible our understanding of the mechanism of PAF and permanent AF has increased dramatically. Patients who were previously told there was no option other than medication, DC cardioversion, and even atrioventricular node ablation, now have an effective cure with ablation procedures. In addition, the tools that physicians have to treat AF are constantly evolving in an attempt to make the procedure safer, more efficacious, simpler, and quicker to perform. The next few years look even more promising with the new technologies discussed.

References

1 Haissaguerre M, Jais P, Shah DC, et al. Spontaneous initiation of atrial fibrillation by ectopic beats originating in the pulmonary veins. *N Engl J Med* 1998;**339**:659–66.

2 Pappone C, Rosanio S, Oreto G, et al. Circumferential radiofrequency ablation of pulmonary vein ostia: a new anatomic approach for curing atrial fibrillation. *Circulation* 2000;**102**:2619–28.

3 Jais P, Weerasooriya R, Shah DC, et al. Ablation therapy for atrial fibrillation (AF): past, present and future. *Cardiovasc Res* 2002;**54**:337–46.

4 Pappone C, Santinelli V, Manguso F, et al. Pulmonary vein denervation enhances long-term benefit after circumferential ablation for paroxysmal atrial fibrillation. *Circulation* 2004;**109**:327–34.

5 Nademanee K, McKenzie J, Kosar E, et al. A new approach for catheter ablation of atrial fibrillation: mapping of the electrophysiologic substrate. *J Am Coll Cardiol* 2004;**43**:2044–53.

6 Jais P, Hsu LF, Rotter M, et al. Mitral isthmus ablation for atrial fibrillation. *J Cardiovasc Electrophysiol* 2005;**16**: 1157–9.

7 Haissaguerre M, Hocini M, Sanders P, et al. Catheter ablation of long-lasting persistent atrial fibrillation: clinical outcome and mechanisms of subsequent arrhythmias. *J Cardiovasc Electrophysiol* 2005;**16**:1138–47.

8 Haissaguerre M, Sanders P, Hocini M, et al. Catheter ablation of long-lasting persistent atrial fibrillation: critical structures for termination. *J Cardiovasc Electrophysiol* 2005;**16**:1125–37.

9 Oral H, Chugh A, Good E, et al. A tailored approach to catheter ablation of paroxysmal atrial fibrillation. *Circulation* 2006;**113**:1824–31.

10 Earley MJ, Abrams DJ, Staniforth AD, Sporton SC, Schilling RJ. Catheter ablation of permanent atrial fibrillation: medium term results. *Heart* 2006;**92**:233–8.

11 Oral H, Pappone C, Chugh A, et al. Circumferential pulmonary-vein ablation for chronic atrial fibrillation. *N Engl J Med* 2006;**354**:934–41.

12 Takahashi Y, Hocini M, O'Neill MD, et al. Sites of focal atrial activity characterized by endocardial mapping during atrial fibrillation. *J Am Coll Cardiol* 2006;**47**:2005–12.

13 Packer DL, Keelan P, Munger TM, et al. Clinical presentation, investigation, and management of pulmonary vein stenosis complicating ablation for atrial fibrillation. *Circulation* 2005;**111**:546–54.

14 Macle L, Jais P, Weerasooriya R, et al. Irrigated-tip catheter ablation of pulmonary veins for treatment of atrial fibrillation. *J Cardiovasc Electrophysiol* 2002;**13**:1067–73.

15 Cox JL, Boineau JP, Schuessler RB, Kater KM, Lappas DG. Five-year experience with the maze procedure for atrial fibrillation. *Ann Thoracic Surg* 1993;**56**:814–23; discussion 823–4.

16 Rostock T, Rotter M, Sanders P, et al. High-density activation mapping of fractionated electrograms in the atria of patients with paroxysmal atrial fibrillation. *Heart Rhythm* 2006;**3**:27–34.

17 Takahashi Y, Jais P, Hocini M, et al. Shortening of fibrillatory cycle length in the pulmonary vein during vagal excitation. *J Am Coll Cardiol* 2006;**47**:774–80.

18 Shah D, Haissaguerre M, Jais P, Hocini M. Nonpulmonary vein foci: do they exist? *Pacing Clin Electrophysiol* 2003;**26**:1631–5.

19 Pappone C, Oreto G, Rosanio S, et al. Atrial electroanatomic remodeling after circumferential radiofrequency pulmonary vein ablation: efficacy of an anatomic approach in a large cohort of patients with atrial fibrillation. *Circulation* 2001;**104**:2539–44.

20 Marom EM, Herndon JE, Kim YH, McAdams HP. Variations in pulmonary venous drainage to the left atrium: implications for radiofrequency ablation. *Radiology* 2004;**230**:824–9.

21 Lin WS, Prakash VS, Tai CT, et al. Pulmonary vein morphology in patients with paroxysmal atrial fibrillation initiated by ectopic beats originating from the pulmonary veins: implications for catheter ablation. *Circulation* 2000;**101**:1274–81.

22 Ho SY, Cabrera JA, Tran VH, et al. Architecture of the pulmonary veins: relevance to radiofrequency ablation. *Heart* 2001;**86**:265–70.

23 Wittkampf FH, Vonken EJ, Derksen R, et al. Pulmonary vein ostium geometry: analysis by magnetic resonance angiography. *Circulation* 2003;**107**:21–3.

24 Hassink RJ, Aretz HT, Ruskin J, Keane D. Morphology of atrial myocardium in human pulmonary veins: a postmortem analysis in patients with and without atrial fibrillation. *J Am Coll Cardiol* 2003;**42**:1108–14.

25 Jongbloed MR, Dirksen MS, Bax JJ, et al. Atrial fibrillation: multi-detector row CT of pulmonary vein anatomy prior to radiofrequency catheter ablation – initial experience. *Radiology* 2005;**234**:702–9.

26 Jongbloed MR, Bax JJ, Lamb HJ, et al. Multislice computed tomography versus intracardiac echocardiography to evaluate the pulmonary veins before radiofrequency catheter ablation of atrial fibrillation: a head-to-head comparison. *J Am Coll Cardiol* 2005;**45**:343–50.

27 Tsao HM, Wu MH, Yu WC, et al. Role of right middle pulmonary vein in patients with paroxysmal atrial fibrillation. *J Cardiovasc Electrophysiol* 2001;**12**:1353–7.

28 Yazar F, Ozdogmus O, Tuccar E, Bayramoglu A, Ozan H. Drainage patterns of middle lobe vein of right lung: an anatomical study. *Eur J Cardiothorac Surg* 2002;**22**:717–20.

29 Ghaye B, Szapiro D, Dacher JN, et al. Percutaneous ablation for atrial fibrillation: the role of cross-sectional imaging. *Radiographics* 2003;**23**(suppl):S19–S33; discussion S48–S50.

30 Dill T, Neumann T, Ekinci O, et al. Pulmonary vein diameter reduction after radiofrequency catheter ablation for paroxysmal atrial fibrillation evaluated by contrast-enhanced three-dimensional magnetic resonance imaging. *Circulation* 2003;**107**:845–50.

31 Meininger GR, Calkins H, Lickfett L, et al. Initial experience with a novel focused ultrasound ablation system for ring ablation outside the pulmonary vein. *J Interv Cardiac Electrophysiol* 2003;**8**:141–8.

32 Nakagawa H, Aoyama H, Pitha JV, et al. Pre-clinical canine testing of a novel high intensity, forward-focused ultrasound balloon catheter for pulmonary vein isolation. *PACE* 2003;**26**:954.

33 Nakagawa H, Antz M, Kuck KH, et al. Initial clinical experience with high intensity focused ultrasound balloon catheter for pulmonary vein antrum isolation in patients with atrial fibrillation. *Circulation* 2004;**110**:II–459.

34 Markus K, Sinha A, Karla D, Hanrath P, Stellbrink C. Initial experience with pulmonary vein isolation using a high intensity focused ultrasound balloon catheter. *Heart Rhythm Meeting* 2005;05-AB-4812-HRS.

35 Mahapatra S, Bunch T, Miller D, Johnson S, Packer D. Critical analysis of the efficacy and safety of a novel steerable high intensity focused ultrasound (HIFU) balloon in pulmonary vein isolation in a canine model. *Heart Rhythm Society* 2005.

36 Wong T, Markides V, Peters NS, Davies DW. Anatomic left atrial circumferential ablation to electrically isolate pulmonary veins using a novel focused ultrasound balloon catheter. *Heart Rhythm* 2006;**3**:370–1.

37 Antz M, Chun KJ, Ouyang F, Kuck KH. Ablation of atrial fibrillation in humans using a balloon-based ablation system: identification of the site of phrenic nerve damage using pacing maneuvers and CARTO. *J Cardiovasc Electrophysiol* 2006;**17**:1242–5.

38 Sacher F, Monahan KH, Thomas SP, et al. Phrenic nerve injury after atrial fibrillation catheter ablation: characterization and outcome in a multicenter study. *J Am Coll Cardiol* 2006;**47**:2498–503.

39 Pappone C, Oral H, Santinelli V, et al. Atrio-esophageal fistula as a complication of percutaneous transcatheter ablation of atrial fibrillation. *Circulation* 2004;**109**:2724–6.

40 Yokoyama K, Nakagawa H, Pitha JV, Lazzara R, Jackman WM. Can high intensity focused ultrasound applications very close to esophagus produce left atrial-esophageal fistula? *Heart Rhythm* 2006;**3**:AB27–34.

41 Nakagawa H, Antz M, Wong T, et al. Initial experience using a forward directed, high-intensity focused ultrasound balloon catheter for pulmonary vein antrum isolation in patients with atrial fibrillation. *J Cardiovasc Electrophysiol* 2007;**18**:136–44.

42 Tse HF, Reek S, Timmermans C, et al. Pulmonary vein isolation using transvenous catheter cryoablation for treatment of atrial fibrillation without risk of pulmonary vein stenosis. *J Am Coll Cardiol* 2003;**42**:752–8.

43 Oral H, Veerareddy S, Good E, et al. Prevalence of asymptomatic recurrences of atrial fibrillation after successful radiofrequency catheter ablation. *J Cardiovasc Electrophysiol* 2004;15:920–4.

44 Wong T, Markides V, Peters NS, Davies DW. Percutaneous pulmonary vein cryoablation to treat atrial fibrillation. *J Interv Cardiac Electrophysiol* 2004;**11**:117–26.

45 Liu S, Lin J, Nie Z, et al. A simplified approach to pulmonary vein isolation using an 8F mesh catheter and a pulsed RF controller. *Fourth International Forum on Atrial Fibrillation* 2006.

46 Pitschner HF, Zaltsberg S, Kuniss D, et al. Circular mapping and PV isolation of the antrum by a new 32-pole foldable umbrella catheter powered by pulsed RF-energy delivery. *Heart Rhythm* 2006;**3**(5):S240–S241.

47 Arruda MS, He DS, Friedman P, et al. A novel mesh electrode catheter for mapping and radiofrequency delivery at the left atrium-pulmonary vein junction: a single-catheter approach to pulmonary vein antrum isolation. *J Cardiovasc Electrophysiol* 2007;**18**:206–11.

48 Tops LF, Bax JJ, Zeppenfeld K, et al. Fusion of multislice computed tomography imaging with three-dimensional electroanatomic mapping to guide radiofrequency catheter ablation procedures. *Heart Rhythm* 2005;**2**:1076–81.

49 Dong J, Dickfeld T, Dalal D, et al. Initial experience in the use of integrated electroanatomic mapping with the three-dimensional MR/CT images to guide catheter ablation of atrial fibrillation. *J Cardiovasc Electrophysiol* 2006;**17**:459–66.

50 Takahashi Y, Rotter M, Sanders P, et al. Left atrial linear ablation to modify the substrate of atrial fibrillation using a new nonfluoroscopic imaging system. *PACE* 2005;**28**:S90–S93.

51 Kim YH, Lim HE, Pak HN. Use of three-dimensional mapping systems in the catheter ablation of atrial fibrillation. *J Cardiovasc Electrophysiol* 2006;**17**:S16–S22.

52 Saliba W, Cummings JE, Oh S, et al. Novel robotic catheter remote control system: feasibility and safety of transeptal puncture and endocardial catheter navigation. *J Cardiovasc Electrophysiol* 2006;**17**:1102–5.

53 Pappone C, Vicedomini G, Manguso F, et al. Robotic magnetic navigation for atrial fibrillation ablation. *J Am Coll Cardiol* 2006;**47**:1390–400.

9

CHAPTER 9

Techniques targeting the pulmonary veins

Sabine Ernst, Feifan Ouyang, Matthias Antz, Julian K. R. Chun, Dietmar Bänsch, & Karl-Heinz Kück

Introduction

The curative catheter ablation of atrial fibrillation (AF) has made some important advances during the last few years towards a reproducible and effective procedure. Besides the role of the trigger to induce AF episodes by rapid bursts from within the pulmonary veins (PVs), invasive electrophysiological studies can also demonstrate the importance of the closely surrounding atrial myocardium to sustain the AF. The currently available ablation techniques targeting the PVs are critically reviewed in this chapter.

To overcome some the shortcomings of radiofrequency ablation, new energy sources such as laser, ultrasound, and cryothermia are investigated, to apply "single shot" lesions around the PV ostia. Other new tools, such as the magnetic navigation system, allow complete remote-controlled mapping (and ablation) by combining both three-dimensional (3D) steering and 3D mapping/imaging in a single system. All these devices and technologies still have to prove their effectiveness and their ability to meet high expectations.

Rational for targeting the pulmonary veins

The role of the PVs as the major sites of induction of AF was identified during the attempt to replicate the surgical approach of compartmentalization by linear incisions (Cox's maze operation) [1–3]. During these initial ablation procedures, repetitive initiating extrasystoles from within the PVs were demonstrated and subsequently eliminated by direct ablation. Although this observation had been made also by other investigators, the role of the PV as the dominate site of AF induction only then came to full recognition [4]. These high frequency triggers can induce AF, and the activity of the trigger itself may explain the amount and duration of the induced AF episodes. But the remodeling processes soon change the properties of the atrial myocardium to sustain the once induced arrhythmia. The elimination of the trigger from the PVs (in the absence of non-PV trigger) removes the initiator and allows the atrial myocardium to reconvert by mechanisms of reverse remodeling. In the goat experiment of Allessie and coworkers, the initiator was the implanted pacemaker: in the beginning, rapid burst pacing was "answered" by only short and self-terminating AF episodes [5]. Once remodeling of the myocardium had taken effect, only a few triggers were necessary to induce AF and sustain the arrhythmia. The famous quote of "AF begets AF" was coined, but the opposite, "sinus rhythm (SR) begets SR", could also be true. By elimination of the trigger (by turning of the rapidly stimulating pacemaker) and stable SR, conduction properties could return to pre-stimulation levels. The important question of whether a "point of no return" can be identified in patients – after that, simple trigger elimination would be worthless since the myocardium would sustain the arrhythmia

Catheter Ablation of Atrial Fibrillation Edited by Etienne Aliot, Michel Haïssaguerre and Warren M. Jackman

anyway, despite the absence of a reinitiating trigger – has not been answered yet. An easy differentiation could be proposed by limiting this approach to patients that still can terminate their arrhythmia episodes (spontaneously or under antiarrhythmic medication) and thereby prove their ability to maintain AF; in other words limit the approach to instances where the remodeling process is not advanced too far. At the other end are patients who, despite treatment with antiarrhythmic medication aimed at rhythm control and even conversion attempts such as electrical cardioversion, have undergone such extensive remodeling processes that additional substrate modification attempts should be considered.

The pulmonary vein antrum as a site for the maintenance of atrial fibrillation

Important electrophysiological information has been obtained meanwhile from postoperative [6] procedures – but also after double Lasso® procedures – on the role of the PV–left atrium (LA) area [7]. These so-called "antrum" areas can not only harbor triggers, but are large enough to sustain fast reentries even in the presence of disconnection from the remaining LA.

Anatomic considerations

The underlying morphology of the PVs should be taken into account whenever an ablation attempt targeting the PVs or nearby structures is attempted [8–10]. Atrial myocardium with the ability to rapidly depolarize is found in fiber-like architecture within the PVs with a length, occasionally, up to several centimeters from the PV ostium. Toward the junction of the PV to the LA, the fiber orientation changes to a rather circumferential orientation with several layers of myocardium displaying an almost chaotic criss-cross pattern. The morphology of the ostia of the PVs is highly individual and only in extremely rare cases truly like the tubes of the 3D mapping systems. In most instances, the ostia are rather oval and funnel-shaped, making a clear discrimination of the PV and LA impossible. In light of the varying branching or proximally fusing PVs, quite frequently forming common ostia, 3D mapping in addition to direct contrast injection allows the identification of the individual morphology of a given patient [11]. However, in the absence of 3D imaging (magnetic resonance imaging (MRI), computed tomography (CT)), or at least two-dimensional (2D) angiography, unusual additional PVs might be overlooked that could also be the site of triggers or could be harmed by an unaware ablation attempt. In addition, adjacent structures (such as the LA appendage and the neighboring ridge towards the lateral PVs) should be carefully assessed to tailor the ablation line to the individual patient. Other imaging modalitities such as intracardiac echocardiography (ICE) can help guide the experienced investigator [12].

Critical review of different techniques targeting the pulmonary veins

Direct trigger ablation

Initial reports described the observation of focal firing from within the mostly superior PVs that initiated paroxysmal episodes of AF [1–2]. Catheter ablation of the trigger (Figure 9.1a) was limited by several problems: (i) incidence of the actively "firing" trigger could not be reproducibly influenced; (ii) all provocation maneuvers (pacing or pharmacological) were unreliable; and (iii) even if induction was achieved there was no means to rule out currently "dormant" triggers within the other PVs. Finally, direct ablation of the triggering site required radiofrequency delivery within the PVs, risking PV narrowing or occlusion.

Proximal disconnection by segmental pulmonary vein isolation

Following the introduction of a multipolar, circular catheter positioned at the ostium of the PVs, an ablation technique aiming at electrical disconnection of muscular fibers between the PVs and the LA was described again by the Bordeaux group [13] (Figure 9.1b). The circular catheter allowed the recording of PV potentials around the PV circumference to guide ablation at the site of earliest activation, even in the absence of an active trigger since a characteristic PV potential could be recorded. Radiofrequency delivery at the site of LA–PV connections resulted in electrical isolation of the PVs,

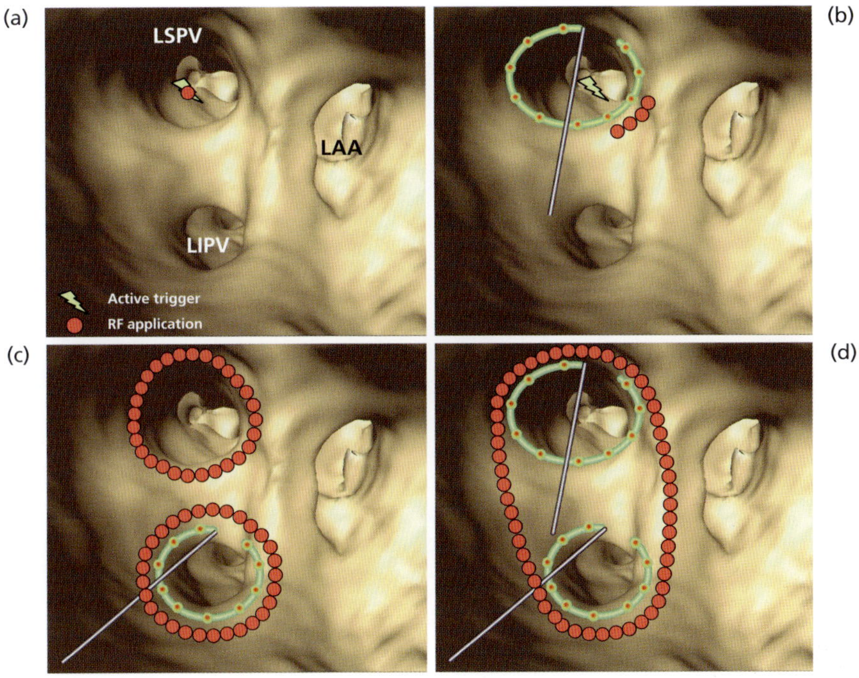

Figure 9.1 Schematic depiction of different ablation techniques targeting the lateral PVs. (a) Focal or direct ablation (red dot) of an active trigger within the lateral superior PV (LSPV). (b) Segmental ostial isolation of an active trigger in the LSPV. (c) "One-by-one" linear ablation of the PVs with (left inferior PV, LIPV) or without the endpoint of complete electrical disconnection (LSPV) as proven by a simultaneous recording from a circular PV mapping catheter. (d) Simultanous isolation of the ipsilateral PVs by a long "point-by-point" lesion encircling the antrum area of the lateral PVs. LAA, left atrial appendage, RF, radio frequency.

preventing further AF induction by trigger isolation [14–20]. A limitation of this technique is the rather high recurrence rate due to transient LA–PV block [21–23].

Pulmonary vein ablation

Circumferential PV ablation using 3D electroanatomic mapping was first described by Pappone et al. [24] (Figure 9.1c). Initially, the lesion set was limited to wide (> 0.5 cm outside the PV ostia) circumferential lesions around and outside the PV ostia, but over time it was modified with wider (1–2 cm outside PV ostia) circumferential lesions [25]. Additional effects such as vagal denervation and additional linear lesions such as posterior lines connecting the PVs and the mitral isthmus line were added [26]. Patients with a vagal reflex during radiofrequency application were reported to have a better clinical outcome. The acute endpoint of the ablation was either amplitude reduction by < 80% or an absolute value of < 0.1 mV within the ablation area.

The double/single Lasso technique

The initial rational for the development of a technique with two circular catheters in both ipsilateral PVs was to prevent PV ostial narrowing by isolating the PVs more ostially. It was initially performed by fluoroscopically guided, extensive, encircling isolation of the ipsilateral superior and inferior PVs [27] (Figure 9.1d). The combination of 3D electroanatomic mapping information of the LA and the so-called "double Lasso" technique led to an ablation strategy that encircles the ipsilateral PVs at the so-called "antrum" level with the endpoint of PV isolation [7]. This ablation approach combines the advantages of both the segmental and circumferential ablation approaches, namely the ease of endpoint validation as assessed by elimination of the PV potentials and the ablation line outside

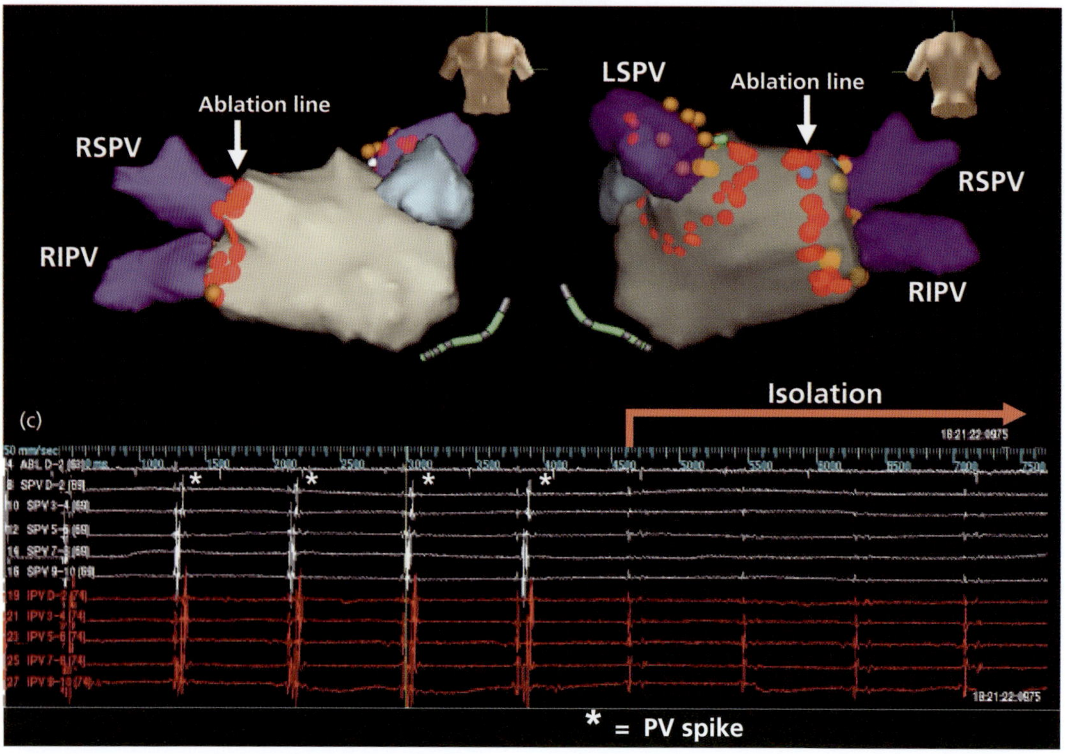

Figure 9.2 Electrical isolation of pulmonary veins (PVs) using NavX®. Posterioanterior (a) and anterioposterior (b) projection of the LA and the adjacent PVs reconstructed using NAVx technology (St. Jude Medical). (c) Recording from the two circumferential PV mapping catheters during radiofrequency delivery resulting in the simultaneous elimination of the typical PV potential (asterisk) after closure of the last conduction gap along the isolation line. LSPV, left superior PV; RIPV, right inferior PV; RSPV, right superior PV.

the PV–LA junction with a low risk of PV injury. After 3D reconstruction of the LA, an angiographic visualization is performed of both the superior and inferior ipsilateral PVs in right and left anterior oblique (RAO and LAO, respectively) projections using injection contrast medium. Special attention should be given to precisely identify the ostia of the PVs by implementing ostial markers into the 3D LA reconstruction. Subsequently, the ablation is performed guided by the 3D mapping system and validated by a simultaneous recording from the two PV mapping catheters to identify gaps along the ablation line (Figure 9.2). Since this technique requires three catheters within the LA for simultaneous recording from both PVs plus ablation, a modified approach is limited to only one circular catheter, which is moved between the ipsilateral PVs. Further precision can be achieved through the fusion of a previously acquired 3D MRI or CT scan with the 3D reconstruction of the mapping system, which has the potential to reduce overall radiation exposure.

Pulmonary vein antrum isolation guided by intracardiac echocardiography

The rationale of using ICE during ablation for AF relies on the ability to identify individual anatomy in real time, overcoming the visualization limitation associated with fluoroscopy [12]. At the moment available systems only depict 2D images, but instant 3D ICE is nearly ready to be introduced in to the "visualization" armamentarium. Two-dimensional ICE is valuable in positioning the mapping circular catheter around the PV opening, and provides an opportunity to optimize energy titration by following the generation of microbubbles, which reflect tissue overheating. However, this is only possible when using non-irrigated ablation catheters, since the saline flow during irrigated-tip ablation excludes this assessment. By monitoring the changes of the target tissue during lesion formation directly, this approach can potentially avoid complications such as perforation, tissue disruption, charring, and clot formation, as well as atrial esophageal fistula. Delineated by ICE, a linear lesion is deployed by a roving ablation electrode that includes both the ostia of the ipsilateral PVs and larger portions of the LA posterior wall. At each location, ablation is performed based on the electrograms recorded on the circular catheter. The endpoint of such a procedure is the electrical isolation of the antrum of all PVs, demonstrated by moving a circular mapping catheter into various positions.

New tools for ablation

The majority of reports on ablation procedures targeting the PVs describe the deployment of radiofrequency current applications. The ablation techniques differ according to the size of the ablation electrode, the amount of deployed energy, and the use of irrigation. The most important problem, which exists for all radiofrequency catheter types, is reconduction across a previously complete lesion or – in other words – the rather high level of transientonly ablation effects [21–23]. In addition, the point-by-point delineation of linear lesions is a time-consuming method which is more susceptible to conduction gaps the longer the designed line is.

Balloon-based techniques

To achieve complete isolation of the PVs with a limited number of applications, several new ablation energies have been investigated – such as (highly intensified) ultrasound, laser, microwave, or cryothermia [28–31]. The majority of techniques are delivered via a balloon, which is positioned at or inside the PV ostium. Depending on the applied catheter design, either circular or arc-shaped energy applications are delivered to achieve electrical disconnection. Further studies are needed to verify if the expectations of an easy-to-use, "single shot", and time-efficient PV isolation tool are met by currently investigated devices.

Remote catheter navigation

As an additional tool to perform catheter ablation procedures, magnetic navigation was introduced nearly 3 years ago. It is based on two permanent magnets that create a uniform magnetic field (0.08 T) [32]. The ablation catheter has three small permanent magnets positioned at the tip that align with the direction of the external magnetic field. By changing the orientation of the outer magnets, the orientation of the magnetic field changes and thereby leads to deflection of the catheter. In addition, a catheter advancer system (Cardiodrive® unit, Stereotaxis, Inc.) is used to allow remote catheter navigation without the need for manual manipulation. Thus, the system allows remote-controlled mapping and ablation from the control room [33].

In general, the feasibility of this system to perform remote-controlled ablation of AF has been demonstrated [34]. Further investigation and technical improvements of the magnetically steerable catheters are, however, needed to prove the effectiveness and applicability in larger patient populations beyond initial single-center study protocols. The system allows the integration of both electroanatomic mapping information (including merging with 3D imaging) and navigation on a single screen, which should at least theoretically facilitate the procedure (Figure 9.3).

Conclusion

The PVs and the adjacent atrial myocardium play an important role in the initiation, but also in the maintenance, of AF. The challenges for an optimal technique targeting the PVs are the reliable identification of the so-called "antrum" area, followed by a "tailored" energy deployment that achieves (with as few applications as possible) a long-term isolating lesion around the antrum area that avoids extracardiac damage. The definition of an acute endpoint for the energy delivery of a given ablation technique allows peers to replicate the technique and thereby prove the applicability to a larger patient cohort beyond single-center experiences. In addition, the results of the follow-up period should be carefully monitored in short-term intervals, and "strong" endpoints such as stable sinus rhythm in the absence of any antiarrhythmic medication,

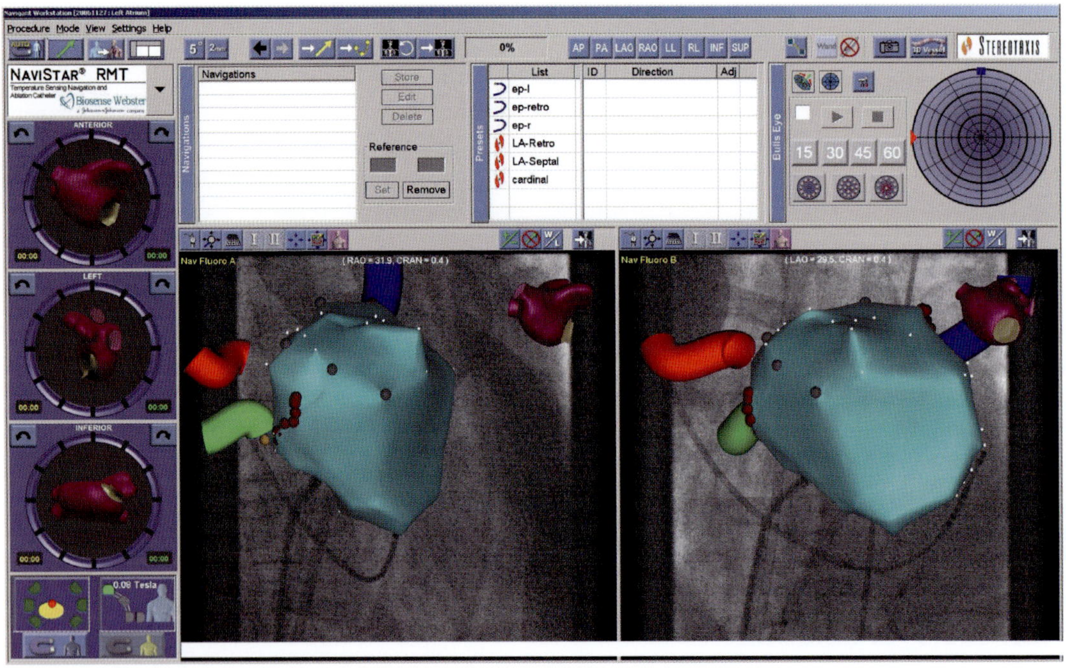

Figure 9.3 New tools for catheter ablation. Screenshot from a workstation of the Niobe® magnetic navigation system (Stereotaxis, Inc.) displaying a 3D electroanatomic reconstruction of the CARTO RMT system (Biosense Webster) within the corresponding right anterior oblique (RAO) and left anterior oblique (LAO) fluoroscopic images. Changing the orientation of the outer magnetic field (0.08 T) results in the movement of a magnetically equipped catheter with real-time depiction.

rather than "free of AF" (which could also mean constant pacing, atrial tachycardia, or junctional escape), must be demanded. The potential complications of any ablation technique should also be carefully assessed since recent consequences have taught us to consider structures beyond the transmural myocardial lesion itself.

References

1 Jais P, Haissaguerre M, Shah DC, Chouairi S, Gencel L, Honcini M, Clementy J. A focal source of atrial fibrillation treated by discrete radiofrequency ablation. *Circulation* 1997;**95**:572–6.

2 Haissaguerre M, Jais P, Shah DC, et al. Spontaneous initiation of atrial fibrillation by ectopic beats originating in the pulmonary veins. *N Engl J Med* 1998;**339**(10):659–66.

3 Cox JL, Boineau JP, Schuessler RB, Kater KM, Lappas DG. Five-year experience with the maze procedure for atrial fibrillation. *Ann Thoracic Surg* 1993;**56**(4):814–23.

4 Hatala R, Weiss C, Koschyk DH, Siebels J, Cappato R, Kuck KH. Radiofrequency catheter ablation of left atrial tachycardia originating within the pulmonary vein in a patient with dextrocardia. *Pacing Clin Electrophysiol* 1996;**19**(6):999–1002.

5 Wijffels MCEF, Kirchhof CJHJ, Dorland R, Allessie MA. Atrial fibrillation begets atrial fibrillation: a study in awake chronically instrumented goats. *Circulation* 1995; **92**:1954–68.

6 Todd DM, Skanes AC, Guiraudon G, Guiraudon C, Krahn AD, Yee R, Klein GJ. Role of the posterior left atrium and pulmonary veins in human lone atrial fibrillation: electrophysiological and pathological data from patients undergoing atrial fibrillation surgery. *Circulation* 2003;**108**(25):3108–14.

7 Ouyang F, Baensch D, Ernst S, et al. Complete isolation of left atrium surrounding the pulmonary veins: new insights from the double lasso technique in paroxysmal atrial fibrillation. *Circulation* 2004;**110**:2090–6.

8 Saito T, Waki K, Becker AE. Left atrial myocardial extension onto pulmonary veins in humans: anatomic observations relevant for atrial arrhythmias. *J Cardiovasc Electrophysiol* 2000;**1**:888–94.

9 Moubarak JB, Rozwadowski JV, Strzalka CT, et al. Pulmonary veins–left atrial junction: anatomic and histological study. *Pacing Clin Electrophysiol* 2000;**23**(11): 1836–8.

10 Ho SY, Cabrera JA, Tran VH, Farre J, Anderson RH, Sanchez-Quintana D. Architecture of the pulmonary veins: relevance to radiofrequency ablation. *Heart* 2001; **86**:265–70.

11 Kato R, Lickfett L, Meininger G, et al. Pulmonary vein anatomy in patients undergoing catheter ablation of atrial fibrillation: lessons learned by use of magnetic resonance imaging. *Circulation* 2003;**107**(15):2004–10.

12 Marrouche NF, Martin DO, Wazni O, et al. Phased-array intracardiac echocardiography monitoring during pulmonary vein isolation in patients with atrial fibrillation: impact on outcome and complications. *Circulation* 2003;**107**(21):2710–16.

13 Haissaguerre M, Jais P, Shah DC, et al. Electrophysiological end point for catheter ablation of atrial fibrillation initiated from multiple pulmonary venous foci. *Circulation* 2000;**101**(12):1409–17.

14 Chen SA, Tai CT, Tsai CF, Hsieh MH, Ding YA, Chang MS. Radiofrequency catheter ablation of atrial fibrillation initiated by pulmonary vein ectopic beats. *J Cardiovasc Electrophysiol* 2000;**11**:218–27.

15 Schneider MA, Ndrepepa G, Zrenner B, Karch MR, Schreieck J, Deisenhofer I, Schmitt C. Noncontact mapping-guided catheter ablation of atrial fibrillation associated with left atrial ectopy. *J Cardiovasc Electrophysiol* 2000;**11**(4):475–9.

16 Oral H, Knight BP, Ozaydin M, et al. Segmental ostial ablation to isolate the pulmonary veins during atrial fibrillation: feasibility and mechanistic insights. *Circulation* 2002;**106**(10):1256–62.

17 Arentz T, von Rosenthal J, Blum T, et al. Feasibility and safety of pulmonary vein isolation using a new mapping and navigation system in patients with refractory atrial fibrillation. *Circulation* 2003;**108**(20):2484–90.

18 Oral H, Scharf C, Chugh A, et al. Catheter ablation for paroxysmal atrial fibrillation: segmental pulmonary vein ostial ablation versus left atrial ablation. *Circulation* 2003;**108**(19):2355–60.

19 Kistler PM, Sanders P, Fynn SP, et al. Electrophysiological and electrocardiographic characteristics of focal atrial tachycardia originating from the pulmonary veins: acute and long-term outcomes of radiofrequency ablation. *Circulation* 2003;**108**(16):1968–75.

20 Deisenhofer I, Schneider MA, Bohlen-Knauf M, et al. Circumferential mapping and electric isolation of pulmonary veins in patients with atrial fibrillation. *Am J Cardiol* 2003;**91**(2):159–63.

21 Gerstenfeld EP, Callans DJ, Dixit S, Zado E, Marchlinski FE. Incidence and location of focal atrial fibrillation triggers in patients undergoing repeat pulmonary vein isolation: implications for ablation strategies. *J Cardiovasc Electrophysiol* 2003;**14**(7):685–90.

22 Cappato R, Negroni S, Pecora D, et al. Prospective assessment of late conduction recurrence across radiofrequency lesions producing electrical disconnection at the pulmonary vein ostium in patients with atrial fibrillation. *Circulation* 2003;**108**(13):1599–604.

23 Verma A, Kilicaslan F, Pisano E, et al. Response of atrial fibrillation to pulmonary vein antrum isolation is directly related to resumption and delay of pulmonary vein conduction. *Circulation* 2005;**112**(5):627–35.

24 Pappone C, Rosanio S, Oreto G, et al. Circumferential radiofrequency ablation of pulmonary vein ostia: a new anatomic approach for curing atrial fibrillation. Circulation 2000;**102**(21):2619–28.

25 Pappone C, Oreto G, Rosanio S, et al. Atrial electroanatomic remodeling after circumferential radiofrequency pulmonary vein ablation: efficacy of an anatomic approach in a large cohort of patients with atrial fibrillation. *Circulation* 2001;**104**(21):2539–44.

26 Pappone C, Santinelli V, Manguso F, et al. Pulmonary vein denervation enhances long-term benefit after circumferential ablation for paroxysmal atrial fibrillation. Circulation 2004;**109**(3):327–34.

27 Takahashi A, Iesaka Y, Takahashi Y, et al. Electrical connections between pulmonary veins: implication for ostial ablation of pulmonary veins in patients with paroxysmal atrial fibrillation. *Circulation* 2002;**105**(25):2998–3003.

28 Antz M, Chun KJ, Ouyang F, Kuck KH. Ablation of atrial fibrillation in humans using a balloon-based ablation system: identification of the site of phrenic nerve damage using Pacing maneuvers and CARTO. *J Cardiovasc Electrophysiol* 2006;**17**(11):1242–5.

29 Natale A, Pisano E, Shewchik J, et al. First human experience with pulmonary vein isolation using a through-the-balloon circumferential ultrasound ablation system for recurrent atrial fibrillation. *Circulation* 2000;**102**(16): 1879–82.

30 Fried NM, Tsitlik A, Rent KC, Berger RD, Lardo AC, Calkins H, Halperin HR. Laser ablation of the pulmonary veins by using a fiberoptic balloon catheter: implications for treatment of paroxysmal atrial fibrillation. *Lasers Surg Med* 2001;**28**(3):197–203.

31 Vogt J, Dorszewski A, Luong Thanh L, Heintze J, Buschler H, Horstkotte D. Isolation of pulmonary veins with a new 28/23 mm cryoballoon in atrial fibrillation – first experience. *Eur Heart J* 2006;**27**:A5073.

32 Faddis MN, Blume W, Finney J, et al. Novel, magnetically guided catheter for endocardial mapping and radiofrequency catheter ablation. *Circulation* 2002;**106**:2980–5.

33 Ernst S, Ouyang F, Linder C, et al. Initial experience with remote catheter ablation using a novel magnetic navigation system. *Circulation* 2004;**109**(12):1472–5.

34 Pappone C, Vicedomini G, Manguso F, et al. Robotic magnetic navigation for atrial fibrillation ablation. *J Am Coll Cardiol* 2006;**47**(7):1390–400.

10

CHAPTER 10

Techniques of linear lesion for atrial fibrillation ablation

Mélèze Hocini, Kang Teng Lim, Prashanthan Sanders, Pierre Jaïs, Mark D. O'Neill, Yoshihide Takahashi, Anders Jönsson, Seiichiro Matsuo, Sébastien Knecht, Leonardo Arantès, Jacques Clémenty, & Michel Haïssaguerre

Introduction

Catheter ablation of atrial fibrillation (AF) has emerged from being an experimental therapy to a potentially curative option for patients with AF over the last decade. The discovery that the pulmonary veins (PVs) act as a dominant source of triggers and drivers of AF, and the subsequent success of the PV isolation procedure to cure paroxysmal AF and significantly reduce AF burden, have revitalized the search for other catheter ablation strategies/techniques to cure not only paroxysmal but persistent and chronic AF [1]. There are three principal techniques for catheter ablation of AF: PV isolation, ablation of left atrial electrophysiological targets, and left linear ablation. Although these steps have been shown to be effective individually, combining these approaches is optimal and has led to improved clinical outcome in most cases of persistent/permanent AF.

While left atrial linear ablation is clearly indicated in the case of macroreentrant tachycardia, the respective place and order of linear lesion and ablation of left atrial electrophysiological targets to modify the left atrium (LA) substrate during AF is under evaluation. The addition of linear lines compared to PV isolation alone has been shown to increase the efficacy of catheter ablation for both paroxysmal and persistent AF [1–5]. The technical difficulty of linear lesion argues against the use of this technique early in the course of catheter ablation procedures. Furthermore, inability to achieve a complete line may be proarrhythmic.

This chapter describes currently used techniques to perform and evaluate linear lesions by catheter ablation. In addition, the consequences of linear lesion are discussed in detail.

Pulmonary vein ablation

In our institution, electrical isolation of all PVs and ablation of cavotricuspid isthmus is performed in all patients undergoing catheter ablation of AF. The techniques used for PV ablation involve the use of a circular catheter (Lasso®, Biosense Webster, Diamond Bar, CA, USA) to map and guide ablation as previously described [2]. In our experience, power can be limited to 30 W, using irrigation rates of 5–20 ml/min to achieve the desired power delivery, and is generally sufficient with temperature limited to 50°C. Electrical isolation of the PV is confirmed by either elimination or dissociation of PV potentials. Depending on operator preference, adjunctive modalities – including three-dimensional

Catheter Ablation of Atrial Fibrillation Edited by Etienne Aliot, Michel Haïssaguerre and Warren M. Jackman

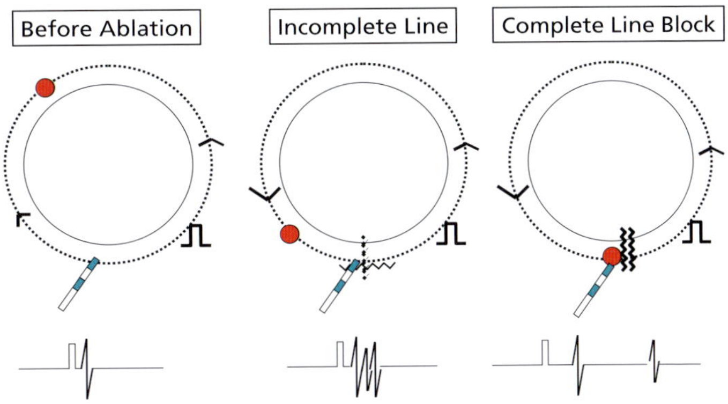

Figure 10.1 Schematic diagram showing the principles of assessing linear blocks after ablation. Before ablation, wavefronts from the pacing stimulus propagate in a clockwise and anticlockwise direction to converge at the high lateral atrium. In the presence of an incomplete line, the latest activation is anticipated lateral to the ablation line. Following complete linear block, the activation detour occurs in the opposite direction resulting in a corridor of widely spaced double potential and the longest delay recorded on the line. The sites of latest activation during pacing from the stimulus site are indicated by red dots. Local on-line electrograms are given below.

electroanatomic mapping (Carto®, Biosense Webster), Ensite NavX® (St. Jude Medical, St. Paul, MN, USA), or intracardiac echo – may be use to guide PV isolation with the aim of achieving electrical disconnection of PVs from the LA.

Cavotricuspid isthmus ablation is performed using a linear dragging technique with an endpoint of bidirectional conduction block in sinus rhythm, a corridor of double potentials on the line, demonstration of an activation detour in the opposite direction, and confirmation with pacing techniques. Assessment techniques for cavotricuspid isthmus ablation represent the paradigm for complete linear ablation and are illustrated in Figure 10.1.

Indications for linear lesion

Linear ablation is considered during AF ablation if AF persists after PV isolation and electrogram-based LA ablation or if macroreentrant tachycardia develops around the mitral annulus or the left PVs [3]. Used in this context, linear ablation is performed in up to 40% of patients with paroxysmal AF and almost all patients with persistent or permanent AF. While this is the approach that we have used to guide the extent of ablation, another acceptable approach in patients with paroxysmal AF would be to reserve substrate modification to those with clinical recurrence after PV isolation. In addition, the relative roles of linear ablation compared to the use of ablation targeting complex fractionated electrograms in an individual patient may still evolve with progress of AF mapping and ablation technology increasing the rate of achieving linear block.

Technical approach to linear ablation

The following catheters are introduced: (1) the quadripolar steerable catheter (Xtrem®, Ela Medical, Montrouge, France) in the coronary sinus, and (2) a 3.5 mm tip externally irrigated ablation catheter (Celsius Thermocool®, Biosense Webster). The ablation catheter is introduced into the LA through the long sheath. The long sheath is continuously flushed with heparinized saline and maintained within the right atrium whenever it is not required for stability in the LA. A variety of navigation tools, such as LocaLisa® (Medtronic, Minneapolis, MN, USA), NavX® (Endocardial Solution, Inc., St. Paul, MN, USA), or the electroanatomic mapping system Carto (Biosense, Webster), can be used adjunctively to fluoroscopy to assist with the procedure [6,7]. These techniques may help determine the position of the ablation catheter (anterior, posterior) relative to the mapping electrodes and potentially aid in evaluating the completeness of linear lesion. These have been demonstrated to significantly reduce the fluoroscopic exposure during linear ablation [6–8]. Whether the use of such tools is required for all patients is debatable as they are costly.

Post-ablation management

In the absence of concurrent indications, all antiarrhythmic drugs should be stopped following ablation in paroxysmal AF but are continued for 1–3 months in patients with permanent AF. Oral anticoagulation is maintained for at least 3 months in patients with paroxysmal AF and 6 months in patients with persistent/permanent AF. After this period, in the absence of arrhythmia, cessation of anticoagulation is considered. The clinical success of the procedure was evaluated at 3, 6, 9 and 12 months. A successful outcome is defined as the absence of *any* atrial arrhythmia after the third month (AF, atrial tachycardia, or flutter) without the use of *any* antiarrhythmic agents.

Left atrial linear ablation for substrate modification

Limited linear ablation within the LA is performed as a means of substrate modification. The aim is to join anatomic structures within the LA to form barriers to fibrillatory wave propagation. Although several sequences have been performed, presented below are linear lesions that have been recently evaluated at our institution: mitral isthmus ablation, ablation at the LA roof, and ablation of the anterior LA. It is necessary to confirm the completeness of these lines by validated electrophysiological methods, which will be discussed below. An incomplete line may not only be ineffective but may result in proarrhythmia [9–12].

Mitral isthmus ablation

Procedure

Mitral isthmus ablation is performed by creating a linear ablation line joining the lateral mitral annulus to the left inferior PV (LIPV) [2]. To undertake this line, the coronary sinus (CS) catheter is positioned to bracket the potential linear lesion between its proximal and distal bipoles. The ablation catheter is introduced through the long sheath to achieve stability, it is bent with a 90–180° curve, and ablation is commenced at the ventricular edge of the lateral mitral annulus where the atrioventricular electrogram shows a 1 : 1 to 2 : 1 ratio. The sheath and catheter assembly is then rotated clockwise to extend the lesion to the LIPV ostium. Occasionally the proximal end of this ablation line needs to be anchored to a more anterior site and is extended to the posterior root of the left atrial appendage (LAA). Ablation in general is commenced at around 3 or 4 o'clock on the mitral annulus and reaches 2 to 3 o'clock at the upper end of the line (Figure 10.2). Radiofrequency (RF) energy is delivered for 90–120 s at each site. Endocardial ablation is performed with a flow rate of 17–60 ml/min, a target temperature of 50°C, and power of 30–37 W. The stability of the catheter needs to be monitored during RF applications using electrograms and intermittent fluoroscopy to avoid inadvertent displacement, which can result in high energy delivery within the LIPV or LAA.

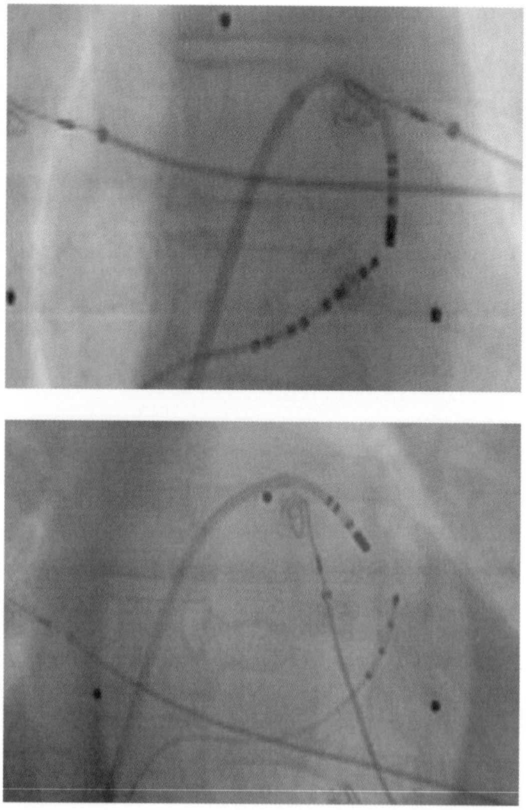

Figure 10.2 These radiographs show the motion utilized to move the ablation catheter along the mitral isthmus from the mitral annulus to the left inferior PV.

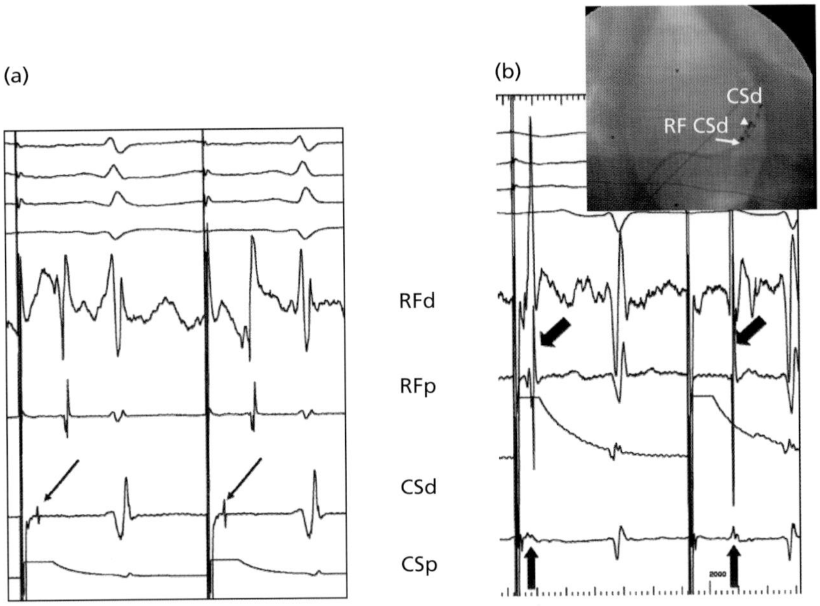

Figure 10.3 (a) The conduction delay recorded at the mitral isthmus ablation line (RFd and RFp) during coronary sinus proximal (CSp) pacing. Persisting epicardial conduction is observed in the coronary sinus distal (CSd). (b) Radiofrequency (RF) delivery through the CS (epicardial approach) results in complete mitral isthmus block.

The effect of each RF application is assessed on the local electrogram during pacing from the proximal bipole of the CS catheter (located immediately septal of the line) to maximize conduction delay.

Splitting of the local potentials, resulting in an increase in the delay from the pacing artefact, is considered evidence of an effective local lesion. After the initial attempt to create this line, mapping is performed to identify and ablate gaps. If the initial attempt failed to produce complete block, ablation needs to be performed more laterally, near the base of the appendage. Persisting epicardial conduction is suspected when linear ablation results in an endocardial delay but not in the adjacent bipole of the CS catheter (lateral of the line) (Figure 10.3a). In this scenario, to achieve complete block, RF application is also required within the CS enface with the endocardial application site (Figure 10.3b). Ablation within the CS is required in approximately two-thirds of patients, that is, the success rate of endocardial ablation alone is 40%. CS ablation is performed with a flow rate of 17–60 ml/min, a target temperature of 50 °C, and power of 20–25 W. The potential risk of circumflex artery injury and cardiac tamponade related to CS ablation, nevertheless this is outweighed by the proarrhythmic risk associated with incomplete mitral isthmus block. CS ablation represents a new paradigm for linear ablation in that epicardial ablation is required to complete the endocardial lines; perhaps this may apply to roof or anterior lines too.

Endpoint of ablation

The endpoint of ablation is the achievement of a bidirectional mitral isthmus conduction block, demonstrated using criteria similar to those previously described for cavotricuspid isthmus block:

1 The presence of widely separated, "on-line" double potentials along the length of the ablation line during CS pacing septal of the line.

2 Mapping the activation detour during pacing from either side of the line.

3 Differential pacing to distinguish slow conduction across the isthmus from complete block.

The techniques used for differential pacing have been described elsewhere. In brief, the distal bipole of the CS catheter is placed just septal to the linear lesion and the ablation catheter is positioned lateral

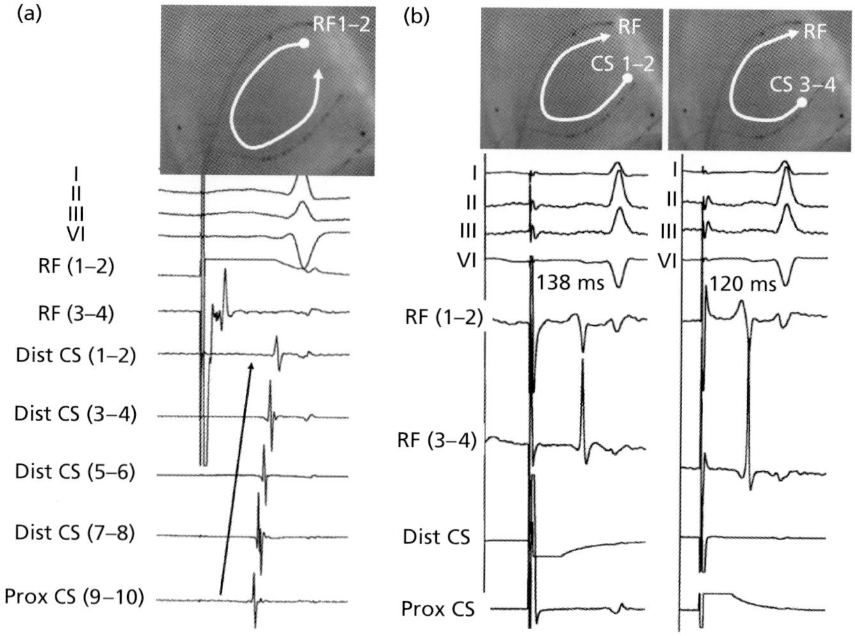

Figure 10.4 Demonstration of mitral isthmus block. (a) During pacing lateral to the ablation line (RF1-2 positioned in the left appendage), the coronary sinus (CS) is activated proximally to distally while being distal-to-proximal with persistent conduction. (b) Pacing from the distal CS results in a delay of 138 ms and represents perimitral activation (shown by the white lines). If the pacing site is switched to the proximal CS it results in a shorter perimitral activation time (120 ms).

to the line on the endocardial surface. Without moving any of the catheters, the pacing site is changed from the distal to proximal bipole of the CS catheter and the stimulus-to-electrogram (endocardial) timing on the ablation catheter is measured. With complete block, the stimulus-to-electrogram timing shortens after shifting the pacing site from the distal to the proximal bipole (Figure 10.4), while it lengthens in the presence of slowed conduction. The average conduction delay after achieving complete block has been 151 ± 26 ms during CS pacing. The conduction delay around the mitral annulus varies according to individuals and is related to LA dimension and LA conduction velocity [13]. A delay of 200 ms does not necessarily mean that a block has been achieved and caution has to be exercised with differential pacing (proximal and distal CS pacing septal to the line while recording LAA delay) as well as pacing lateral to the line (LAA pacing while recording CS activation). However, we have not observed conduction block with a short delay of < 110 ms.

What to do if linear block is not achieved

During ablation, the persistence of high voltage electrograms or the inability to decrease electrogram amplitude is perceived as indicating thick, resistant atrial tissue more prone to persistent gaps.

When mitral isthmus ablation fails to terminate perimitral flutter, mapping again of the mitral annulus and post pacing interval maneuvers should be performed to ensure that the tachycardia mechanism has not changed. If perimitral flutter is still confirmed without obvious gaps along the endocardium, ablation is required within the distal CS to ablate the epicardial side opposite the initial mitral line. Ablation performed along an approximately 1 cm segment of the distal CS, targeting either fractionated or sharp potential, results in termination of perimitral flutter in most cases. Otherwise, we perform pace termination of the tachycardia because mapping during sinus rhythm (pacing from CS) allows much easier identification of conduction gaps than during tachycardia.

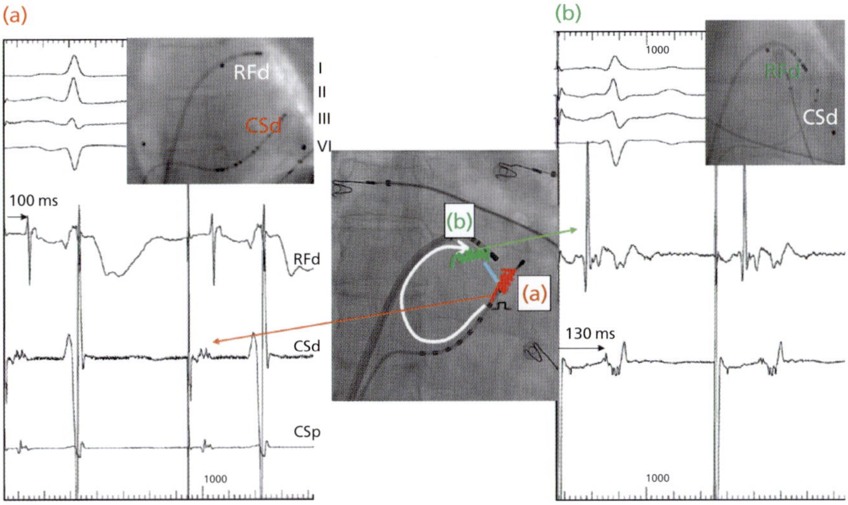

Figure 10.5 Conduction gaps can be seen either at the top or bottom of the mitral isthmus line, with the corresponding electrograms, during an assessment of linear block.

To search for conduction gaps during pacing, we map again carefully along the line at the endocardium, and compare the local delay (spike to local potential) between the two ends of the line, the shortest delay indicating the location of the gaps (Figure 10.5). Sometimes, this is marked by a long fractionated electrogram while in some cases only a local discrete spike is present.

The most frequent gap site is the ostium of the LIPV, presumably because of catheter instability at this location [14]. In addition, an underemphasized part of the left isthmus is the junction between the LIPV and base of the LAA. Its ablation often requires a different movement of the catheter, being nearly horizontal in contrast to the vertical movement initially performed (Figure 10.6).

In cases of resistant mitral isthmus (usually after 30 min of RF application), we defer the procedure to allow edema regression. Linear block is achieved in > 80% of cases after the second procedure.

Validation

We have previously reported the success of this technique in patients with paroxysmal AF [4].

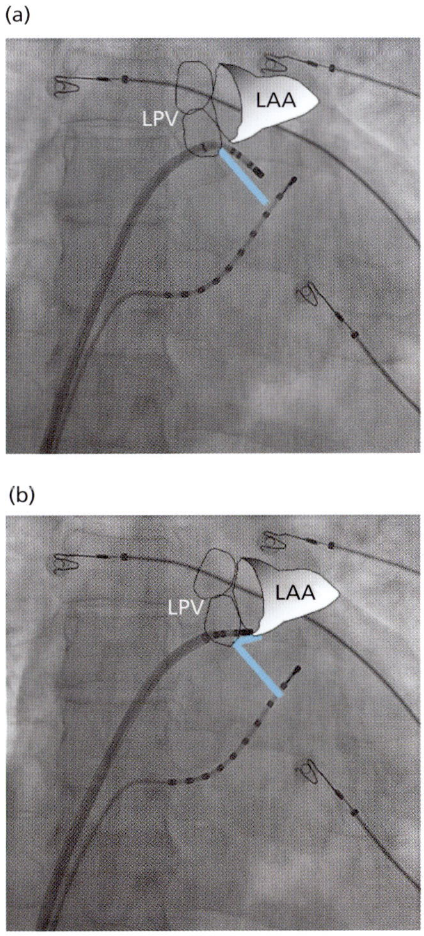

Figure 10.6 (*opposite*) Diagrams illustrating conduction through the posterior ridge responsible for an incomplete mitral isthmus block. LAA, left atrial appendage; LPV, left posterior pulmonary vein.

When 100 consecutive patients with paroxysmal AF underwent PV isolation together with mitral isthmus ablation, and were compared to an equal number of consecutive patients undergoing PV isolation alone, mitral isthmus block was achieved in 92% of the patients. This was required after 20 ± 10 min of endocardial RF, and an additional 5 ± 4 min of epicardial RF application from within the CS in 68%. One year following the last procedure, 87% of patients with mitral isthmus ablation and 69% without ($P = 0.002$) were arrhythmia-free in the absence of antiarrhythmics. The procedure and fluoroscopic durations were 156 ± 47 min and 43 ± 23 min, respectively. In a recent randomized study, Fassini et al. reported a higher success rate in patients with complete than incomplete linear lesion at the mitral isthmus in addition to PV isolation (76% versus 62%, respectively) [11]. In a randomized study of 62 patients undergoing catheter ablation for persistent AF, substrate modification techniques comprising of linear roof and mitral isthmus ablation were associated with significant reduction in the recurrence of AF compared to PV isolation alone (44% versus 77%, respectively; $P = 0.002$) [15].

Roofline ablation

Procedure

Ablation of the LA roof is performed by creation of a contiguous line of ablation lesions joining the superior PVs. RF ablation is performed using an externally irrigated ablation catheter with temperature limited to 50°C. When the catheter is positioned perpendicular to the tissue interface, a delivered power of 25–28 W is used; and when positioned parallel, a delivered power of 30–32 W is used. Irrigation rates vary from 20 to 50 ml/min to deliver the desired power.

To perform this ablation, the ablation catheter is introduced through a long sheath to achieve stability and allow orientation of the catheter tip towards the LA roof. Commencing at the encircling lesion at the left superior PV, the sheath and catheter assembly is rotated clockwise posteriorly and dragged towards the right superior PV (Figure 10.7a). To avoid the risk of atrioesophageal fistula, as recently described [16], ablation is performed cranially at the LA roof. To achieve stability along the cranial LA roof, the catheter may be directed towards the

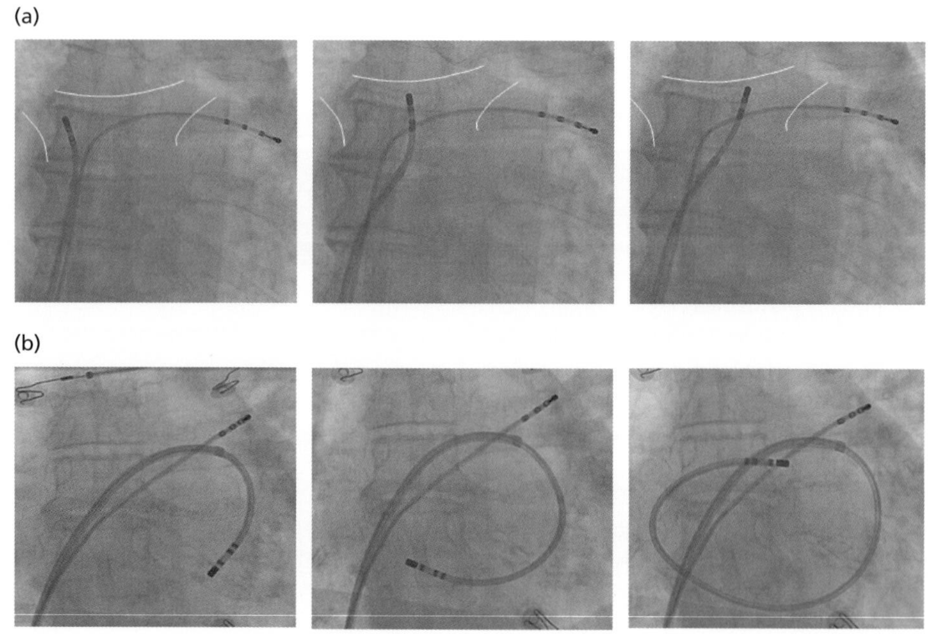

Figure 10.7 (a) A series of radiographs showing the motion utilized to move the ablation catheter along the LA roof from the left to right PV with the pacing catheter placed in the LAA. (b) The ablation catheter looped around the lateral, inferior, septal, and then cranial walls, thus allowing dragging of the catheter by withdrawal from the left to the right superior PV ostia.

left superior PV and the sheath rotated to face the right PVs, or vice versa. Two alternative methods could also be used to reach the LA roof for ablation:

1 The catheter can be looped around the lateral, inferior, septal, and then cranial walls, laying the catheter down along the cranial wall of the LA to allow dragging of the catheter by withdrawal from the left to the right superior PV ostia (Figure 10.7b).

2 The catheter can be maximally deflected to form a tight loop near the left superior PV with the tip facing the right PVs. Releasing the curve positions the catheter tip adjacent to the right superior PV ostia and allows dragging back to the left PV.

Regardless of the technique utilized, ablation is preferably performed cranially rather than posteriorly. RF energy is delivered for 60–120 s at each point while monitoring the on-line potentials. Local potential elimination or formation of double potentials, during pacing or AF, signifies effectiveness of the ablation locally. The stability of the catheter is monitored during RF applications using proximal electrograms, intermittent fluoroscopy, and/or a navigation system to recognize inadvertent displacement of the catheter.

Endpoint of ablation

The electrophysiological endpoint of ablation is achieved when a complete line of block joining the two superior PVs is demonstrated. Evaluation of complete linear block is performed after the restoration of sinus rhythm to allow pacing of the anterior LA adjacent to the line. Anterior LA pacing is achieved by pacing the LAA. Complete linear block is defined by the following criteria:

1 Demonstration by point-by-point mapping of an on-line corridor of double potentials along the entire length of the roof during pacing of the anterior LA (Figure 10.8).

2 Demonstration of an activation detour circumventing first the left PVs, then the right PVs, and activating the posterior wall caudocranially with no conduction through the LA roof (Figure 10.9).

The latter is demonstrated by point-by-point sequential mapping, either conventionally or utilizing electroanatomic mapping (Figure 10.10). In some cases it is difficult to record both double potentials along the ablation line; thus, the second potential is measured at the posterior LA close to the ablation line.

What to do if linear block is not achieved

In situations where there are difficulties achieving linear block, conduction gaps should be searched systematically. This includes:

1 Carefully perform mapping again along the line (at three portions of the roofline near the left superior PV, the middle of the roofline, and near the right superior PV) to determine local delay on the line while pacing the LAA.

2 When no conduction gap is identified, ablation is performed more anteriorly to the previous line (Figure 10.11), in a manner similar to cavotricuspid isthmus ablation.

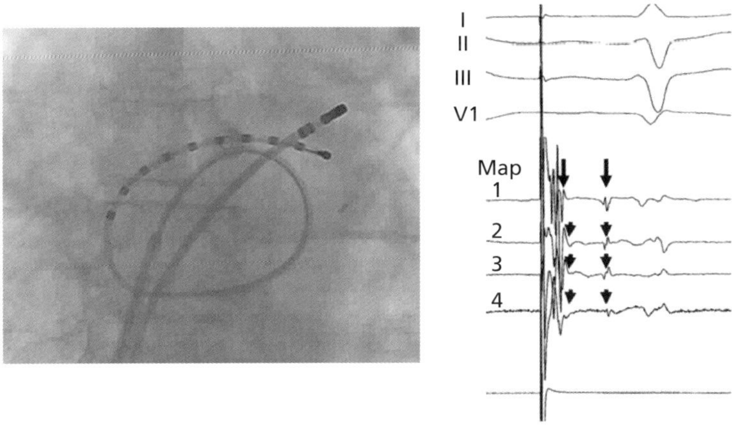

Figure 10.8 Corridor of double potentials during LAA pacing recorded at various sites on the line using a decapolar catheter looped into the LA.

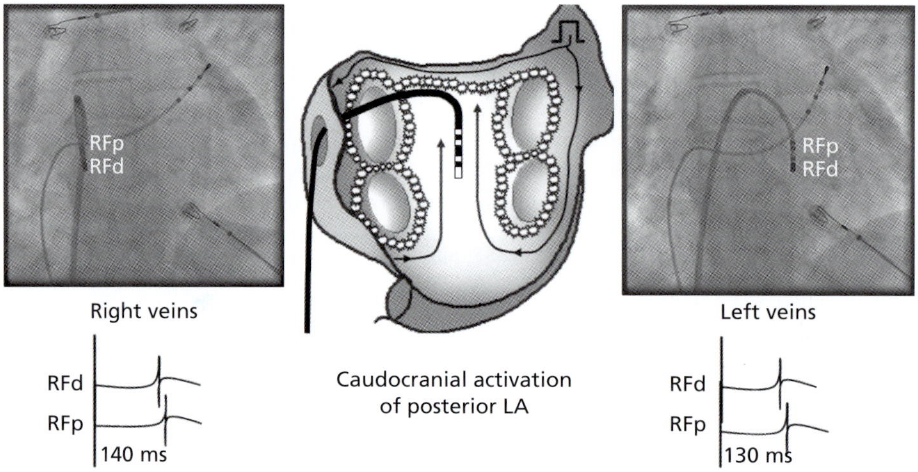

Figure 10.9 A schematic drawing of activation of the posterior left atrium (LA) in a caudocranial way. The left and right panels show a series of radiographs with the catheter placed in the right and left side of the posterior LA, with the expected activation patterns below, shown for a block at the LA roof.

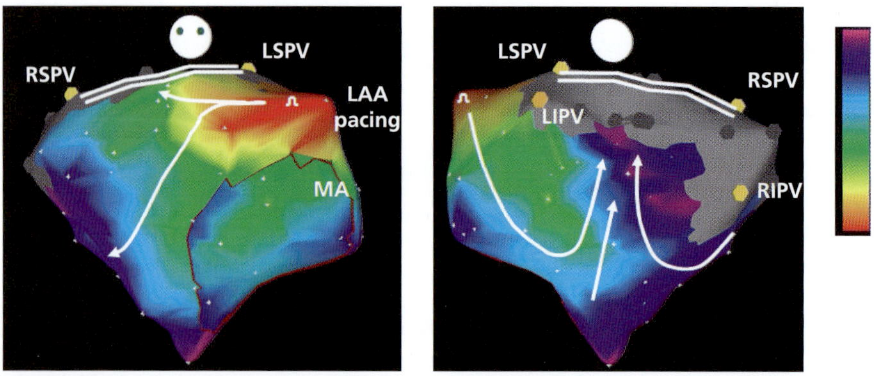

Figure 10.10 Electroanatomic activation maps during LA appendage (LAA) pacing demonstrating the activation detour to the posterior LA wall. LSPV, left superior pulmonary vein; MA, mitral annulus; RIPV, right inferior pulmonary vein; RSPV, right superior pulmonary vein.

Validation

We have previously reported the success of this technique in patients with paroxysmal AF [17]. In this prospective randomized study, 90 patients with drug-refractory paroxysmal AF underwent either PV isolation alone or PV isolation in combination with roofline ablation. Roofline ablation required 12 ± 6 min of RF energy delivery with a fluoroscopic duration of 7 ± 2 min and was performed in 19 ± 7 min. Complete block was confirmed in 43 patients (96%) and resulted in an activation delay that was shorter circumventing the left PVs than the right PVs during LAA pacing (138 ± 15 ms versus 146 ± 25 ms, respectively; $P = 0.01$). At 15 ± 4 months, 87% of the roofline group and 69% of the group with PV isolation alone were arrhythmia-free without antiarrhythmics ($P = 0.04$). Importantly, these results were achieved without significant complications.

Ablation of the anterior left atrial line

Procedure

In our early experience, we attempted an earlier configuration attempted to transect the anterior LA because it was thought at the time that Bachmann's bundle had a special perpetuating role [18]. Linear ablation of the anterior LA is achieved by the following configuration of linear ablation (Figure 10.12):

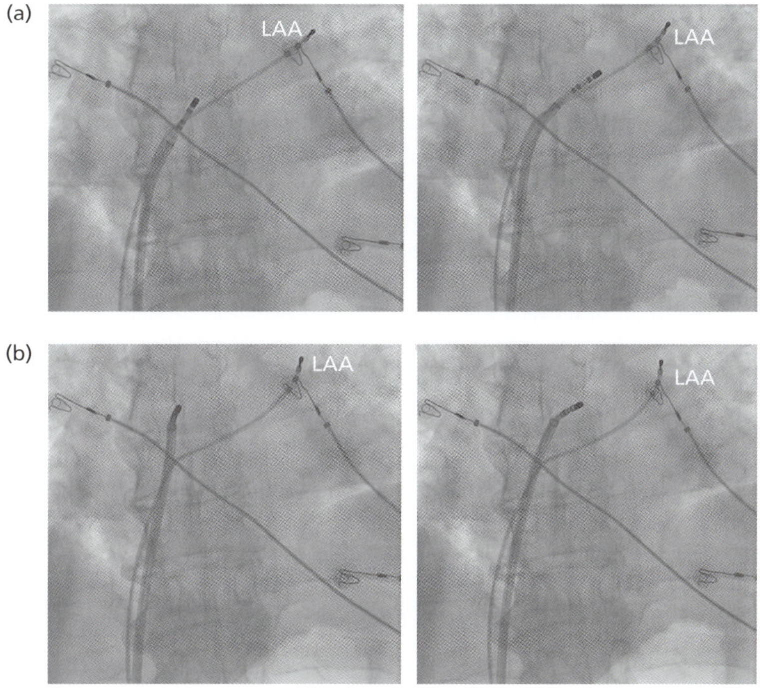

Figure 10.11 (a) A series of radiographs showing the motion utilized to move the ablation catheter along the anterior LA from the anterior mitral to the LA roof. (b) Electroanatomic activation maps during LA appendage (LAA) pacing with a complete block at the anterior LA.

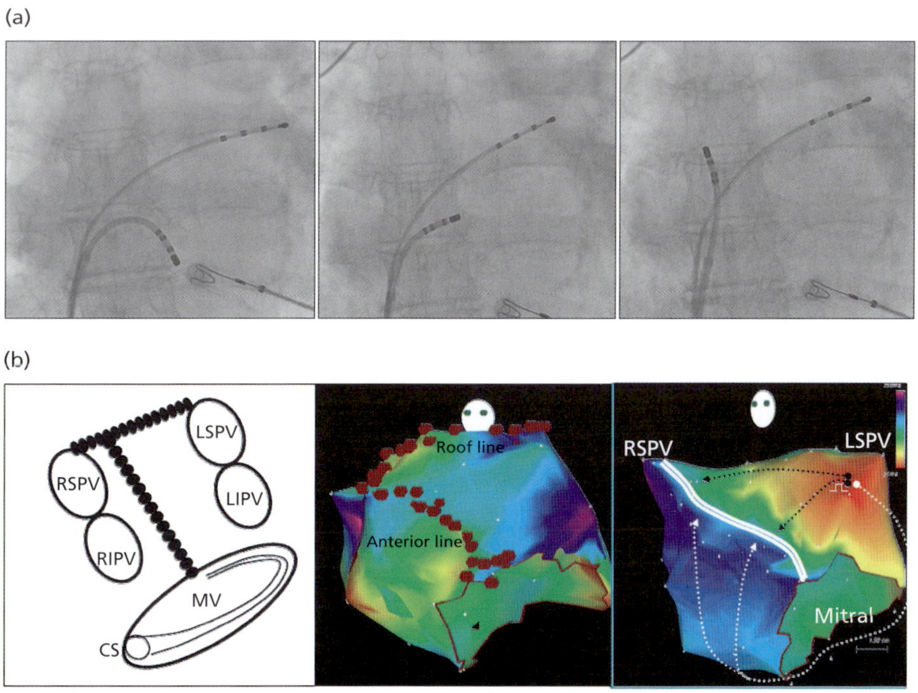

Figure 10.12 (a) Radiographic images of a sequence taken when performing ablation of the anterior LA line. (b) Electroanatomic mapping illustrating the line drawn from the anterior mitral annulus joining the roofline, and assessment of the linear block during LAA pacing. CS, coronary sinus; LIPV, left inferior pulmonary vein; LSPV, left superior pulmonary; MV, mitral valve; RIPV, right inferior pulmonary vein; RSPV, right superior pulmonary vein.

(i) joining the two superior PVs (roofline); and (ii) joining the roofline, as septally as possible, to the anterior mitral annulus (anterior line).

Anterior line ablation is typically performed following ablation of the roofline. The ablation catheter is curved and is advanced to the anterior mitral annulus and ablation is commenced where the atrioventricular electrogram shows a 1 : 1 to 2 : 1 ratio. Gradual anticlockwise torque of the sheath with release of the catheter curvature is used to drag the catheter to the roofline (Figure 10.12a). Further application is performed if mapping suggests the presence of a gap at these sites. RF energy is delivered with power limited to 40–45 W, using irrigation rates of 17–60 ml/min to achieve the desired power delivery, and the temperature limited to 50°C.

Validation

Complete linear block is validated by: (i) demonstrating a corridor of double potentials along the line during pacing lateral to the line; (ii) differential pacing techniques by pacing lateral to the line, as previously described; and (iii) activation mapping to demonstrate an activation detour during either pacing the LA lateral to the ablation line (Figure 10.12b) or during high septal, right atrial pacing when the earliest LA activation is anteroseptal to the ablation line.

This configuration of lesions has been found to be highly effective in termination of AF (up to 60% of patients who were in AF at the time of the procedure). However, anterior line ablation is technically very challenging, with complete linear block confirmed in only 58% of patients. This lesion set resulted in only 64% of patients being arrhythmia-free without the use of antiarrhythmic agents at 28 ± 4 months after the last procedure. In addition, 29% of these patients required further ablation for macroreentry due to recovered gaps in these long ablation lines. In addition, this lesion set was associated with significantly prolonged and altered activation of the LA during sinus rhythm and has thus led to its limited use. As a consequence, we no longer perform this line as part of our catheter ablation strategy.

Conclusion

Linear ablation is the specific treatment for macroreentrant arrhythmia and is an integral part of the strategy to modify the atrial substrate responsible for perpetuating AF. The addition of linear lines has been associated with improved clinical outcomes for patients undergoing catheter ablation. Among the three techniques for catheter ablation, linear ablation is the most technically challenging, justifying its use at the end of AF ablation procedures or when macrorentrant tachycardia occurs. Nevertheless, complete linear block can be achieved in ~90% of patients with operator persistence and ablation within the CS for the mitral isthmus line. Linear lesion at the LA roof is easier to complete and safer, although a little more complex to evaluate. On the other hand, mitral isthmus ablation is more difficult to complete although its evaluation is easier. It is therefore left as the last step in the sequential ablation approach for substrate modification. These lesions represent a "closed chest" surgical procedure and result in a significant improvement in the clinical suppression of arrhythmia. However, further improvement in ablation tools is needed to facilitate a higher achievement of linear block.

References

1 Sheikh I, Krum D, Cooley R, et al. Pulmonary vein isolation and linear lesions in atrial fibrillation ablation. *J Interv Cardiac Electrophysiol* 2007;**17**(2):103–9.

2 Jais P, Hocini M, Hsu LF, et al. Technique and results of linear ablation at the mitral isthmus. *Circulation* 2004; **110**(19):2996–3002.

3 Willems S, Klemm H, Rostock T, et al. Substrate modification combined with pulmonary vein isolation improves outcome of catheter ablation in patients with persistent atrial fibrillation: a prospective randomized comparison. *Eur Heart J* 2006;**27**(23):2871–8.

4 Kottkamp H, Tanner H, Kobza R, et al. Time courses and quantitative analysis of atrial fibrillation episode number and duration after circular plus linear left atrial lesions: trigger elimination or substrate modification: early or delayed cure? *J Am Coll Cardiol* 2004;**44**(4):869–77.

5 Jais P, Hocini M, Sanders P, et al. Long-term evaluation of atrial fibrillation ablation guided by noninducibility. *Heart Rhythm* 2006;**3**(2):140–5.

6 Macle L, Jais P, Scavee C, et al. Pulmonary vein disconnection using the LocaLisa three-dimensional nonfluoroscopic catheter imaging system. *J Cardiovasc Electrophysiol* 2003;**14**:693–7.

7 Rotter M, Takahashi Y, Sanders P, et al. Reduction of fluoroscopy exposure and procedure duration during

ablation of atrial fibrillation using a novel anatomical navigation system. *Eur Heart J* 2005;**26**:1415–21.

8 Takahashi Y, Rotter M, Sanders P, et al. Left atrial linear ablation to modify the substrate of atrial fibrillation using a new nonfluoroscopic imaging system. *Pacing Clin Electrophysiol* 2005;**28**:S90–S93.

9 Ernst S, Ouyang F, Lober F, Antz M, Kuck KH. Catheter-induced linear lesions in the left atrium in patients with atrial fibrillation: an electroanatomic study. *J Am Coll Cardiol* 2003;**42**(7):1271–82.

10 Pappone C, Manguso F, Vicedomini G, et al. Prevention of iatrogenic atrial tachycardia after ablation of atrial fibrillation: a prospective randomized study comparing circumferential pulmonary vein ablation with a modified approach. *Circulation* 2004;**110**(19):3036–42.

11 Fassini G, Riva S, Chiodelli R, et al. Left mitral isthmus ablation associated with PV isolation: long-term results of a prospective randomized study. *J Cardiovasc Electrophysiol* 2005;**16**(11):1150–6.

12 Karch MR, Zrenner B, Deisenhofer I, et al. Freedom from atrial tachyarrhythmias after catheter ablation of atrial fibrillation: a randomized comparison between 2 current ablation strategies. *Circulation* 2005;**111**(22):2875–80.

13 Rotter M, Hsu L, Prashanthan S, et al. Correlation between atrial size and conduction delay during ablation of the tricuspid and mitral isthmuses. *Heart Rhythm* 2004;**1** (Issue 1S).

14 Rostock T, O'Neill M, Sanders P, et al. Characterization of conduction recovery across left atrial linear lesions in patients with paroxysmal and persistent atrial fibrillation. *J Cardiovasc Electrophysiol* 2006;**17**(10):1106–11.

15 Willems S, Klemm H, Rostock T, et al. Substrate modification combined with pulmonary vein isolation improves outcome of catheter ablation in patients with persistent atrial fibrillation: a prospective randomized comparison. *Eur Heart J* 2006;**27**(23):2871–8.

16 Pappone C, Oral H, Santinelli V, et al. Atrio-esophageal fistula as a complication of percutaneous transcatheter ablation of atrial fibrillation. *Circulation* 2004;**109**(22): 2724–6.

17 Hocini M, Jais P, Sanders P, et al. Techniques, evaluation and consequences of linear block at the left atrial roof in paroxysmal atrial fibrillation. A prospective randomized study. *Circulation* 2005;**112**:3688–96.

18 Sanders P, Jais P, Hocini M, et al. Electrophysiologic and clinical consequences of linear catheter ablation to transect the anterior left atrium in patients with atrial fibrillation. *Heart Rhythm* 2004;**1**(2):176–84.

11

CHAPTER 11

Ablation strategies in paroxysmal atrial fibrillation

Isabel Deisenhofer & Claus Schmitt

Introduction

The paroxysmal form of atrial fibrillation (AF) is a fascinating subset of this chameleonic arrhythmia. It might be regarded as an intermediate step in the transition from focal atrial tachycardia to sustained AF. Episodes are often preceded by repetitive focal atrial activity which finally degenerates into AF. There seems to be a general consensus that the triggering initiator is the prevailing arrhythmia feature in the genesis of paroxysmal AF, whereas the substrate maintaining AF seems to play only a secondary role.

Focal approaches to ablate paroxysmal atrial fibrillation using global mapping tools

Right atrium basket mapping

Based on work with mapping right atrial tachycardias [1] our group tried to characterize the onset and activation patterns of paroxysmal AF. Multisite mapping of the right atrium (RA) was performed using a 64-electrode basket catheter (Figure 11.1) [2]. Three-dimensional activation patterns were analyzed using computerized systems (Figures 11.2 and 11.3). According to the criteria introduced by Konings et al. [3,4], AF was classified into three types (Figure 11.2). In contrast to persistent AF, paroxysmal AF had significantly longer AF cycle lengths, less disorganized type III AF, and a smaller number of endocardial breakthroughs from the left atrium (LA) to the RA. In general, the lateral RA wall showed the highest degree of organization, and the septal region the lowest. Coexistence of reentrant and apparently focal activation patterns was documented in paroxysmal AF [2].

Left atrium basket mapping

To better characterize episodes of paroxysmal AF, we performed basket mapping in the LA [5]. Interestingly, specific activation patterns were recorded

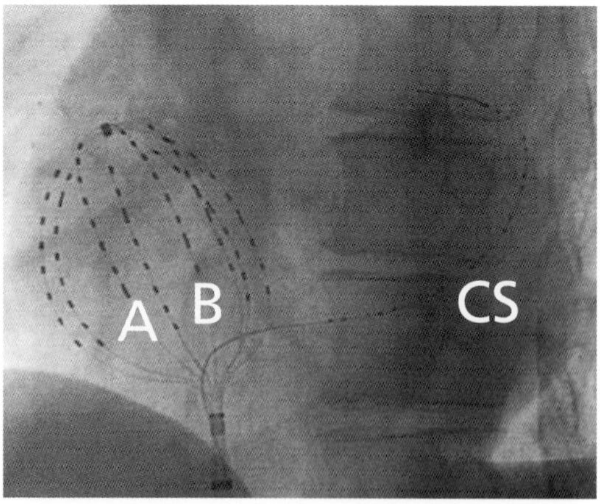

Figure 11.1 Fluoroscopic appearance of a basket catheter and coronary sinus (CS) catheter in a left anterior oblique 45° projection. Spline A and B can be identified by longer marker electrodes in position 8 (spline A) and 7 (spline B). (Reproduced from [2] with permission)

Catheter Ablation of Atrial Fibrillation Edited by Etienne Aliot, Michel Haïssaguerre and Warren M. Jackman
© 2008 Blackwell Publishing, ISBN: 978-1-4501-6349-1.

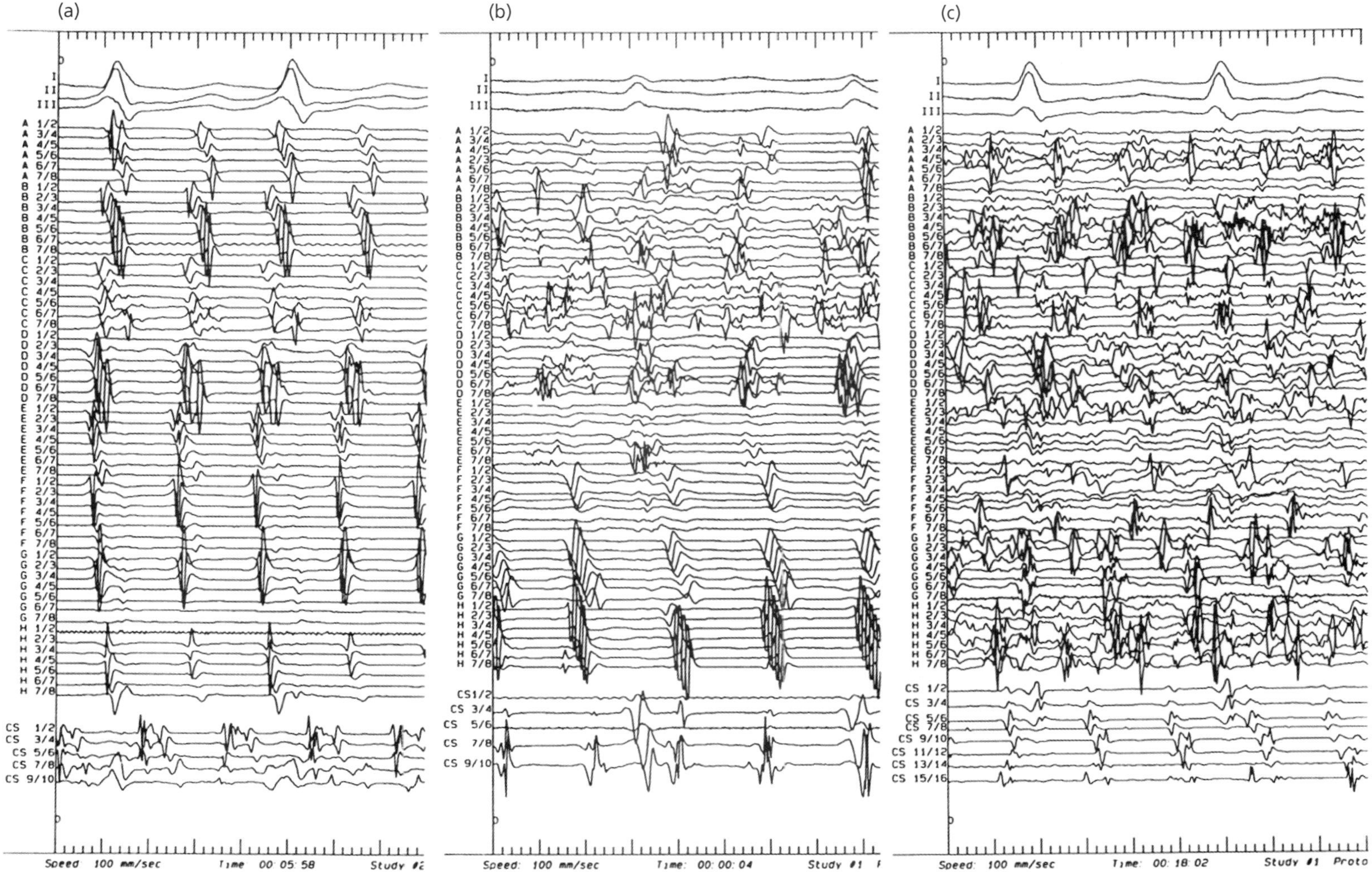

Figure 11.2 Three types of activation observed in the right atrium (RA). Three surface ECG leads, 56 bipolar basket catheter electrograms, and the CS electrograms are shown. (a) Homogeneously regular activation: during a homogeneously regular pattern, the entire RA was activated from a single wavefront emerging from the high anteroseptal area (electrode B1/2). (b) Non-homogeneous activation: types II and III AF are observed along the posterior and septal regions of the RA (splines A–D), whereas the lateral wall (splines G and H) is activated by type I AF. (c) Homogeneously irregular activation: complex activity (AF types II and III) is observed throughout the RA. Splines E and F were located across the tricuspid annulus. (Reproduced from [2] with permission)

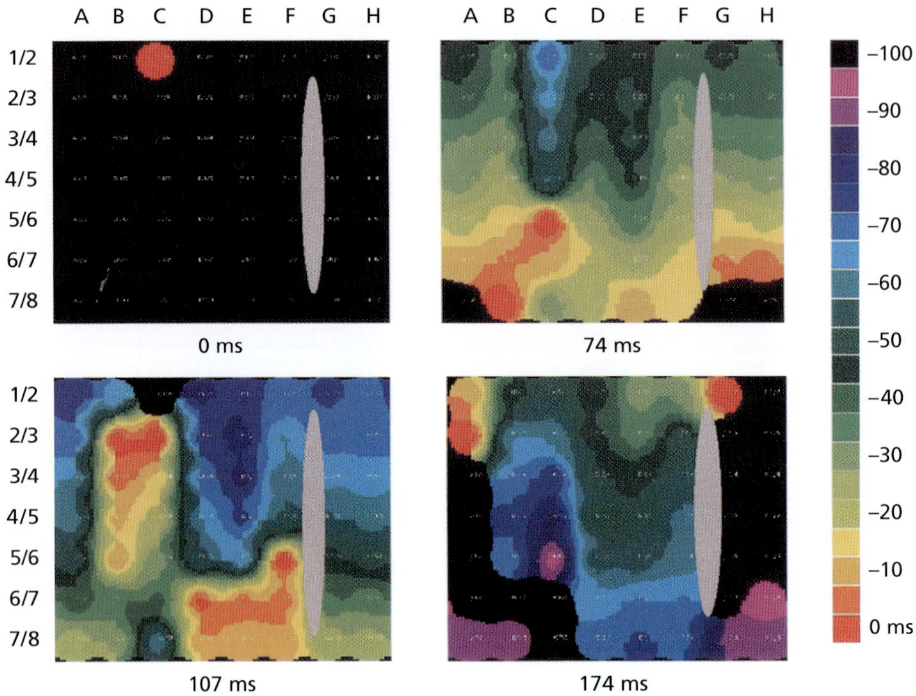

Figure 11.3 Three-dimensional activation patterns in a patient with paroxysmal AF. Isochrones are drawn every 5 ms. Splines A and B are located in the posterior wall, splines B–D in the septal wall, spline E across the tricuspid annulus, and splines G and H in the lateral wall of the RA. Electrode pairs 1/2 are located in the upper RA, whereas electrode pairs 7/8 are located in the lower RA. Gray ellipses show the position of the tricuspid valve. Red represents the head of the activation front. At time 0, an early breakthrough is observed in the high septal region. After 74 ms, almost the entire RA was activated from that spot. At the level of electrode pair B6/7 (low posterior region), the main wavefront is divided into two wavefronts heading toward the low posterior (electrode B7/8) and posteroseptal (electrode C5/6) regions. After 107 ms, the lateral wavefront crossed the isthmus region and emerged at the low septal region, whereas the posteroseptal wavefront activated most of the posteroseptal area. At 174 ms, two wavefronts are just reentering the posterior and the lateral regions again. (Reproduced from [2] with permission)

in different LA regions (Figure 11.4). The previous observation from the RA that paroxysmal AF had longer AF cycle lengths was confirmed. Furthermore, paroxysmal AF showed more pronounced regional differences compared to persistent AF. Another important observation was the occurrence of fairly organized intermediary rhythms followed by fibrillatory activity recorded in the initiation phase of paroxysmal AF (Figure 11.5). These earliest generators of AF were located more frequently at the posterior wall of the LA.

Right atrium and left atrium basket mapping

To achieve a global mapping strategy, we performed simultaneous biatrial basket mapping studies during AF [6] that revealed interesting phenomena. An example is shown in Figure 11.6 which shows a 2 : 1 left-to-right conduction block (Figure 11.6a, basket recordings from the RA) and a 2 : 1 conduction block within the LA (Figure 11.6b, basket recordings from the LA).

Non-contact mapping

In a similar fashion, we and others performed non-contact mapping studies from the RA and LA during the initiation of AF [7,8]. As a simultaneous mapping tool, non-contact mapping theoretically allows the determination of AF onset by delineating the origin of the first atrial premature complex leading to AF. However, as shown in another publication from our group, non-contact mapping has

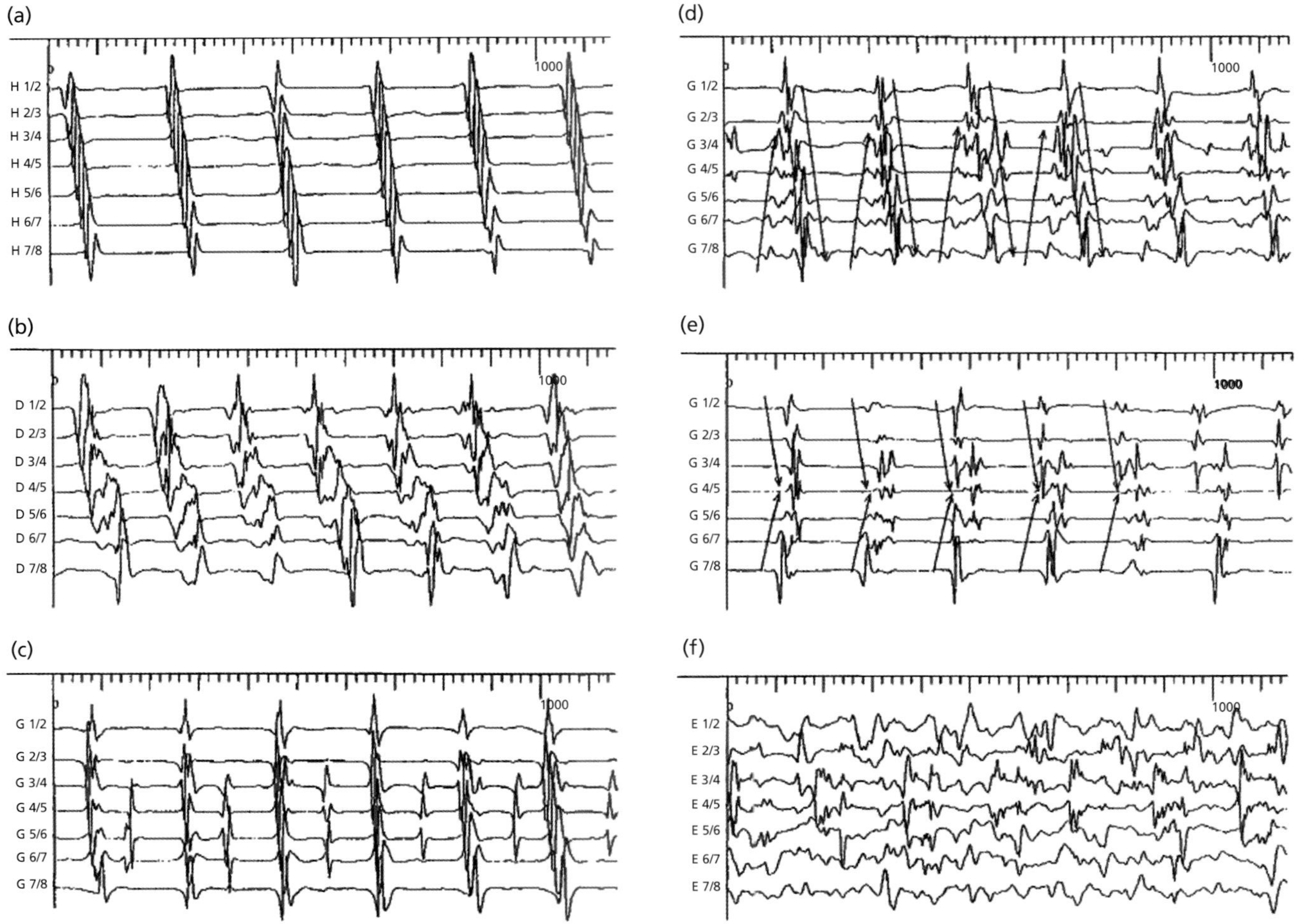

Figure 11.4 Atrial fibrillation types observed in different regions of the LA. (a) Type I AF, one wavefront with rapid conduction. (b–e) Different patterns of type II AF: (b) one wavefront with slow conduction; (c–e) examples of two wavefronts (f) Type III AF. (Reproduced from [5] with permission)

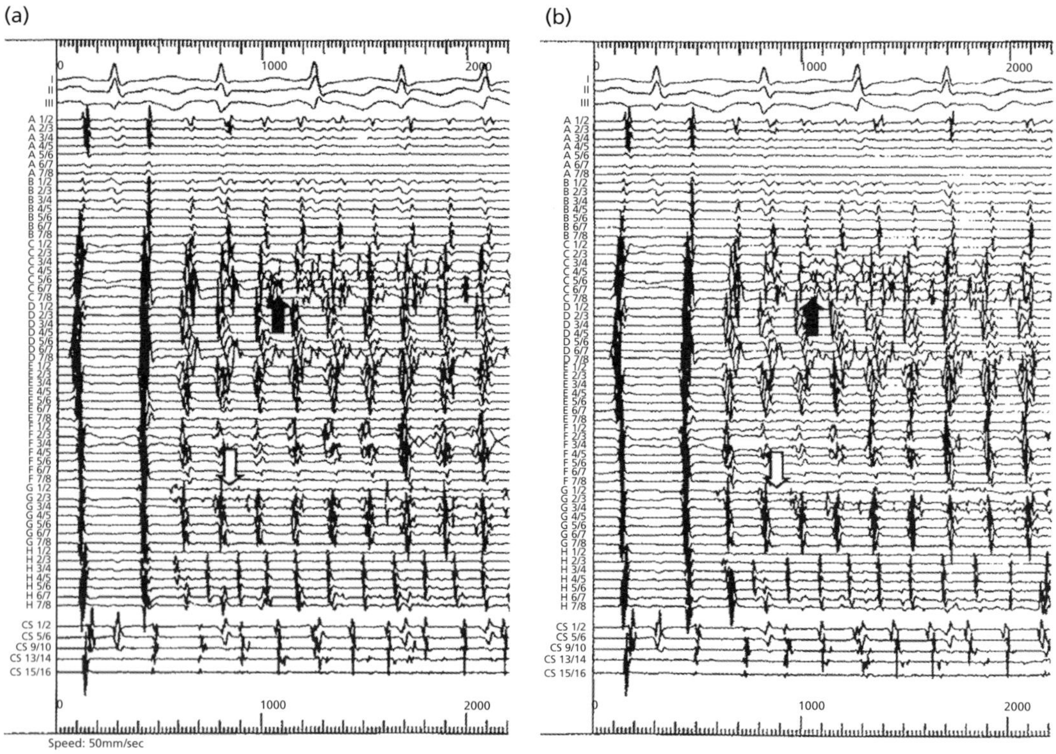

Figure 11.5 Comparison of two initiation episodes in the same patient separated in time by 39 min. Shown are three ECG leads, 56 basket bipolar electrograms, and the coronary sinus (CS) recordings. (a) The first beat is a sinus beat. Following the third beat of the intermediary rhythm, the electrode pairs G1/2 and G2/3 located in the posterior wall (white arrow) and electrode pairs C3/4 to C7/8 located in the anterior wall of the left atrium (black arrow) generated the earliest fibrillatory activity. (b) During the repeated episode, the same regions again produced the earliest fibrillatory activity. There were four more AF episodes that followed exactly the same pattern of initiation. All episodes were triggered by monomorphic atrial premature complexes originating from the left superior PV. The triggering atrial premature complex and the subsequent beats of intermediary rhythm preserved the same sequence of activation, although slowed conduction was observed starting with the second beat of the intermediary rhythm. Splines A and B in both recordings were located over the mitral annulus and recorded farfield ventricular signals. (Reproduced from [5] with permission)

limitations regarding its accuracy that depends on selected filter settings [9].

Ablation strategies and lessons learned from global biatrial mapping

In a combined approach of either biatrial basket mapping (Figure 11.7) or consecutive RA/LA non-contact mapping (Figure 11.8) we tried to trace the onset of 94 AF onsets in 45 patients [10]. The results of this focal mapping approach encircling the site of origin were disappointing. A main reason was probably that the concept of the importance of isolating the pulmonary veins (PVs) was not understood at that time (see next section). The global mapping tools did not allow one to look inside the PVs nor did they cover the LA regions equally (e.g. the LA basket only incompletely covers the LA septum or the mitral annulus). However, two lessons were learned. First, the onset of AF varied and was bifocal in nearly 30%. Second, with the limited accuracy of these mapping tools in mind, the role of an extrapulmonary origin of AF onset was not a "quantité négligeable" – more than 40% of ectopic foci triggering AF onset were located in extravenous parts of the RA and LA. This importance of extrapulmonary AF sources was confirmed by Lin et al. [11].

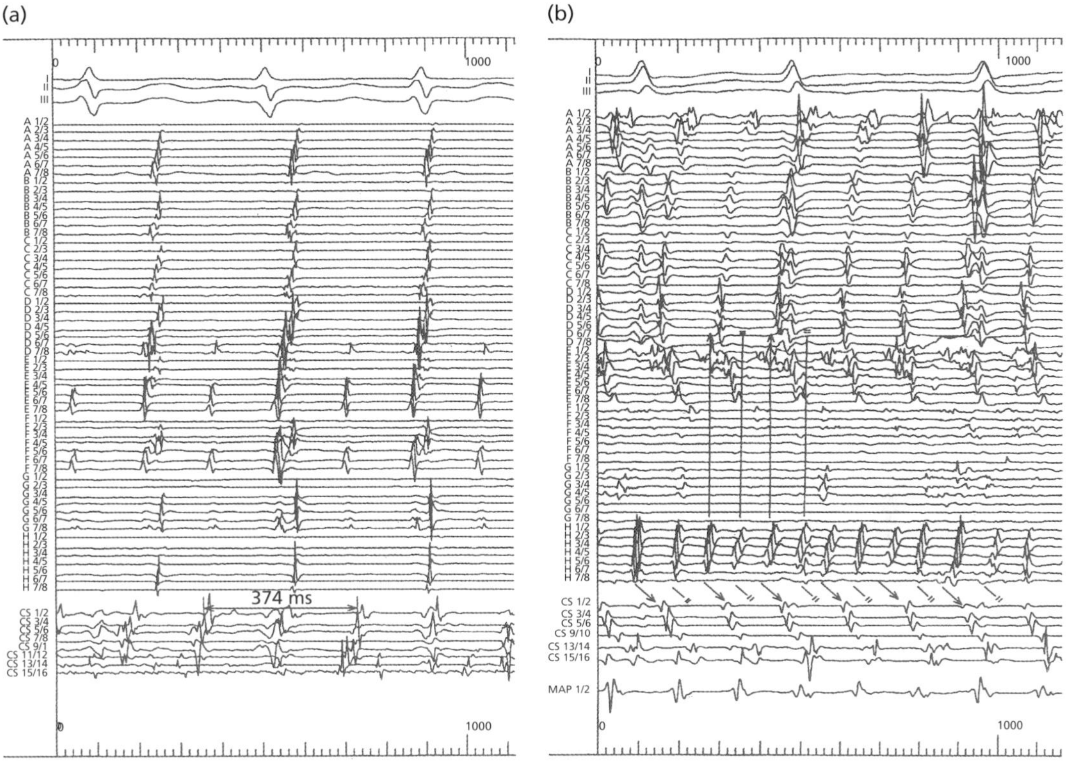

Figure 11.6 A left-to-right atrial conduction block during AF (a) and a rotor fibrillatory activity in the posterior wall of the LA (b). (a) Three surface ECG leads and the recordings from the basket catheter and the coronary sinus (CS) are shown. Every second impulse that enters the RA is blocked, leading to a regular activation of the RA with a cycle length of 374 ms. The entire RA is activated from the low inferoposterior pathway. The earliest activity is observed in the electrode pairs F7/8 located in the low posteroinferior region of the RA. Low amplitude signals in electrode pairs G5/6 to G7/8 represent farfield signals from the left side of the interatrial septum. (b) Regular activity with a cycle length of 80 ms recorded in the posterior wall of the LA. Shown from top to bottom are three surface ECG leads, 56 bipolar electrograms from the basket catheter, CS electrograms, and recordings from the left inferior PV (MAP1/2). A 2 : 1 block between the posterior wall and the rest of LA, the CS, and the left inferior PV is seen. The same conduction ration was also observed for the remaining three PVs. An area of low potentials (splines F and G) is recorded over the roof of the LA. The recordings in (a) and (b) are from different patients. (Reproduced from [6] with permission)

Strategies focusing on the pulmonary veins

Michel Haïssaguerre and coworkers from the Bordeaux group were the first to describe the tracing of an arrhythmogenic focus to a PV [12]. From this and other observations, they derived the groundbreaking idea that a PV could be the predominant focal source initiating AF episodes [13] (Figure 11.9). They deduced that the elimination of focal PV activity or (to avoid local PV damage) electrical isolation of the PV from the LA could prevent PV focal activity entraining the atria into the arrhythmia [13,14].

Ostial pulmonary vein isolation

Electrical PV isolation was established as a therapeutic concept after it became clear that identifiable strands of myocardial tissue enter the PV from the LA [15,16]. Identification and ablation of the conducting part of the PV–LA interface allow electrical PV isolation by ablating a part of or the whole PV circumference. An indispensable tool for this approach is the correct and reliable identification of local PV potentials corresponding to myocardial strands that enter into the PV. High density circumferential mapping of the PV ostia is necessary and a variety of catheters with distal electrodes

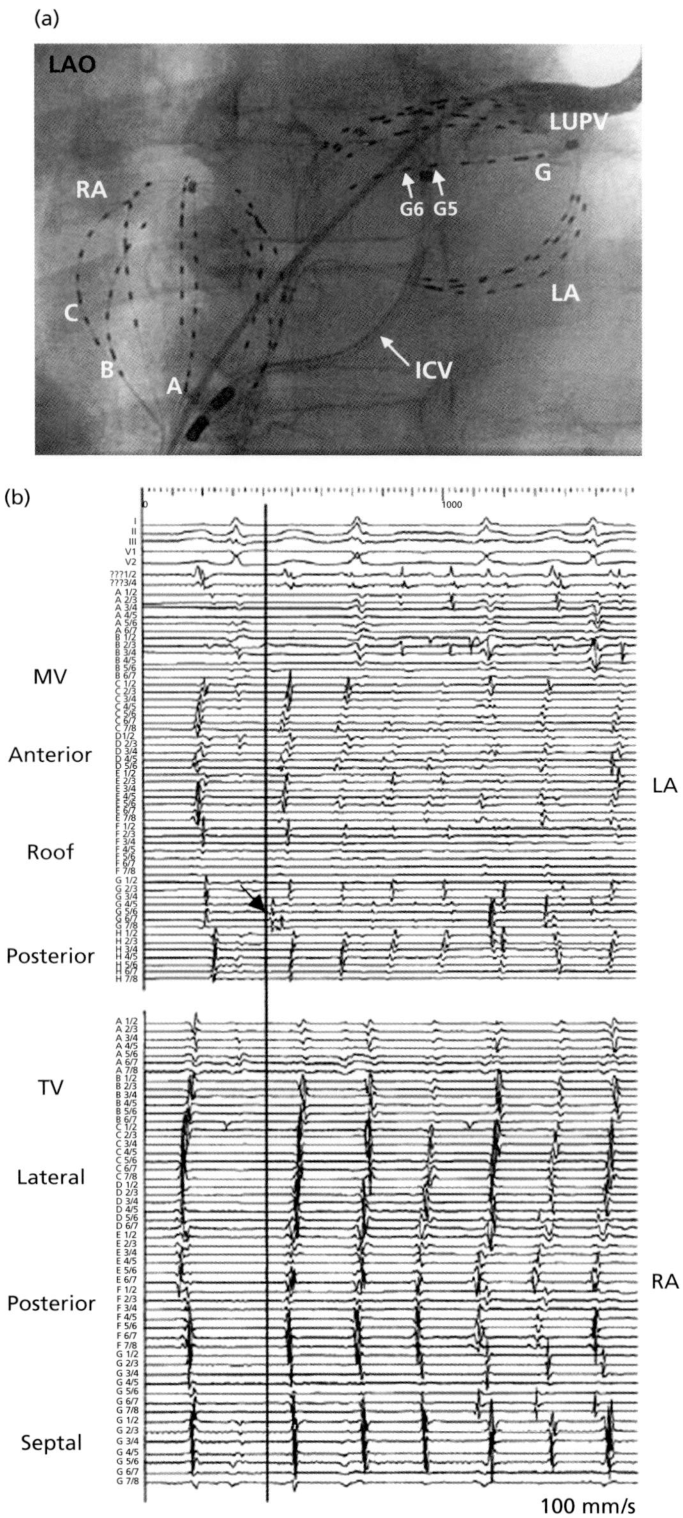

Figure 11.7 (a) Fluoroscopic view of basket catheters placed in the right and left atria in the left anterior oblique (LAO) position and angiography of the left upper pulmonary vein (LUPV). The letters A, B, and C mark the splines with a fluoroscopic identifier on electrodes 8 (A), 7 (B), and 6 (C) in the right atrium (RA). The remaining splines are oriented in a clockwise direction with the basket as seen from the proximal aspect. For the left atrial basket, electrode pair G5/6, which is located in the mid-posterior area of the left atrium (LA), marks the location of a focus that induced an AF episode (B). Angiography of the LUPV showed a close basket–tissue contact at the ostial region of this vein.
(b) Spontaneous onset of an AF episode. Simultaneous recordings from five surface electrocardiographic leads, two intracardiac electrograms from the mapping catheter placed in the LUPV, and 128 bipolar electrograms from the right and left atria are presented. Annotations on the left side of the figure denote the anatomic position of the splines. The first beat is a sinus rhythm beat. The second beat is an atrial premature complex inducing an AF episode. The earliest electrical activity is displayed in the electrode pair G5/6, which corresponds to the position shown in (a). The electrical activity recorded in the mapping catheter is late compared with the earliest spot of activation. ICV, internal cardioversion catheter; MV, mitral valve; TV, tricuspid valve. (Reproduced from [10] with permission)

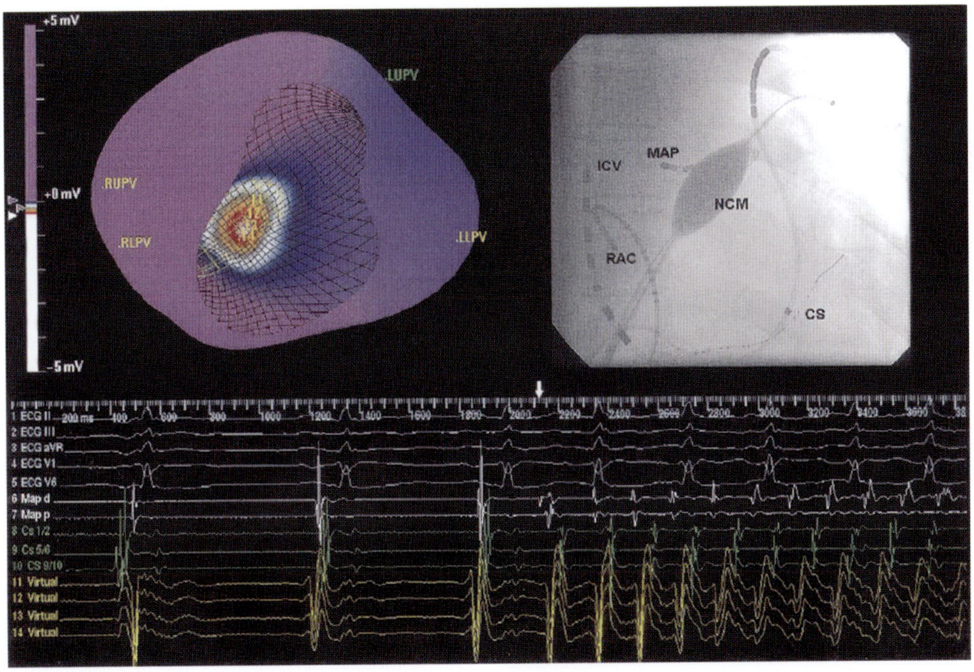

Figure 11.8 Documentation of the ectopic focus inducing an AF episode in the mid-posterior wall of the LA. (Above) Half-opened ED map of the LA (left), and a fluoroscopic view of the non-contact mapping balloon and other catheters in the right and left atria (right). In the virtual map of the LA, the earliest spot of activation was located in the mid-posterior wall of the LA far from all four PV ostia. The tip of the mapping (MAP)/ablation catheter was steered at the point of earliest activity guided by the non-contact mapping system (NCM). (Below) Conventional and virtual electrograms obtained during the onset of AF. Five electrocardiographic leads, intracardiac electrograms recorded from the mapping catheter (map d, map p), coronary sinus (CS1/2, CS5/6, CS9/10), and four virtual electrograms are shown. The first three beats are sinus beats. The fourth beat is an atrial premature complex that initiated the AF. The electrogram recorded by the mapping/ablation catheter displayed a double spike morphology. The white arrow marks the first spike of the electrogram recorded by the mapping/ablation catheter. CS, coronary sinus catheter; ICV, internal cardioversion catheter; LLPV, left lower pulmonary vein; LUPV, left upper pulmonary vein; RAC, right atrial catheter; RLPV, right lower pulmonary vein; RUPV, right upper pulmonary vein. (Reproduced from [10] with permission)

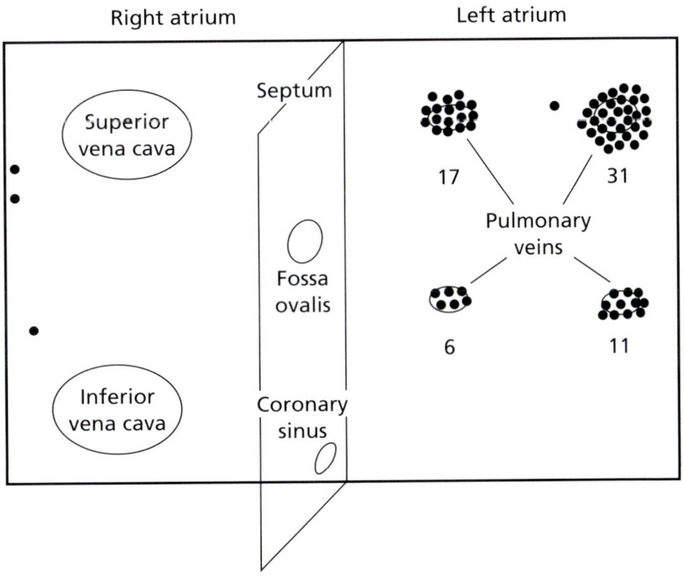

Figure 11.9 Diagram of the sites of 69 foci triggering atrial fibrillation in 45 patients. Note the clustering in the PVs, particularly in both superior PVs. The numbers indicate the distribution of foci in the PVs. (Reproduced from [13] with permission)

(a)

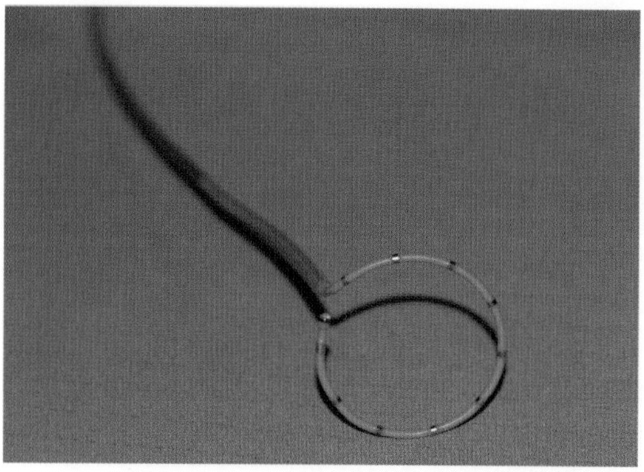

(b)

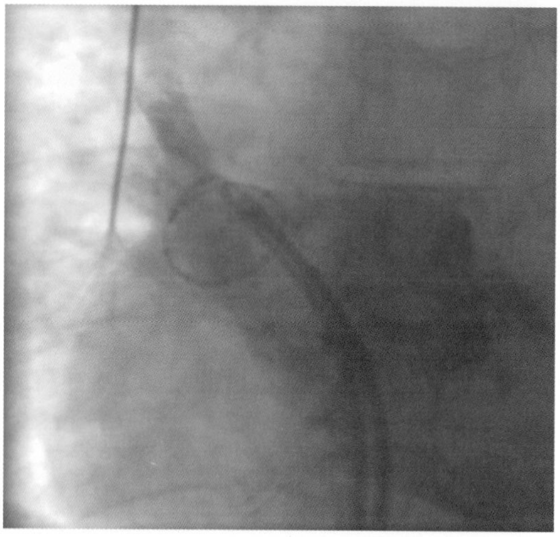

Figure 11.10 (a) The decapolar Lasso® catheter (Cordis-Webster) as an example of a distally circular-shaped catheter designed to map circumferentially the PV ostia. (b) Angiography of the right superior PV, with the Lasso catheter placed at the ostium of the PV, is performed by hand injection of 10 ml of contrast medium (anteroposterior projection). A variety of similar catheters from other manufacturers is available.

mounted in a circular manner are available for this purpose [17] (Figures 11.10 and 11.11).

There are some advantages to this approach. Ablation can be performed regardless of the prevailing atrial rhythm and does not require an active focus at the moment of the electrophysiological study. One might call it a "round up the usual suspects" technique: no matter if you actually *observe* a PV being arrhythmogenic during the electrophysiological study, isolating *all* PVs is helpful and causes – in the hands of an experienced operator – probably no or only little harm. Using PV isolation, Haïssaguerre and coworkers achieved stable sinus rhythm in 73% of patients with paroxysmal AF. Other operators report success rates between 51% and 82% [16,18–26].

General considerations

Published studies using PV isolation (PVI) have revealed some important points [16–37]:

1 The rate of patients that need more than one procedure to reach a good clinical outcome varies between 15% and 40%. During virtually all repeat ablation procedures, reconduction of one or more PV is observed [27–29].

2 The danger and the clinical sequelae of severe ablation – induced PV stenosis-like coughing, dyspnea, and hemoptisis – should not be underestimated. Scanning for post-ablation PV stenosis should always be part of the follow-up after PVI [30–31].

3 AF relapse after PVI is rather common, but relapse during the first month does not necessarily predict clinical outcome after 3 or more months. Therefore a "blanking period" of at least 1 month after PVI could make sense. Another consequence concerns the timing of a repeat ablation. In our experience, repeat ablation > 3 months after initial PVI tends to result in a better outcome than early repeat ablation (< 3 months after initial PVI) [32–33].

4 There is a learning curve to this approach. Only a few centers were able to reach the Bordeaux group success rates in 2000 to 2001 and, at the same time, complication rates were rather higher. In our own experience, early results were sobering [20]. This changed gradually with an increase in patient numbers and a better understanding of the complex LA anatomy.

Pulmonary vein isolation: an evolving technique

The PVI technique has evolved over the last years. In the beginning it seemed almost impossible to reach all PVs, especially the right inferior PV [19–21]. In early publications only a small percentage of right inferior PVs were isolated. Today, most centers include the right inferior PV in their ablation set from the beginning [26,32,33].

Distinguishing local PV potentials from left atrial farfield electrograms also presented a challenge. A variety of pacing maneuvers have been

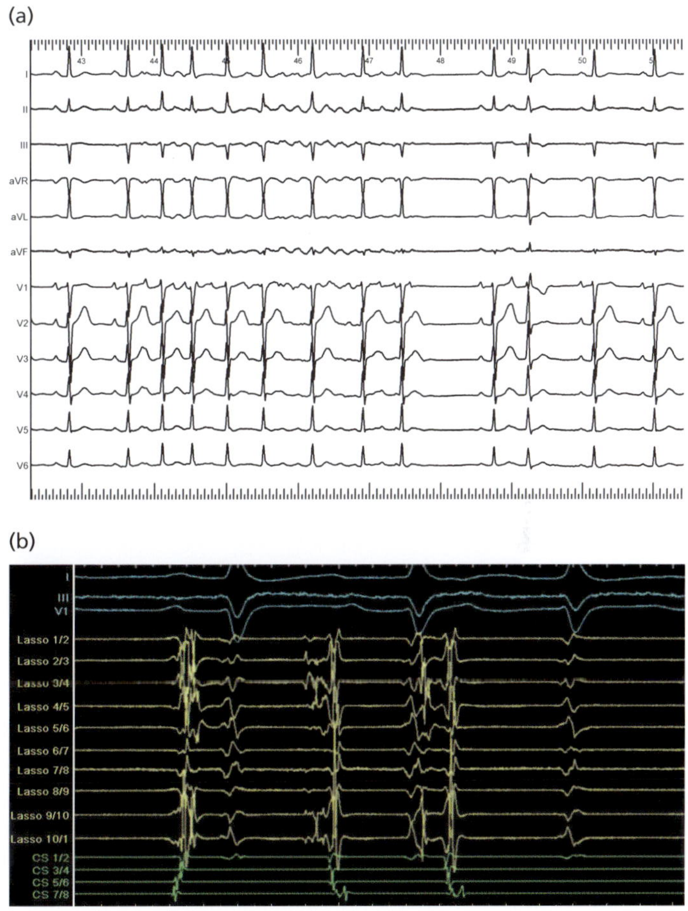

Figure 11.11 Focal activity with frequent ectopic beats and short bursts originating from the left superior PV (LSPV) in a patient with frequent short episodes of AF. (a) The surface ECG recording shows focal discharges initiating even a very short episode of AF (paper speed 25 mm/s). (b) The corresponding intracardiac recordings. The circular mapping catheter (Lasso 1/2 to 10/1) is placed at the ostium of the LSPV. A normal sinus beat with coronary sinus (CS) activation from proximal to distal (7/8 to 1/2) and fused LA farfield potential and PV potential (PVP) in the Lasso recordings is followed by two ectopic beats originating from inside the LSPV. During the ectopic beats the PVP in the Lasso recordings occurs markedly before the LA farfield activity (inversion of PVP and LA potential) and the CS is activated from distal to proximal. Note that the earliest electrical signal in the Lasso catheter precedes the P wave in the surface ECG recordings by almost 100 ms. Paper speed is 100 mm/s; the tracings from top to bottom are: ECG I, III, and V1 (light blue); Lasso 1/2 to 10/1 (yellow); CS 1/2 to 7/8 (green).

developed to improve correct discrimination, including pacing in the distal and proximal coronary sinus (CS) and in the left atrial appendage (LAA) [34–36].

Regarding the anatomic ablation target, a move from an isolation level almost inside the PV to more ostial or antral isolation sites has been observed over the years. Initially, only fluoroscopy-based PV angiographies were used to judge the localization of the catheter(s) in relation to the PV ostia. Soon, more advanced visualization tools were used. Non-fluoroscopic three-dimensional (3D) mapping tools like the electroanatomic mapping system (Carto®, Biosense Webster) or, especially, the NavX® system (St. Jude Medical) are extremely helpful as the PV ostia are shown in 3D space. The relationship of the ablation catheter and (for the NavX system) even the mapping catheters are also shown (Figure 11.12). By using these systems, a significant reduction in fluoroscopy time and procedure duration is achieved [37,38].

Intracardiac echocardiography may help to better define the actual ostium of the PV. It has also been used to titrate the ablation power and to monitor the ablation effect [39]. Ablation power was increased up to 50 W until scattered microbubbles (type 1 bubbles) occurred. If a brisk shower of dense microbubbles (type 2 bubbles) was observed, ablation was stopped immediately. Excellent clinical outcome (90% of patients in stable sinus rhythm) was reported with this technique [39].

Recently, it has become possible to display synchronically, or fuse, the computer tomography (CT) or magnetic resonance imaging (MRI) derived 3D reconstruction of the LA with the catheter-created mapping surface of the LA. This feature is even more important in anatomically guided ablation approaches [40] (Figures 11.13 and 11.14).

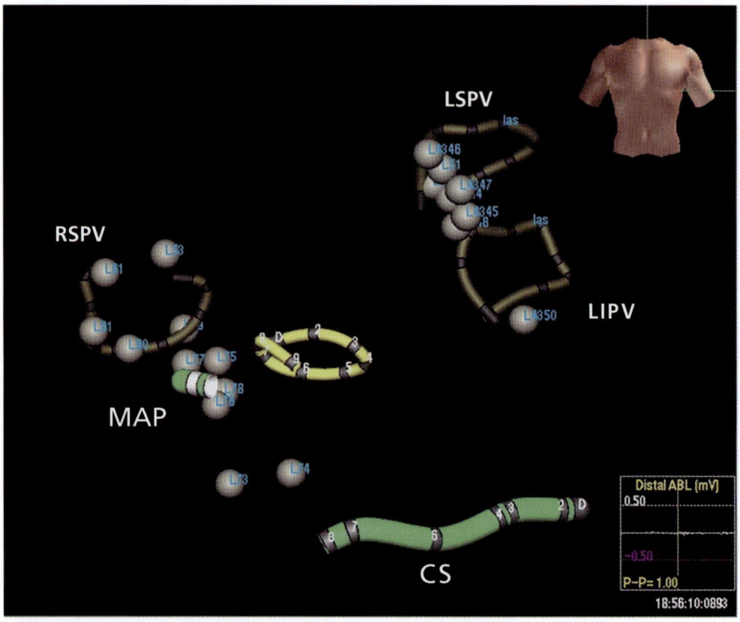

Figure 11.12 Screen capture of NavX catheter navigation during segmental PVI for paroxysmal AF. The former positions of the circular mapping catheter at the ostia of both the left and the right superior PV (LSPV, RSPV, respectively) are displayed as light yellow "shadows" of the catheter. The gray tags indicate the respective ablation sites at the PV ostia, showing clearly that it was enough to ablate only small segments of the ostial circumference to isolate the PV. Coronary sinus (CS) and map catheters, as well as the circular mapping catheter in darker yellow, are displayed in real time at their respective actual position. To spare time, the 3D anatomic reconstruction of the whole LA was skipped. LIPV, left inferior pulmonary vein; LSPV, left superior pulmonary vein.

There has also been a significant evolution regarding ablation catheters as well as power and temperature settings. In the beginning, PVI was performed using solid tip, 4 mm, standard ablation catheters. To avoid charring or thrombus formation and to reduce the occurrence of PV–LA reconduction, a shift towards cooled-tip catheters occurred [22,26]. Due to cardiac perforation and (audible) steam pop occurrence, the maximum power settings for the irrigated-tip ablation catheters were subsequently reduced over the years from up to 50 W to 30–35 W nowadays [41].

Circular ostial pulmonary vein isolation: balloons and similar ablation tools

Ostial PVI aims at electrically isolating the PV from the LA. This may necessitate lesions all around the PV ostia. To overcome the sometimes cumbersome task of applying circumferential lesions in a point-by-point manner, circumferentially ablating catheters were developed. Using these catheters, a complete PV isolation with a single or few applications might be possible, superseding the exact analysis where conductive strands connect the LA with the PV. Most of these tools are balloon-shaped catheters, working with diverse energy sources that are advanced to the PV ostium and then deployed to their full size.

Balloons working with microwave (Atrionix® balloon), high focused ultrasound energy, or cryoenergy have been developed [42–44]. Alternatively, a cone-shaped ablation catheter applying radiofrequency energy with a mesh-like surface has been used in clinical trials [45] (Figure 11.15). Laser energy-delivering balloons have also been tested in bench testing and with animals [46].

The microwave tool has been abandoned because of severe side effects, such as permanent phrenic nerve palsy, PV perforation, and severe PV stenosis, and its very limited steering capability [42]. The high focused ultrasound tool has been tested with promising preliminary results, but will probably need further improvement in steering capacities and reduction of the shaft size [44]. The most

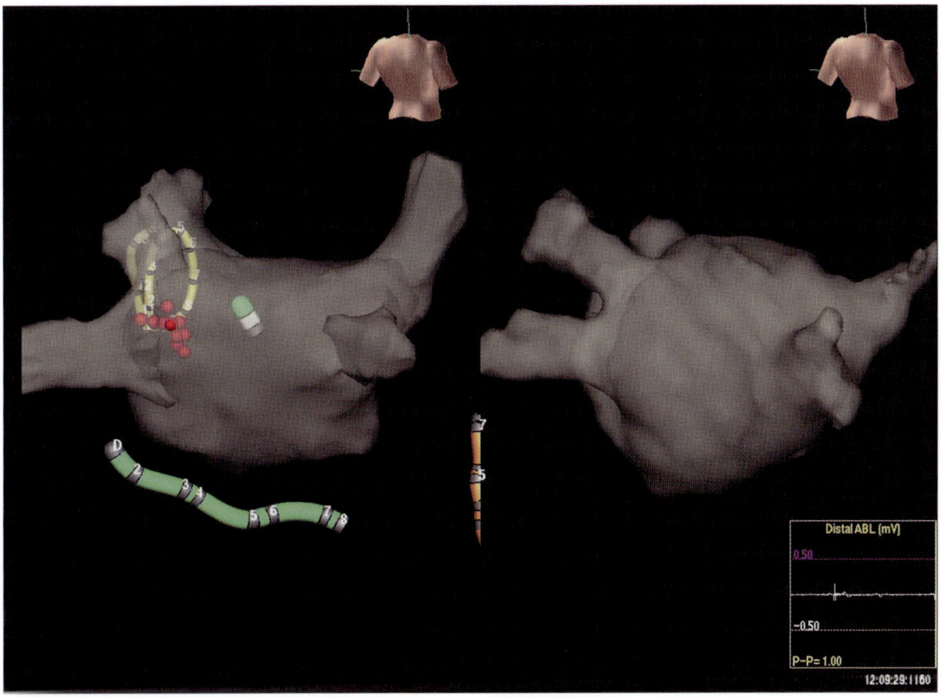

Figure 11.13 NavX catheter navigation with side-by-side display of the LA anatomy from a multislice CT scan (right side) and the 3D reconstruction obtained by catheter data processing via the NavX system (left side). The ablation catheter, circular-shaped mapping catheter, and the CS catheter are displayed in their actual position throughout the procedure. A modified posteroanterior view of the LA is shown. The circular-shaped mapping catheter and the ablation catheter are positioned at the ostium of the left superior PV; the CS catheter is in green. The red tags mark prior ablation positions.

promising of the balloon technologies might be the cryoballoon, which has been shown to offer quite good isolation capacities and good clinical results regarding the complete elimination of AF [43] (Figure 11.16).

The three most important limitations of the above-mentioned balloon tools are:

1 There is no possibility to map the PV ostium, i.e. the actual isolation of the PV has to be shown with an additional (circular) mapping catheter. The cone-shaped Mesh® (C.R. Bard, Lowell, MA, USA) catheter (ablating with "conventional" radiofrequency energy) with its 36 recording electrodes overcomes this limitation and even exists as a "pure" mapping catheter without ablation capabilities [45].

2 In many cases, the balloons fail to achieve a complete PVI. Thus, so-called touch-up ablations with a (second, conventional) ablation catheter are necessary. This increases the possible danger of air embolism because of repetitive catheter withdrawing and advancing through the transseptal sheath and increases the costs of the whole procedure considerably [43].

3 "Collateral damage", such as phrenic nerve palsy and lung tissue injury, is a relatively frequent observation and is not easy to avoid [44].

Circumferential pulmonary vein ablation

In contrast to a mapping-guided ostial PVI, which may necessitate only segmental energy applications or the balloon-based circular ostial ablation in some instances, more antral or "extra-ostial" ablation methods have been described. Of these, circumferential PV ablation (CPVA) is the most widespread ablation technique in paroxysmal AF ablation. The first description of this technique was published by its "inventor", Carlo Pappone from Milan (San Raffaele University Hospital) [47].

With this approach, wide encircling lesions placed outside the ostia of the ipsilateral PV (0.5–1 cm away from the ostium) aim to modify the substrate

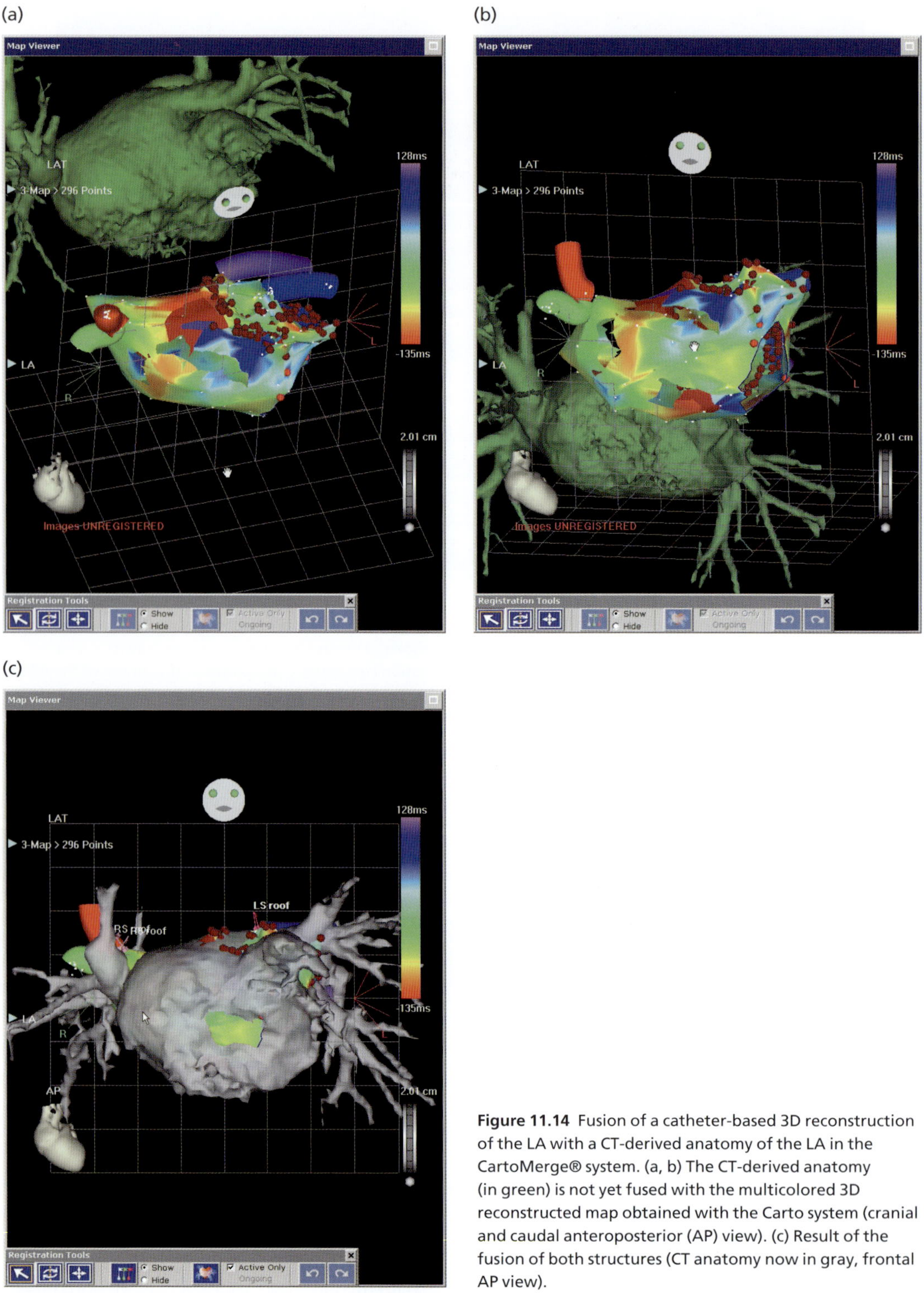

Figure 11.14 Fusion of a catheter-based 3D reconstruction of the LA with a CT-derived anatomy of the LA in the CartoMerge® system. (a, b) The CT-derived anatomy (in green) is not yet fused with the multicolored 3D reconstructed map obtained with the Carto system (cranial and caudal anteroposterior (AP) view). (c) Result of the fusion of both structures (CT anatomy now in gray, frontal AP view).

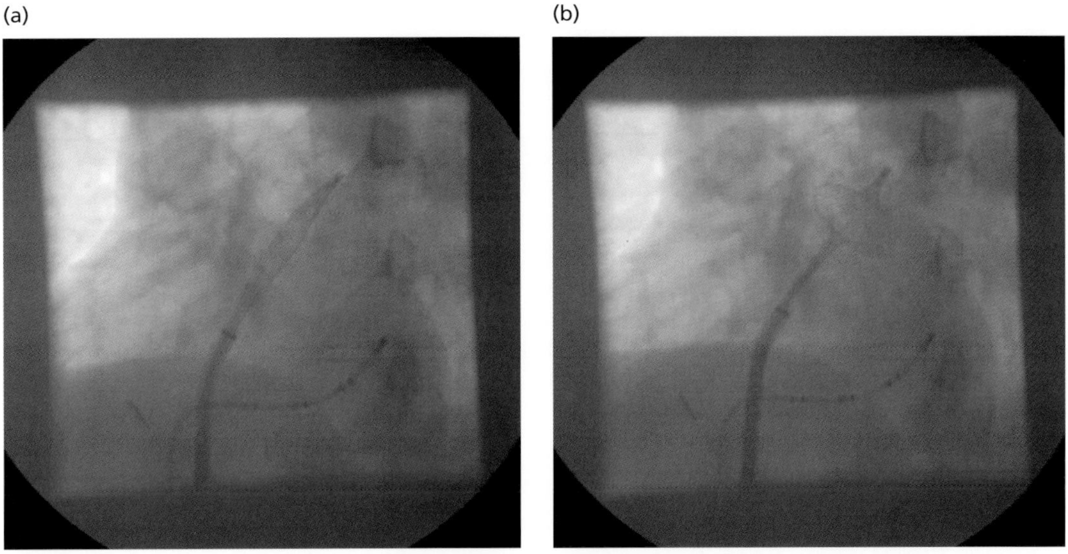

Figure 11.15 Fluoroscopic appearance of the Mesh catheter in an anteroposterior view. (a) The Mesh catheter is advanced via a long sheath in the LA and its tip points in the direction of the left superior PV (LSPV). It is not yet deployed. (b) The Mesh catheter is unfolded and covers with its cone-like shape the circumference of the LSPV ostium. With the parts of the mesh that are directed forward and touch the ostial tissue of the PV, radiofrequency energy delivery is possible.

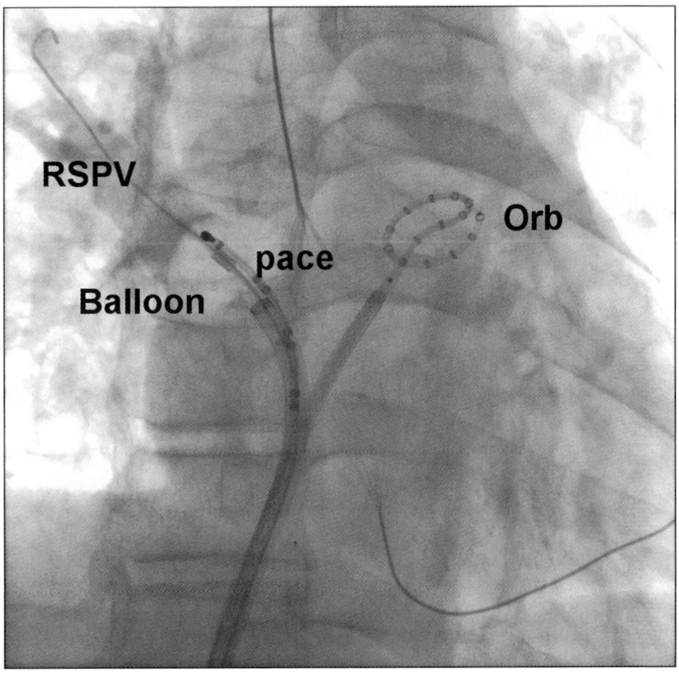

Figure 11.16 Anteroposterior fluoroscopic view during cryoballoon (Arctic Front®, CryoCath, Montreal, Canada) isolation of the right superior PV (RSPV). The cryoballoon is advanced over the wire to the ostium of the RSPV and is inflated there. A small amount of contrast medium is administered through the inner lumen of the cryoballoon catheter shaft distally inside the PV to control the total occlusion of the PV by the cryoballoon and thus an optimal circumferential contact of the ablating balloon and the ostial PV tissue. To monitor for phrenic nerve damage, which occurs rather frequently while isolating the RSPV with a balloon tool, stimulation of the right phrenic nerve is performed with a right atrial pacing catheter (pace) placed in the high right atrium/superior vena cava region. The circumferential mapping catheter (Orb; Orbiter PV®, C.R. Bard) is in "parking position" close to the left superior PV. It will be advanced after cryoablation into the RSPV to check electrical isolation of the PV.

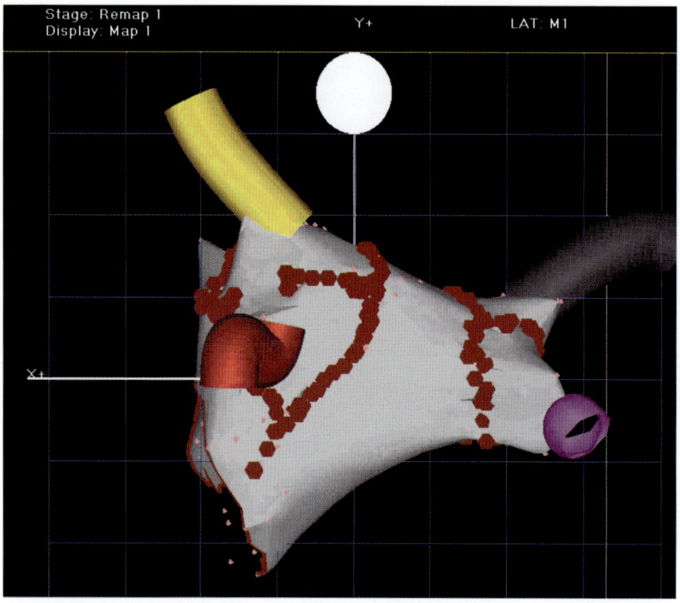

Figure 11.17 Electroanatomic Carto map of the LA in posteroanterior view during CPVA. The PVs are represented by colored tubes. An anatomically guided encircling of the PV by lesions placed in linear manner around the PV ostia was performed around the left and right PVs; in this case lines in between the ipsilateral PV were added. According to the technique described by Pappone et al., an additional line joining the lateral mitral annulus with the inferior portion of the left PV encircling lesion was added. Ablation points are highlighted as red tags.

for AF and to delay LA–PV conduction. A reduction of local bipolar electrogram amplitude of ≥ 80% or ≤ 0.1 mV and a conduction delay over the ablation line are the endpoint of this technique [47,48,49]. It is important to note that complete electrical PVI is not a requirement for ablation and is not checked routinely. In fact, it has been demonstrated that 45–80% of the encircled PVs are not electrically isolated [50,51]. In addition to the two encircling lesions, at least one line connecting the inferioposterior part of the left circle with the posterolateral mitral annulus should be deployed (the so-called left isthmus line or mitral isthmus line) (Figure 11.17).

The most important distinction of ostial PVI is that the primary objective in PVI is to *eliminate* the AF-initiating trigger. In CPVA, a deep change in the AF-maintaining substrate together with *modification* of the trigger is the rationale of the approach. The procedure is performed with the help of a 3D mapping system, in general the Carto system. The reported success rates of the circumferential PV ablation approach in paroxysmal AF vary between 42% and 88% [47–53].

Technique and tricks

Circumferential PV ablation can be at the same time technically easier and more difficult to perform than ostial PVI for the following reasons:

- It requires only one catheter in the LA (the mapping/ablation catheter for the 3D mapping system), but the whole LA has to be explored.
- It is not necessary to map the PV ostium extensively, but it is important to reconstruct the extra-ostial region(s) carefully.
- The risk of PV stenosis seems to be lower than in PVI, although occurrence of PV stenosis has been reported in several studies [50,51,53].
- After CPVA, regular atrial tachycardias are found in 4–30% of patients [53–56]. These new-onset tachycardias may have a focal or reentrant mechanism and tend to be difficult to treat. To prevent atrial macroreentry after CPVA, additional posterior lines connecting both circular lesions around the ipsilateral PV have been added to the initial lesion set [52,56].
- The most severe and almost always fatal complication of CPVA is the formation of a fistula between the posterior LA and the esophagus [57,58]. The actual incidence of this complication is difficult to estimate, but about 60 cases have been reported worldwide so far. To avoid these fistulae, several changes have been made to the ablation technique [59–63]. The maximum power during ablation at the posterior LA wall has been lowered to 30–35 W (cooled-tip ablation catheter) or 60–70 W (8 mm tip ablation catheter). The position of the esophagus in relation to the LA and ablation

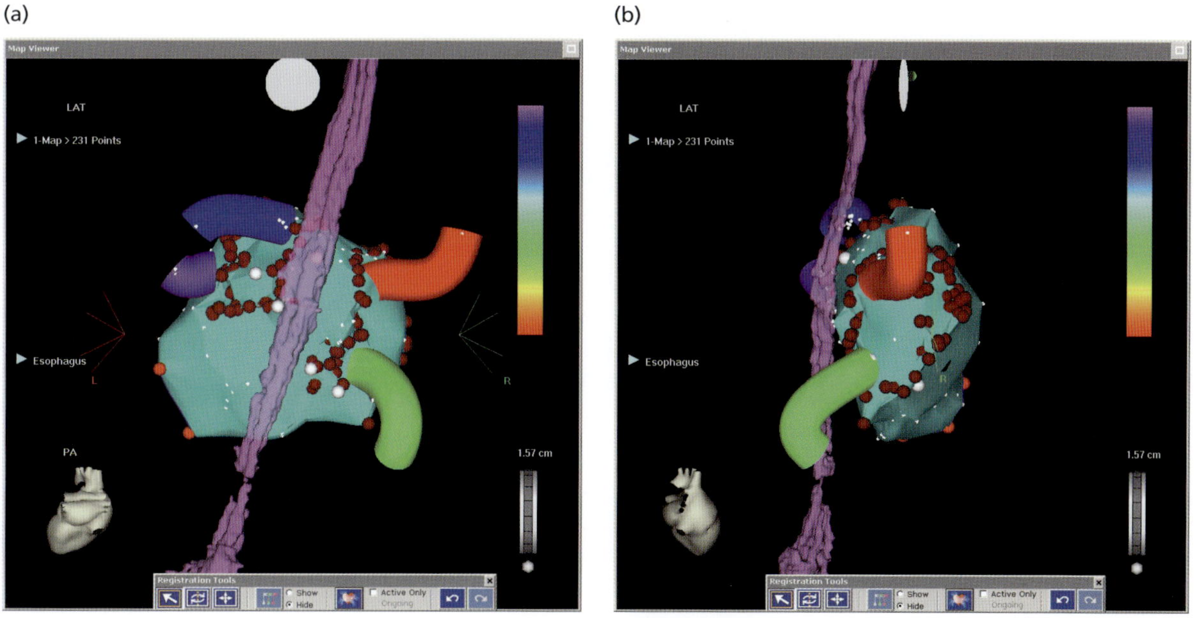

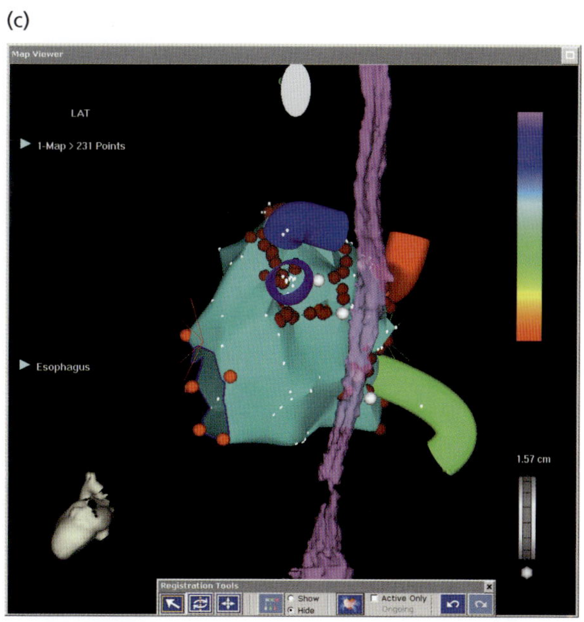

Figure 11.18 CartoMerge view of the LA and the course of the esophagus. Posteroanterior (a), right lateral (b), and left lateral (c) views of the 3D reconstructed map of the LA and its relationship to the position of the esophagus are displayed. Ablation tags are shown in red. The CT-derived anatomy of the LA is hidden to allow a better view of the ablation tags on the electroanatomic map. Note that the linear lesion encircling the left PV is placed in utmost proximity to the course of the esophagus. There are contradictory data regarding the stability of the esophagus position in 3D space during the ablation procedure.

catheter is displayed during the ablation by showing the anatomic reconstruction in the fused anatomy/catheter mapping image or by highlighting the esophagus in fluoroscopy by a small amount of barium contrast (Figure 11.18). Additionally, the intraesophagus temperature has been measured in some studies by a probe placed inside the esophagus lumen. The value of direct temperature measurement is not yet clear, but it seems that even minor changes in temperature (< 1°C) are a sign of significant esophageal damage. Regarding the display of the esophagus in the 3D reconstructed and fused CT- or MRI-derived anatomy, there are data suggesting that within some hours the esophagus moves significantly with respect to the LA [62,63].

Ostial pulmonary vein isolation versus circumferential pulmonary vein ablation

When comparing the clinical success of ostial PV isolation and CPVA, findings have been inconsistent. Oral et al. from Michigan University published a randomized trial [52] comparing segmental ostial PVI (40 patients) and CPVA (40 patients) in paroxysmal AF. At 6 months' follow-up, 67% of the patients treated with PVI and 88% of patients treated with CPVA were free of symptomatic AF (difference between both treatment groups significant at $P = 0.02$).

In a randomized study from our center [53] comparing the PVI approach (50 patients) with the CPVA technique (50 patients), converse results were found: at 6 months, 82% of the PVI-treated patients (41/50) and 54% of the CPVA group patients (27/50) were free of arrhythmia-related symptoms ($P = 0.02$). Analyzing the actual freedom from any atrial tachyarrhythmia in a continuous 7-day Holter electrocardiogram (ECG) 6 months after the ablation procedure, 66% of the PVI patients and 42% of the CPVA patients were free of any tachyarrhythmia ($P < 0.01$).

There are some methodological and procedural differences between the two studies which may explain the contradictory results at least partially. First, different ablation catheters were used. In the Michigan study, 8 mm tip ablation catheters were used for the CPVA with a power limit of 60 W, whereas solid-tip (i.e. non-irrigated tip) catheters with up to 30 W power were used for the PVI. In the Munich study, irrigated-tip catheters were used for most of the PVI patients with a power limit set at 30–35 W, creating probably more transmural lesions in PVI than would be created by a solid-tip catheter. In CPVA, both 8 mm tip and irrigated-tip catheters were used. It may be

(a)

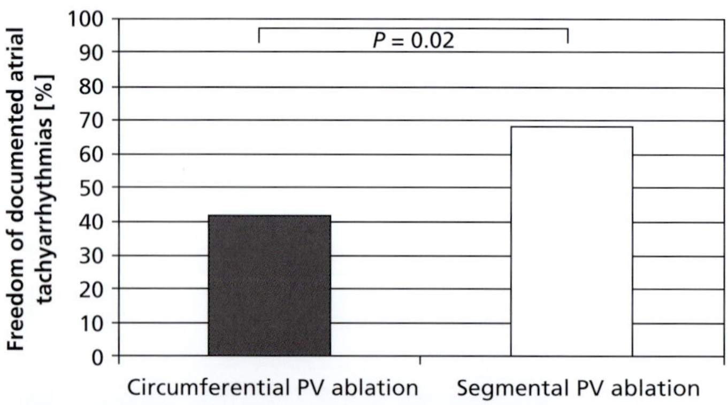

(b)

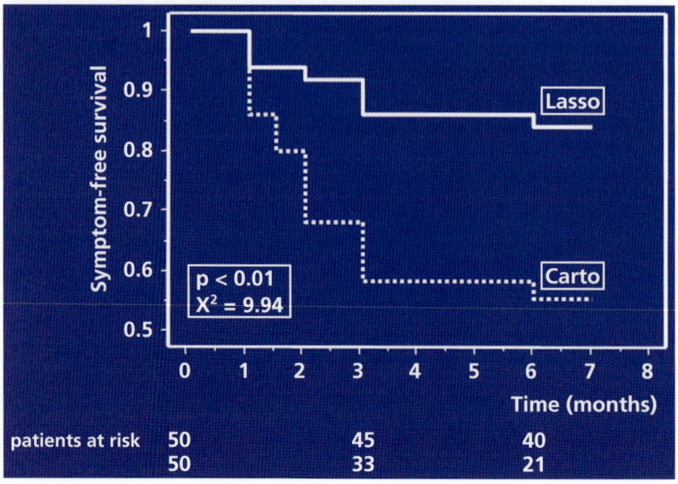

Figure 11.19 (a) Percentage of actual arrhythmia-free patients (assessed with 7-day Holter ECGs) 6 months after segmental and circumferential PV ablation. (b) A Kaplan–Meier graph for both treatment groups regarding the freedom of symptoms. (Reproduced from [53] with permission)

speculated that the 8 mm tip catheter is more appropriate to draw linear lesions than the 4 mm irrigated-tip catheter.

Another important point when comparing both studies is the method of surveying and evaluating the follow-up of the patients. In the Michigan study, patients were seen 4 weeks and 3 or 6 months after the ablation procedure. Patients were questioned for symptoms and received event monitors in case of arrhythmia symptoms; (serial) Holter ECGs were not scheduled. The mean follow-up was 164 ± 100 days (approximately 5 ± 3 months), and the result after 6 months is given only in percentage of patients, without giving the absolute number (i.e. it is not clear how many of the patients actually reached the 6 months' follow-up). In the Munich study, all patients reached at least the 6 months' follow-up and all were seen 1, 3, and 6 months after the ablation procedure. The results are given for both freedom from arrhythmia *symptoms*, as assessed by patient questioning, and freedom from *actual occurrence of arrhythmia*, as assessed by intensive ECG monitoring using a continuous 7-day Holter ECG recording in all patients (Figure 11.19). The results differed significantly between both assessment methods: many patients who are free of arrhythmia symptoms after AF ablation still have (asymptomatic) AF episodes. This has important implications, for example for anticoagulation treatment after AF ablation.

Circumferential pulmonary vein isolation

In the circumferential PV isolation approach, which was first described by Ouyang et al. from the Hamburg/St. Georg group [64], wide encircling lesions comprising both ipsilateral PVs are drawn as in CPVA but with the aim of electrical PVI. Circular linear lesions in the atrial tissue located close to the PV ostia are applied [64,65]. In some respects, this technique is a conjunction of ostial PV isolation and CPVA. A controlled complete isolation of the PVs is achieved with lesions placed in the LA, thus minimizing the risk for PV stenosis. A 3D reconstruction of the LA with the electroanatomic mapping system is used in the same manner as in CPVA. To monitor complete PVI, one or two circular mapping catheters are placed in the ostia of the ipsilateral PV (Figure 11.20). Disappearance of all PV potentials is the endpoint for ablation.

(a)

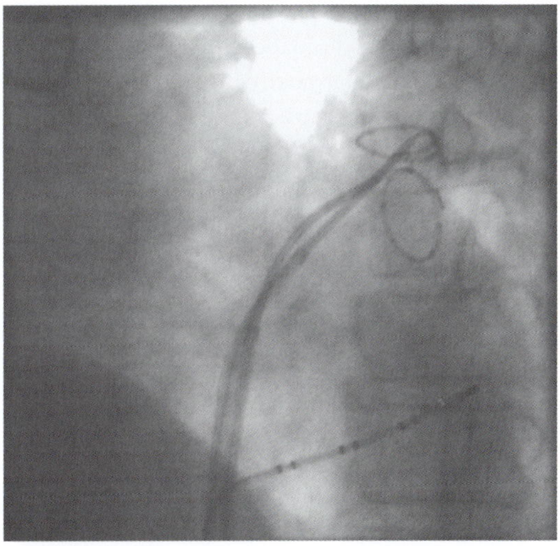

(b)

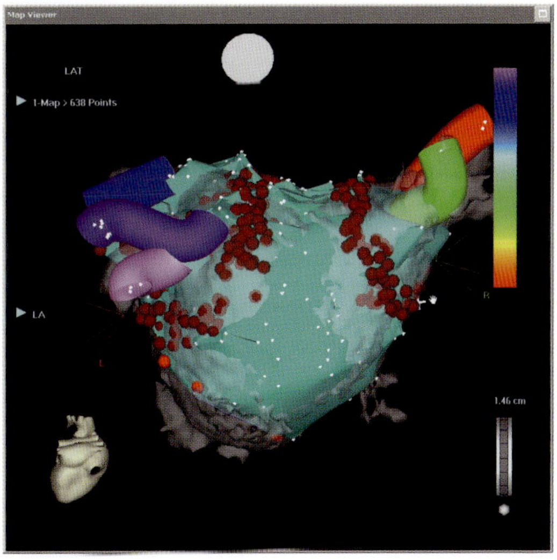

Figure 11.20 The technique of circumferential PV isolation. (a) A left anterior oblique fluoroscopic view of the two circular mapping catheters placed simultaneously in the superior and inferior left PVs. (b) The CartoMerge posteroanterior view of the LA after completing the circumferential lesions around the right and left PVs. The ablation points are shown as red tags, the electroanatomic map is displayed in turquoise (with colored tubes representing the PVs), and the CT-derived anatomy is in gray. In some parts of the circumferential lesions, multiple ablation tags indicate that it was particularly difficult in this region to achieve a complete conduction block over the line.

Ouyang et al. reported a 95% success rate in paroxysmal AF (39/41 patients) with 22% of patients (9/41) needing two ablation procedures [64,65]. Relapse of atrial tachyarrhythmia was in all cases due to conduction gaps across the linear lesions [65]. In a recent study by Cheema et al., less favorable results were observed [66]. A total of 64 patients with paroxysmal (29 patients), persistent (19 patients), or permanent AF (16 patients) were studied in a long-term setting. After a follow-up of 13 ± 1 months, overall, 19 of 29 patients with paroxysmal AF (65%) were arrhythmia-free, with 14 of the 29 patients (42%) arrhythmia-free after a single ablation procedure.

In a recent study by Arentz et al. [67], segmental ostial PVI (small isolation area approach) was compared in a randomized fashion with a more atrially located extra-ostial isolation of both ipsilateral PVs (large isolation area approach) in patients with both paroxysmal AF (67 patients) and persistent AF (43 patients). After a follow-up of 15 ± 4 months, overall 27 of 55 patients (49%) in the small isolation area group and 37 of 55 patients (67%) in the large isolation area group were free of recurrent AF as documented by serial Holter ECGs and repetitive exercise tests ($P \leq 0.05$). Importantly, there was no significant difference in ablation success if only paroxysmal AF patients were compared (19/35 with the small isolation area approach versus 23/32 with the large isolation area approach; $P = 0.1$). Thus, it remains unclear if larger isolating lesions are necessary in paroxysmal AF or if "small" ostial PV isolation might be sufficient for this subgroup of patients.

In conclusion, ablation approaches targeting the PVs, and especially those aiming at PVI, have evolved into a standard therapeutic strategy with good clinical results and acceptable complication rates.

Ablation of fractionated potentials and autonomic nerves

There are ablation approaches that do not intend to eliminate the initiating trigger in paroxysmal AF, but instead target precipitating factors of AF initiation or maintenance. Of these, we want to focus on the ablation of complex fractionated atrial electrograms (CFAEs) and the modulation of epicardially located ganglionated plexuses of autonomic nerves.

Ablation of complex fractionated atrial electrograms

The first description of this technique was published by Koonlawee Nademanee et al. in 2004 [68]. The hypothesis underlying the ablation technique is that complex fractionated electrograms recorded during AF are a marker for areas with electrical wavefront breaking, changes of electrical activation front direction, or slow conduction [3,4]. These areas are thought to be essential for the perpetuation of small fluctuating microreentries sustaining AF. It is assumed that the multiple microreentries during AF cannot persist if all these areas have been ablated. Another hypothesis is that rotors, drivers, or generators of AF, characterized by fractionated potentials, are eliminated with this ablation technique [69] (Figure 11.21). The endpoint of this approach in paroxysmal AF is AF termination during ablation with subsequent non-inducibility [68]. In the first reports, sinus rhythm was achieved during ablation as well as during follow-up in approximately 95% of patients, although many patients had been suffering from chronic AF for years. To date, few publications have described this technique, and most of them have done so in conjunction with other ablation approaches. As to the location of atrial regions with CFAE and preferential ablation sites with termination or organization of AF, findings from our center suggest that areas with CFAE are often located at the PV ostia, the anterior wall of the LA with the opening of the LAA, and the interatrial septum [70]. The decision where to ablate is sometimes difficult and until recently was solely based on the morphology of signals and the intuition of the operator. Recently, new software for the Carto as well as the NavX 3D mapping system provides the possibility of generating color-coded "fragmentation maps" of the atria [71].

The ablation of CFAE has not been used as a stand-alone approach in paroxysmal AF, probably because it is thought to modify the substrate maintaining AF, which is the leading feature in persistent and permanent AF. Its effect on the trigger (and its activity) is more difficult to imagine and might be small(er).

Ablation of autonomic plexuses

Similar to the ablation of CFAE, the ablation approach trying to modify mixed ganglionated

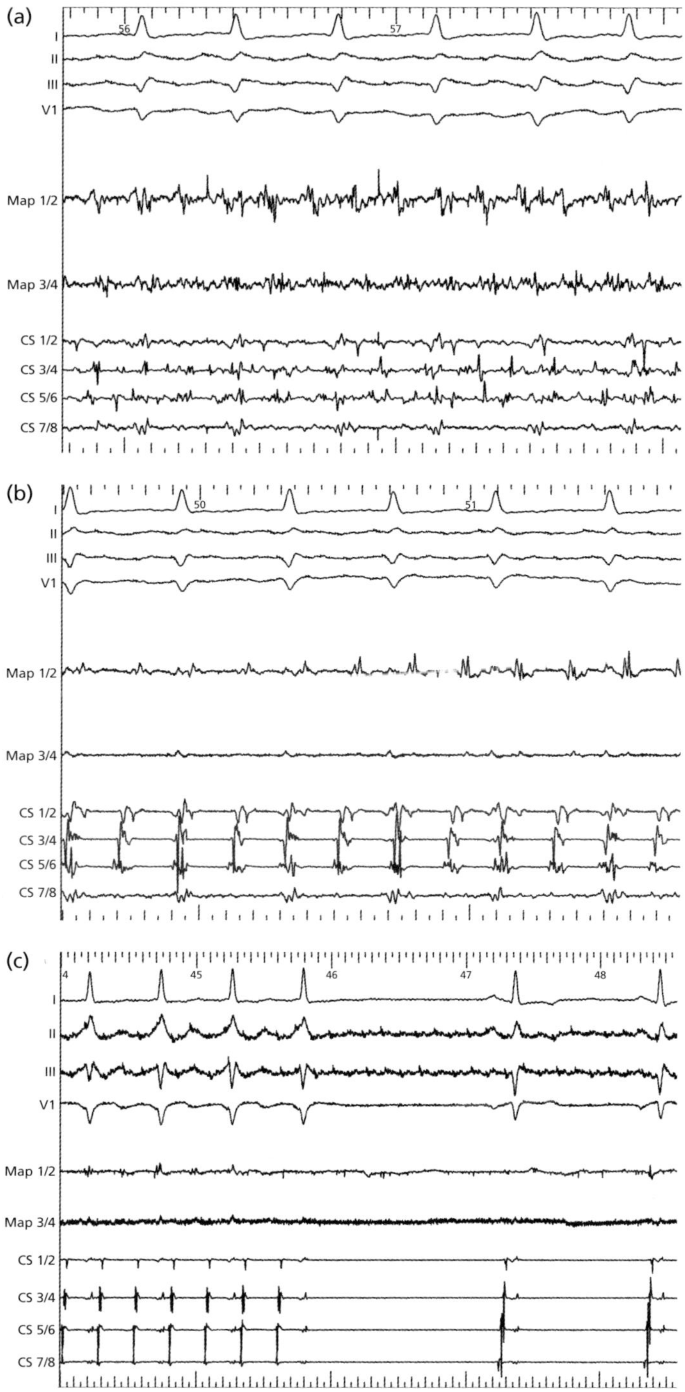

Figure 11.21 Electrogram recordings obtained during an electrogram-guided substrate ablation following the technique described by Nademanee et al. [68] In all three panels, surface ECG leads I, II, III, and V1 are shown at the top, followed by the intracardiac recordings of the ablation catheter (map 1/2 and 3/4) and the four bipolar coronary sinus (CS) recordings 1/2 to 7/8. (a) An example of a typical CFAE is displayed in the map catheter recordings at the beginning of an electrogram-guided substrate modification ablation procedure. Note the typical disorganized and fast electrical activity during AF recorded in the CS catheter (paper speed 100 mm/s). (b) AF is already slowed down in cycle and more organized after some ablations (paper speed 100 mm/s). (c) An even slower, completely regular atrial tachycardia (left part of the tracing) finally stops during ablation to sinus rhythm (paper speed 50 mm/s).

plexuses has not been extensively used [72–74]. In fact, there are only very scarce published data in humans assessing the effect of this technique. The targets of this approach are the so-called "fat pads", which contain mixed vegetative ganglionated plexuses. The localization of the fat pads in humans is slightly variable. Most commonly, four of the fat pads are located close to the four ostia of the PV

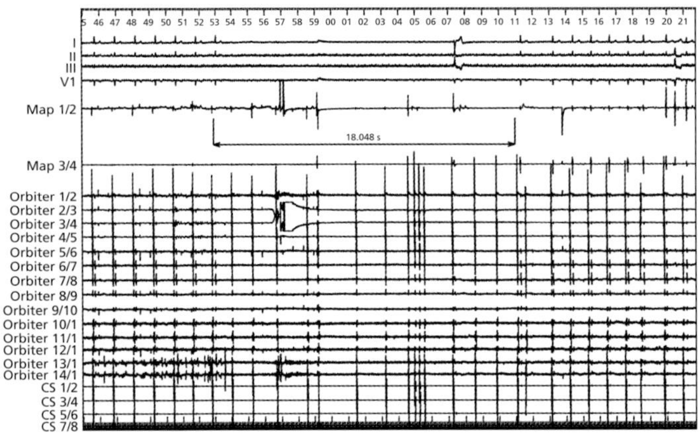

Figure 11.22 Pronounced vagal reaction during ablation at the ostium of the left superior PV (LSPV). The 14-polar circumferential mapping catheter (orbiter 1/2 to 14/1; Orbiter PV) is placed at the ostium of the LSPV. Radiofrequency energy ablation is delivered just proximal to the Orbiter PV catheter (map 1/2 and 3/4). Due to radiofrequency energy delivery, a prononunced vagal reaction is elicited, most likely through interference with the left superior "fat pad". Sinus bradycardia and AV block III° with an asystole of 18 s results. ECG tracings I, II, III, and V1 are displayed at the top, with coronary sinus (CS) recordings below.

[75]. The ganglionated plexuses are thought to influence the heart (especially atrial myocardial refractoriness and the activity of arrhythmogenic foci) by both sympathetic and parasympathetic inputs [76] (Figure 11.22).

The current ablation technique identifies the location of the fat pads by systemic vagal response to local high frequency (> 50 Hz) burst pacing. After ablation, local burst pacing should have no systemic vagal effects anymore.

In a non-randomized study by Scherlag et al. with 60 patients [74], a significant increase in success was achieved by combining fat pad ablation with ostial PVI compared to ostial PVI alone (70% success in PVI alone versus 91% by combining PVI with fat pad ablation). Similarly, Pappone et al. showed in 2004 that by adding a "complete vagal denervation" in 102 of a total of 295 patients with CPVA, they improved the results (sinus rhythm after 1 year) in paroxysmal AF from 85% (166/195 patients with CPVA alone) to 99% (101/102 patients with CPVA and vagal denervation) [77]. Unfortunately, the Milan group never published any further data using this peculiar technique.

In a study recently published by Bauer et al. from our center [78], we analyzed Holter ECG data from a randomized study comparing ostial PVI to CPVA [53] using standard heart rate variability measures and the new "deceleration capacity" parameter. This parameter is a very specific and sensitive Holter ECG measure for vagal activity [79]. Vagal activity decreased immediately after the ablation procedure with both approaches, considering all measured heart rate variability parameters including the deceleration capacity [78]. This vagal "denervation" persisted up to 12 months after ablation in CPVA, whereas in ostial PVI the values had returned to normal 4 weeks after the procedure (Figure 11.23). It is noteworthy that in this randomized study (as pointed out above), the ostial PVI approach was associated with a significantly better outcome compared to the CPVA technique [53].

Overall, there is not much clinical experience with these approaches as a stand-alone therapy for paroxysmal AF.

Combined approaches

Considering the multiple facets of AF it seems only natural that one single ablation technique might not be enough to treat all aspects of this fascinating arrhythmia. Therefore, the application of two or more ablation techniques in varying combinations has been proposed.

Pulmonary vein isolation and ablation targeting other thoracic veins

It became clear quite early that the PVs are not the only great thoracic veins with arrhythmogenic potential. Focal atrial activity from the CS and the superior vena cava (SVC) was also described, although mostly in the form of focal atrial tachycardia [80–84]. In both structures, myocardial muscular strands extending distally into the vein have been observed and mapped in electrophysiological studies.

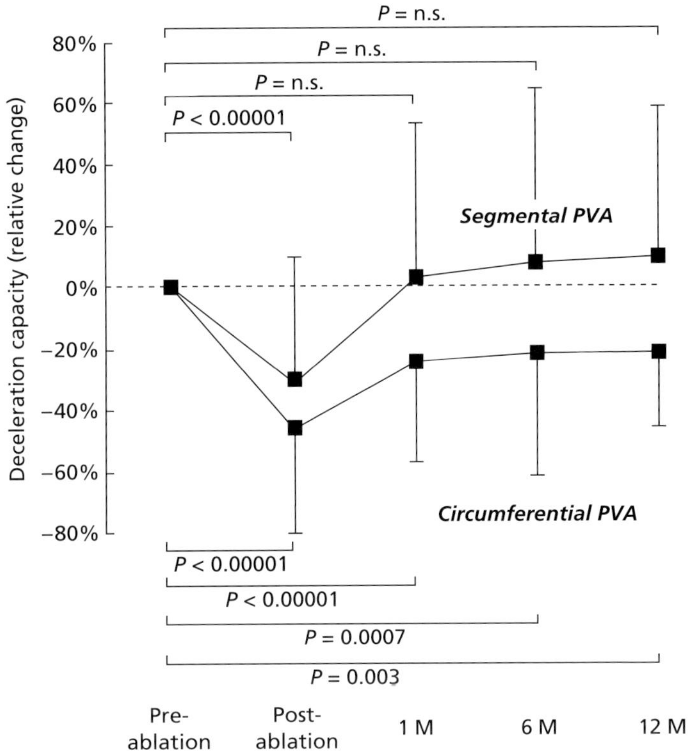

Figure 11.23 Relative change of deceleration capacity after circumferential and segmental pulmonary vein ablation (PVA) the day before ablation, the day after ablation, and 1, 6, and 12 months after ablation. Data are presented as mean standard deviations. The differences between circumferential and segmental PVA were significant at 1, 6, and 12 months after ablation. The results of this same study regarding the ablation success of the two ablation approaches are displayed in Figure 11.19. (Reproduced from [78] with permission)

Vein of Marshall

A tributary of the CS, the so-called vein of Marshall, has been reported to exhibit focal electric activity inducing AF [85,86]. Hwang et al. [85] reported in 2000 that it was possible to retrogradely cannulate this relatively small vein in 17 of 28 patients presenting with paroxysmal AF. In eight of 17 patients, local electric activation could be documented by recording intravenous double potentials; and in six of eight patients, focal electric activity arising distally in the vein of Marshall was found to initiate episodes of AF. By ablating (endocardially) the insertion of the vein of Marshall, focally induced paroxysmal AF was eliminated in four of six patients.

Despite these encouraging results this approach did not get widespread acceptance, mostly because the incidence of arrhythmogenic foci in the vein of Marshall is probably not very high.

Superior vena cava

The second great thoracic vein that has been reported to be a possible target in the ablation of paroxysmal AF is the SVC [87–89]. Tsai et al. from the group in Taipei, Taiwan reported in 2000 that in eight of 130 patients treated for paroxysmal AF, ectopic beats arising from the SVC initiated episodes of AF [87]. By eliminating the arrhythmogenic foci, all eight patients remained in stable sinus rhythm during a mean follow-up of 9 ± 3 months. In 2002, Goya et al. from the Hamburg St. Georg group published a series of 16 patients with ongoing paroxysmal AF after the isolation of all PVs due to focal activity from the SVC [88]. After electrical isolation of the SVC, 82% of the patients (13/16) were free of arrhythmia in a follow-up of 12.6 ± 8 months. Although these data are encouraging, the electrical SVC isolation for arrhythmogenic foci has not (yet) become a standard approach – maybe due to its relatively low incidence.

The inferior vena cava has not been reported to be frequently involved in the initiation or maintenance of AF. This is probably due to the fact that in the majority of patients there are no muscular (myocardial) strands extending to the inferior vena cava.

Inducibility guided additional ablation targeting the substrate

In paroxysmal AF, the central paradigm is the initiating trigger and not the maintaining substrate. Since the concept of trigger elimination has emerged for this entity, ablation approaches aiming at substrate modification have not been used extensively. PVI eliminates the main source of initiating foci. However, there are approximately 25% of patients who continue to experience AF episodes after PVI [18–29]. If these patients were identified during the procedure and were treated with additional (substrate) ablation, the clinical success rate after ablation might increase. It seems that the "differentiation tool" to identify these patients could be the inducibility of sustained AF after PVI. The additional benefit of an inducibility guided differentiated ablation strategy has been demonstrated for both additional linear lesions and ablation of CFAE [90,91]. In 70 patients with paroxysmal AF randomized to PVI alone (35 patients) or PVI + mitral isthmus line ablation, the inducibility of sustained AF was tested after ablation [90]. If sustained AF was not inducible, only 13% of patients (6/46) experienced relapse of AF as compared to 36% (9/24) with still inducible AF. In a similar study comparing PVI alone versus PVI + linear lesion at the septum, LA roof, and anterior LA in 100 patients with paroxysmal AF [91], patients with inducible AF had a significantly less favorable outcome than those with no inducibility after ablation (67% versus 85%).

Adding linear lesions

On the right atrial side, the cavotricuspid isthmus line remains the only commonly used linear lesion. It has some incontestable advantages: it is (relatively) safe, easy to apply, easy to test for completeness, and is only very rarely proarrhythmogenic. Alas, it is not very helpful in most cases of AF. In contrast, left atrial lines have gained increasing attention in the setting of AF.

Mitral isthmus line

In analogy to the right atrial isthmus line, a left atrial isthmus line has been described that extends from the left inferior PV to the lateral mitral annulus. In CPVA, the inferior lateral part of the lesion encircling the left PV is the starting point of this line. In paroxysmal AF, this line after PVI increased the success rate from 69% (69/100 patients) to 87% (87/100) in 200 consecutive (non-randomized) patients [92]. Of note is the fact that the completeness of block over the left isthmus line was tested in this study by: (i) documenting a corridor of widely split double potentials on the line; (ii) an activation detour around the mitral annulus while pacing in the distal CS; and (iii) differential pacing maneuvers. To achieve complete block, epicardial (intra-CS) applications had to be delivered in 62% of patients.

Confusingly, it has been claimed that a conduction delay of more than 120 ms over the line was enough to prevent atrial tachycardia [93].

Roof line

Similar to the above-mentioned study, Hocini et al. of the Bordeaux group compared PVI alone with PVI + roofline connecting both superior PVs in a randomized study [94]. The additional roofline increased the success rate from 69% after PVI alone (31/45 patients) to 87% after PVI + roofline (39/45) during a follow-up of 15 ± 4 months ($P = 0.04$).

A newly designed linear ablation catheter ("flowliner" catheter) has been proposed for roofline creation. It is a radiofrequency-energy-delivering catheter with a very long, two-segmented, open-irrigated tip with an active electrode length of 2.2 cm. Results of the pivotal trial addressing completeness of the roof line, mean ablation, procedure time, and clinical outcome are not yet available.

Pulmonary vein isolation plus complex fractionated atrial electrogram ablation

In a randomized prospective study from our group, PVI alone (48 patients) was compared to the combination of PVI and CFAE ablation (50 patients) in paroxysmal AF [95]. The study protocol stipulated that inducibility of sustained AF was tested in all 98 patients after PVI, but that CFAE ablation was performed only in patients randomized to the combined approach. In both groups AF was still inducible in approximately two-thirds of patients. CFAE ablation was performed in 30 of 50 patients randomized to PVI + CFAE ablation. After a 1-month blanking period, 73% (PVI + CFAE) and 75% of patients (PVI alone) remained arrhythmia-free as assessed by 7-day Holter ECGs. From the results of this study, the value of additional CFAE ablation after PVI is, at the least, questionable.

Combinations of more than two techniques

There are data suggesting that the combination of: (i) PVI; (ii) isolation of the thoracic veins; (iii) CFAE ablation; and (iv) linear lesions, might provide better clinical success [96–98]. The electrical isolation of all PVs and other potentially arrhythmogenic thoracic veins (CS, SVC) is performed first. Afterwards, induction of AF is attempted with aggressive atrial burst pacing (five attempts, maximal pacing output, three different pacing sites). If AF is not inducible or non-sustained, no further ablation is performed. If AF is inducible or persists despite previous ablation, ablation of CFAE is applied, and thereafter – if AF is still inducible – linear lesions in the LA (roofline, left isthmus line) are inserted.

The success rates of this approach are promising, but procedures may be long-lasting and feasible without severe complications only in experienced centers.

Conclusion

The multitude of ablation techniques, cited studies, and results sometimes seem confusing, but reflect the sinuous change of paradigms in the ablative therapy of paroxysmal AF. The central role of triggering foci within the PVs is a stable constant that is generally accepted and, therefore, PVI is the common base of most ablation concepts. The possibility that additional ablative measures are needed or useful has to be evaluated in randomized, large-scale trials.

References

1 Schmitt C, Zrenner B, Schneider M, et al. Clinical experience with a novel multielectrode basket catheter in right atrial tachycardias. *Circulation* 1999;**99**:2414–22.

2 Zrenner B, Ndrepepa G, Karch MR, et al. Electrophysiologic characteristics of paroxysmal and chronic atrial fibrillation in human right atrium *J Am Coll Cardiol* 2001;**38**:1143–9.

3 Konings KTS, Kirchhof CJHJ, Smeets JRLM, et al. High-density mapping of electrically induced atrial fibrillation in humans *Circulation* 1994;**89**:1665–80.

4 Konings KTS, Smeets JLRM, Penn OC, et al. Configuration of unipolar atrial electrograms during electrically induced atrial fibrillation in humans. *Circulation* 1997; **95**:1231–41.

5 Ndrepepa G, Karch MR, Schneider MA, et al. Characterization of paroxysmal and persistent atrial fibrillation in the human left atrium during initiation and sustained episodes. *J Cardiovasc Electrophysiol* 2002;**13**:525–32.

6 Karch MR, Ndrepepa G, Schneider MAE, et al. Single chamber atrial fibrillation involving only the left atrium: implications for maintenance and radiofrequency ablation strategy. *Pacing Clin Electrophysiol* 2003;**26**: 883–91.

7 Schneider MAE, Ndrepepa G, Zrenner B, et al. Noncontact mapping-guided catheter ablation of atrial fibrillation associated with left atrial ectopy. *J Cardiovasc Electrophysiol* 2000;**11**:475–9.

8 Hindricks G, Kottkamp H. Simultaneous noncontact mapping of left atrium in patients with paroxysmal atrial fibrillation. *Circulation* 2001;**104**:297–303.

9 Schneider MA, Ndrepepa G, Weber S, et al. Influence of high-pass filtering on noncontact mapping and ablation of atrial tachycardias. *Pacing Clin Electrophysiol* 2004;**27**: 38–46.

10 Schmitt C, Ndrepepa G, Weber S, et al. Biatrial multisite mapping of atrial premature complexes triggering onset of atrial fibrillation. *Am J Cardiol* 2002;**89**:1381–77.

11 Lin WS, Tai CT, Hsieh MH, et al. Catheter ablation of paroxysmal atrial fibrillation initiated by non-pulmonary vein ectopy. *Circulation* 2003;**107**:3176–83.

12 Jais P, Haissaguerre M, Shah DC, et al. A focal source of atrial fibrillation treated by discrete radiofrequency ablation. *Circulation* 1997;**95**:572–6.

13 Haissaguerre M, Jais P, Shah DC, et al. Spontaneous initiation of atrial fibrillation by ectopic beats originating in the pulmonary veins. *N Engl J Med* 1998;**339**:59–66.

14 Chen SA, Hsieh MH, Tai CT, et al. Initiation of atrial fibrillation by ectopic beats originating from the pulmonary veins: electrophysiological characteristics, pharmacological responses, and effects of radiofrequency ablation. *Circulation* 1999;**100**:1879–86.

15 Saito T, Waki K, Becker A. Left atrial myocardial extensions onto pulmonary veins in humans: anatomic observations relevant for atrial arrhythmias. *J Cardiovasc Electrophysiol* 2000;**11**:888–94.

16 Haissaguerre M, Jais P, Shah DC, et al. Electrophysiological end point for catheter ablation of atrial fibrillation initiated from multiple pulmonary venous foci. *Circulation* 2000;**101**:1409–17.

17 Hocini M, Haissaguerre M, Shah D, et al. Multiple sources initiating atrial fibrillation from a single pulmonary vein identified by a circumferential catheter. *Pacing Clin Electrophysiol* 2000;**23**:1828–31.

18 Haissaguerre M, Shah DC, Jais P, et al. Electrophysiological breakthroughs from the left atrium to the pulmonary veins. *Circulation* 2000;**102**:2462–5.
19 Oral H, Knight BP, Tada H, et al. Pulmonary vein isolation for paroxysmal and persistent atrial fibrillation. *Circulation* 2002;**105**:1077–81.
20 Deisenhofer I, Schneider MA, Bohlen-Knauf M, et al. Circumferential mapping and electric isolation of pulmonary veins in patients with atrial fibrillation. *Am J Cardiol* 2003;**91**:159–63.
21 Arentz T, von Rosenthal J, Blum T, et al. Feasibility and safety of pulmonary vein isolation using a new mapping and navigation system in patients with refractory atrial fibrillation. *Circulation* 2003;**108**:2484–90.
22 Macle L, Jais P, Weerasooriya R, et al. Irrigated tip catheter ablation of pulmonary veins for treatment of atrial fibrillation. *J Cardiovasc Electrophysiol* 2002;**13**:1067–73.
23 Oral H, Knight BP, Ozaydin M, et al. Segmental ostial ablation to isolate the pulmonary veins during atrial fibrillation: feasibility and mechanistic insights. *Circulation* 2002;**106**:1256–62.
24 Seshadri N, Marrouche NF, Wilber D, et al. Pulmonary vein isolation for treatment of atrial fibrillation: recent updates. *Pacing Clin Electrophysiol* 2003;**26**:1636–40.
25 Marchlinski FE, Callans D, Dixit S, et al. Efficacy and safety of targeted focal ablation versus PV isolation assisted by magnetic electroanatomic mapping. *J Cardiovasc Electrophysiol* 2003;**14**:358–65.
26 Vasamreddy CR, Lickfett L, Jayam VK, et al. Predictors of recurrence following catheter ablation of atrial fibrillation using an irrigated-tip ablation catheter. *J Cardiovasc Electrophysiol* 2004;**15**:692–7.
27 Gerstenfeld EP, Callans DJ, Dixit S, et al. Incidence and location of focal atrial fibrillation triggers in patients undergoing repeat pulmonary vein isolation: implications for ablation strategies. *J Cardiovasc Electrophysiol* 2003;**14**:685–90.
28 Oral H, Knight BP, Ozaydin M, et al. Clinical significance of early recurrences of atrial fibrillation after pulmonary vein isolation. *J Am Coll Cardiol* 2002;**40**:100–4.
29 Nanthakumar K, Plumb VJ, Epstein AE, et al. Resumption of electrical conduction in previously isolated pulmonary veins: rationale for a different strategy? *Circulation* 2004;**109**:1226–9.
30 Scanavacca MI, Kajita LJ, Vieira M, Sosa EA. Pulmonary vein stenosis complicating catheter ablation of focal atrial fibrillation. *J Cardiovasc Electrophysiol* 2000;**11**:677–81.
31 Packer DL, Keelan P, Munger TM, et al. Clinical presentation, investigation, and management of pulmonary vein stenosis complicating ablation for atrial fibrillation. *Circulation* 2005;**111**:546–54.
32 Callans DJ, Gerstenfeld EP, Dixit S, et al. Efficacy of repeat pulmonary vein isolation procedures in patients with recurrent atrial fibrillation. *J Cardiovasc Electrophysiol* 2004;**15**:1050–5.
33 Deisenhofer I, Böhlen-Knauf M, Estner H, et al. Success of early versus late repeat ablation after electric pulmonary vein isolation for atrial fibrillation. *Heart Rhythm* 2005;**2**:S233
34 Shah D, Haissaguerre M, Jais P, et al. Left atrial appendage activity masquerading as pulmonary vein potentials. *Circulation* 2002;**105**:2821–5.
35 Hocini M, Shah DC, Jais P, et al. Concealed left pulmonary vein potentials unmasked by left atrial stimulation. *Pacing Clin Electrophysiol* 2000;**23**:1832–5.
36 Asirvatham SJ. Pulmonary vein related manoeuvres: Part I. *Heart Rhythm* 2007;**4**:538–45.
37 Estner H, Deisenhofer I, Luik A, et al. Electrical isolation of pulmonary veins in patients with atrial fibrillation: reduction of fluoroscopy exposure and procedure duration by the use of a non-fluoroscopic navigation system (NavX®). *Europace* 2006;**8**:583–7.
38 Rotter M, Takahashi Y, Sanders P, et al. Reduction of fluoroscopy exposure and procedure duration during ablation of atrial fibrillation using a novel anatomical navigation system. *Eur Heart J* 2005;**26**:1415–21.
39 Marrouche NF, Martin DO, Wazni O, et al. Phased-array intracardiac echocardiography monitoring during pulmonary vein isolation in patients with atrial fibrillation: impact on outcome and complications. *Circulation* 2003;**107**:2710–16.
40 Dong J, Dickfeld T, Dalal D, et al. Initial experience in the use of integrated electroanatomic mapping with three-dimensional MR/CT images to guide catheter ablation of atrial fibrillation. *J Cardiovasc Electrophysiol* 2006;**17**:459–66.
41 Hsu LF, Jais P, Hocini M, et al. Incidence and prevention of cardiac tamponade complicating ablation for atrial fibrillation. *Pacing Clin Electrophysiol* 2005;**28**(S1): S106–S109.
42 Natale A, Pisano E, Shewchik J, et al. First human experience with pulmonary vein isolation using a through-the-balloon circumferential ultrasound ablation system for recurrent atrial fibrillation. *Circulation* 2000;**102**:1879–82.
43 Van Belle Y, Janse P, Rivero-Ayerza MJ, et al. Pulmonary vein isolation using an occluding cryoballoon for circumferential ablation: feasibility, complications, and short-term outcome. *Eur Heart J* 2007;**28**:2231–7.
44 Schmidt B, Antz M, Ernst S, et al. Pulmonary vein isolation by high-intensity focused ultrasound: first-in-man study with a steerable balloon catheter. *Heart Rhythm* 2007;**4**:575–84.
45 Arruda MS, He DS, Friedman P, et al. A novel mesh electrode catheter for mapping and radiofrequency delivery at the left atrium-pulmonary vein junction: a

single-catheter approach to pulmonary vein antrum isolation. *J Cardiovasc Electrophysiol* 2007;**18**:206–11.

46 Reddy VY, Houghtaling C, Fallon J, et al. Use of a diode laser balloon ablation catheter to generate circumferential pulmonary venous lesions in an open-thoracotomy caprine model. *Pacing Clin Electrophysiol* 2004;**27**:52–7.

47 Pappone C, Rosanio S, Oreto G, et al. Circumferential radiofrequency ablation of pulmonary vein ostia: a new anatomic approach for curing atrial fibrillation. *Circulation* 2000;**102**:2619–28.

48 Pappone C, Oreto G, Rosanio S, et al. Atrial electroanatomic remodelling after circumferential radiofrequency pulmonary vein ablation: efficacy of an anatomic approach in a large cohort of patients with atrial fibrillation. *Circulation* 2001;**104**:2539–44.

49 Pappone C, Augello G, Sala S, et al. A randomized trial of circumferential pulmonary vein ablation versus antiarrhythmic drug therapy in paroxysmal atrial fibrillation: the APAF Study. *J Am Coll Cardiol* 2006;**48**:2340–7.

50 Hocini M, Jais P, Hsu LF, et al. Prevalence of pulmonary vein disconnection after anatomical ablation for atrial fibrillation: consequences of wide atrial encircling of the pulmonary veins. *Eur Heart J* 2004;**26**:696–704.

51 Vasamreddy CR, Dalal D, Eldadah Z, et al. Safety and efficacy of circumferential pulmonary vein catheter ablation of atrial fibrillation. *Heart Rhythm* 2005;**2**:42–8.

52 Oral H, Scharf C, Chugh A, et al. Catheter ablation for paroxysmal atrial fibrillation: segmental pulmonary vein ostial ablation versus left atrial ablation. *Circulation* 2003;**108**:2355–60.

53 Karch MR, Zrenner B, Deisenhofer I, et al. Freedom from atrial tachyarrhythmias after catheter ablation of atrial fibrillation: a randomized comparison between 2 current ablation strategies. *Circulation* 2005;**111**:2875–80.

54 Mesas CE, Pappone C, Lang CC, et al. Left atrial tachycardia after circumferential pulmonary vein ablation for atrial fibrillation: electroanatomic characterization and treatment. *J Am Coll Cardiol* 2004;**44**:1071–9.

55 Deisenhofer I, Estner H, Zrenner B, et al. Left atrial tachycardia after circumferential pulmonary vein ablation for atrial fibrillation: incidence, electrophysiological characteristics and results of radiofrequency ablation. *Europace* 2006;**8**:572–83.

56 Pappone C, Manguso F, Vicedomini G, et al. Prevention of iatrogenic atrial tachycardia after ablation of atrial fibrillation: a prospective randomized study comparing circumferential pulmonary vein ablation with a modified approach. *Circulation* 2004;**110**:3036–42.

57 Pappone C, Oral H, Santinelli V, et al. Atrio-esophageal fistula as a complication of percutaneous transcatheter ablation of atrial fibrillation. *Circulation* 2004;**109**:2724–6.

58 Cummings JE, Schweikert RA, Saliba WI, et al. Brief communication: atrial-esophageal fistulas after radiofrequency ablation. *Ann Intern Med.* 2006;**144**:572–4.

59 Sanchez-Quintana D, Cabrera JA, Climent V, et al. Anatomic relations between the esophagus and left atrium and relevance for ablation of atrial fibrillation. *Circulation* 2005;**112**:1400–5.

60 Redfearn DP, Trim GM, Skanes AC, et al. Esophageal temperature monitoring during radiofrequency ablation of atrial fibrillation. *J Cardiovasc Electrophysiol* 2005; **16**:589–93.

61 Cummings JE, Schweikert RA, Saliba WI, et al. Assessment of temperature, proximity, and course of the esophagus during radiofrequency ablation within the left atrium. *Circulation* 2005;**112**:459–64.

62 Cury RC, Abbara S, Schmidt S, et al. Relationship of the esophagus and aorta to the left atrium and pulmonary veins: implications for catheter ablation of atrial fibrillation. *Heart Rhythm* 2005;**2**:1317–23.

63 Kottkamp H, Piorkowski C, Tanner H, et al. Topographic variability of the esophageal left atrial relation influencing ablation lines in patients with atrial fibrillation. *J Cardiovasc Electrophysiol* 2005;**16**:146–50.

64 Ouyang F, Bansch D, Ernst S, et al. Complete isolation of left atrium surrounding the pulmonary veins: new insights from the double-Lasso technique in paroxysmal atrial fibrillation. *Circulation* 2004;**110**:2090–6.

65 Ouyang F, Antz M, Ernst S, et al. Recovered pulmonary vein conduction as a dominant factor for recurrent atrial tachyarrhythmias after complete circular isolation of the pulmonary veins: lessons from double Lasso technique. *Circulation* 2005;**111**:127–35.

66 Cheema A, Dong J, Dalal D, et al. Long-term safety and efficacy of circumferential ablation with pulmonary vein isolation. *J Cardiovasc Electrophysiol* 2006;**17**:1080–5.

67 Arentz T, Weber R, Burkle G, et al. Small or large isolation areas around the pulmonary veins for the treatment of atrial fibrillation? Results from a prospective randomized study. *Circulation* 2007;**115**:3057–63.

68 Nademanee K, McKenzie J, Kosar E, et al. A new approach for catheter ablation of atrial fibrillation: mapping of the electrophysiologic substrate. *J Am Coll Cardiol* 2004;**43**:2044–53.

69 Jalife J. Rotors and spiral waves in atrial fibrillation. *J Cardiovasc Electrophysiol* 2003;**14**:776–80.

70 Schmitt C, Estner H, Hecher B, et al. Radiofrequency ablation of complex fractionated atrial electrograms (CFAE): preferential sites of acute termination and regularisation in paroxysmal and persistent atrial fibrillation. *J Cardiovasc Electrophysiol* 2007;**18**:1039–46.

71 Wu J, Deisenhofer I, Luik A, et al. Automatic 3D mapping of complex fractionated atrial electrograms (CFAE) in

patients with paroxysmal and persistent atrial fibrillation. *Heart Rhythm* 2007;**4**:S346.

72 Schauerte P, Scherlag BJ, Pitha J, et al. Catheter ablation of cardiac autonomic nerves for prevention of vagal atrial fibrillation. *Circulation* 2000;**102**:2774–80.

73 Scherlag BJ, Yamanashi W, Patel U, et al. Autonomically induced conversion of pulmonary vein focal firing into atrial fibrillation. *J Am Coll Cardiol* 2005;**45**:1878–86.

74 Scherlag BJ, Nakagawa H, Jackman WM, et al. Electrical stimulation to identify neural elements on the heart: their role in atrial fibrillation. *J Intervent Cardiac Electrophysiol* 2005;**13**:37–42.

75 Scherlag BJ, Po S. The intrinsic cardiac nervous system and atrial fibrillation. *Curr Opin Cardiol* 2006;**21**: 51–4.

76 Armour JA, Richer LP, Pagé P, et al. Origin and pharmacological response of atrial tachyarrhythmias induced by activation of mediastinal nerves in canine. *Auton Neurosci* 2005;**118**:68–78.

77 Pappone C, Santinelli V, Manguso F, et al. Pulmonary vein denervation enhances long-term benefit after circumferential ablation for paroxysmal atrial fibrillation. *Circulation* 2004;**109**:327–34.

78 Bauer A, Deisenhofer I, Schneider R, et al. Effects of circumferential or segmental pulmonary vein ablation for paroxysmal atrial fibrillation on cardiac autonomic function. *Heart Rhythm* 2006;**3**:1428–35.

79 Bauer A, Kantelhardt JW, Barthel P, et al. Deceleration capacity as a predictor of mortality after myocardial infarction. *Lancet* 2006;**267**(9523):1674–81.

80 Dong J, Schreieck J, Ndrepepa G, Schmitt C. Ectopic tachycardia originating from the superior vena cava. *J Cardiovasc Electrophysiol* 2002;**13**:620–4.

81 Shah DC, Haissaguerre M, Jais P, Clementy J. High-resolution mapping of tachycardia originating from the superior vena cava: evidence of electrical heterogeneity, slow conduction, and possible circus movement reentry. *J Cardiovasc Electrophysiol* 2002;**13**:388–92.

82 Pak HN, Lim HE, Kim YH. Atrial tachycardia originating from the coronary sinus ostium dissociated with fibrillatory activity inside persistent left superior vena cava. *Heart Rhythm* 2005;**2**:333.

83 Yamane T, Miyanaga S, Inada K, et al. A focal source of atrial fibrillation in the superior vena cava: isolation and elimination by radiofrequency ablation with the guide of basket catheter mapping. *J Interv Cardiac Electrophysiol* 2004;**11**:131–4.

84 Tada H, Naito S, Meguro K, et al. Persistent tachycardia originating from the superior vena cava as a driver for atrial fibrillation. *Pacing Clin Electrophysiol* 2004;**27**: 252–5.

85 Hwang C, Wu TJ, Doshi RN, et al. Vein of Marshall cannulation for the analysis of electrical activity in patients with focal atrial fibrillation. *Circulation* 2000;**101**:1503–5.

86 Kamanu S, Tan AY, Peter CT, Hwang C, Chen PS. Vein of Marshall activity during sustained atrial fibrillation. *J Cardiovasc Electrophysiol* 2006;**17**:839–46.

87 Tsai CF, Tai CT, Hsieh MH, et al. Initiation of atrial fibrillation by ectopic beats originating from the superior vena cava: electrophysiological characteristics and results of radiofrequency ablation. *Circulation* 2000;**102**:67–74.

88 Goya M, Ouyang F, Ernst S, et al. Electroanatomic mapping and catheter ablation of breakthroughs from the right atrium to the superior vena cava in patients with atrial fibrillation. *Circulation* 2002;**106**:1317–20.

89 Liu TY, Tai CT, Lee PC, et al. Novel concept of atrial tachyarrhythmias originating from the superior vena cava: insight from noncontact mapping. *J Cardiovasc Electrophysiol* 2003;**14**:533–9.

90 Haissaguerre M, Sanders P, Hocini M, et al. Changes in atrial fibrillation cycle length and inducibility during catheter ablation and their relation to outcome. *Circulation* 2004;**109**:3007–13.

91 Oral H, Chugh A, Lemola K, et al. Noninducibility of atrial fibrillation as an end point of left atrial circumferential ablation for paroxysmal atrial fibrillation. A randomized study. *Circulation* 2004;**110**:2797–801.

92 Jais P, Hocini M, Hsu LF, et al. Technique and results of linear ablation at the mitral isthmus. *Circulation* 2004; **110**:2996–3002.

93 Pappone C, Augello G, Mazzone P, et al. Complete mitral isthmus block is not required to prevent atrial tachycardia after circumferential pulmonary vein ablation. *Heart Rhythm* 2005;**2**:S16

94 Hocini M, Jais P, Sanders P, et al. Techniques, evaluation, and consequences of linear block at the left atrial roof in paroxysmal atrial fibrillation – a prospective randomized study. *Circulation* 2005;**112**:3688–96.

95 Deisenhofer I, Schmitt C, Estner HL, et al. Additional ablation of complex fractionated atrial electrograms (CFAE) after pulmonary vein isolation in paroxysmal atrial fibrillation: results of a controlled randomized study. *Heart Rhythm* 2007;**4**:S115.

96 Haissaguerre M, Sanders P, Hocini M, et al. Catheter ablation of long-lasting persistent atrial fibrillation: critical structures for termination. *J Cardiovasc Electrophysiol* 2005;**16**:1125–37.

97 Oral H, Chugh A, Good E, et al. A tailored approach to catheter ablation of paroxysmal atrial fibrillation. *Circulation* 2006;**113**:1824–31.

98 Jais P, Hocini M, Sanders P, et al. Long-term evaluation of atrial fibrillation ablation guided by noninducibility. *Heart Rhythm* 2006;**3**:140–5.

12

CHAPTER 12

Ablation strategies in chronic atrial fibrillation

Mark D. O'Neill, Kang Teng Lim, Pierre Jaïs, Mélèze Hocini, Yoshihide Takahashi, Anders Jönsson, Frédéric Sacher, Prashanthan Sanders, Sathish Kodali, Leonardo Arantès, Seiichiro Matsuo, Sébastien Knecht, Thomas Rostock, Martin Rotter, Jacques Clémenty, George J. Klein, & Michel Haïssaguerre

Introduction

Atrial fibrillation (AF) is arguably the most challenging arrhythmia facing physicians today and accounts for approximately one-third of hospitalizations for cardiac rhythm disturbances [1]. It is common, increases with age, and is associated with increased morbidity and mortality [2,3]. Safe and effective pharmacological therapy is not available. Despite being a relatively new treatment, catheter ablation has advanced rapidly both in terms of the numbers and success of procedures performed worldwide [4]. Although catheter ablation may now be considered early in the management of a patient with paroxysmal AF, the treatment of chronic AF poses a significant challenge. We will discuss contemporary ablation strategies for chronic AF and describe in detail the catheter ablation approach practiced in Bordeaux.

Catheter Ablation of Atrial Fibrillation Edited by Etienne Aliot, Michel Haïssaguerre and Warren M. Jackman

Definition of atrial fibrillation

The ACC/AHA/ESC (American College of Cardiology/American Heart Association/European Society of Cardiology) 2006 guidelines for the management of patients with atrial fibrillation [5] classified AF into:

- Paroxysmal AF defined as recurrent AF with two or more episodes and terminating spontaneously within 7 days.
- Persistent AF defined as AF that is sustained beyond 7 days but necessitates pharmacological or electrical cardioversion.
- Permanent AF defined as AF in which cardioversion has either failed or not been attempted.

There have been criticisms that the term "permanent AF" is not appropriate in the context of patients undergoing catheter or surgical AF ablation since it refers to a group of patients where a decision has been made not to pursue restoration of sinus rhythm. In a recent publication, Oral et al. used an alternative classification of AF that included chronic AF, defined as AF lasting ≥ 6 months [6]. In contrast, our definition of chronic AF is AF lasting ≥ 1 month based on a previous classification by Levy et al. [7].

Surgical origins of catheter ablation strategies for atrial fibrillation

Early attempts at catheter ablation of AF were inspired largely by the success of the maze surgical procedure (and its subsequent modifications) in treating both paroxysmal and persistent AF [8]. Cox devised the procedure based on his assumption that reentrant circuits were necessary for maintenance of AF, and that "channeling" the cardiac impulse through a pathway (maze) of insufficient width to sustain reentry would preserve sinus rhythm. This surgery was subsequently modified and the current maze III iteration of the procedure now incorporates four critical lesion sets: (1) encirclement and effective electrical isolation of the pulmonary veins (PVs); (2) a line joining the circumferential PV lesion to the mitral annulus; (3) a circumferential lesion in the coronary sinus; (4) cryoablation of the cavotricuspid isthmus. Other iterations of this surgery using similar lesion strategies with other ablative tools (especially radiofrequency) have been reported with good success. Melo et al. [9] proposed ipsilateral paired PV encirclement, while Sueda et al. [10] described en bloc PV isolation (PVI) with success rates in the order of 55–75%. All incorporate the PV region with the addition of linear lesions as per the maze III prototype required in patients with "complex" AF, that is AF that is chronic and frequently associated with significant cardiac comorbidity. The parallels with current ablation strategies for chronic AF are striking.

Although surgical treatment of AF dominated early attempts to cure AF, percutaneous catheter ablation has usurped much of its role. The indication for surgical AF ablation according to the latest HRS/EHRA/ECAS (Heart Rhythm Society/European Heart Rhythm Society/European Cardiac Arrhythmia Society) expert consensus comprises patients undergoing cardiac surgery who have symptomatic AF or selected asymptomatic patients in whom the ablation can be performed with minimal risk. Stand-alone surgery can be considered for AF patients who prefer a surgical approach, have one or more failed attempts at catheter ablation, or who are not candidates for catheter ablation.

From linear ablation to pulmonary vein isolation

Coincident with early surgical work was the development and emergence of radiofrequency energy as a means to target selectively endocardial structures for ablation [11]. The encouraging developments in surgical treatment of AF outlined above prompted a parallel evolution in catheter-based attempts at achieving a similar outcome [12]. The first catheter-based attempt to recreate the maze III lesion set was accomplished by Swartz et al. in 1993 [13]. Kay, Packer, and Swartz published their experience of this approach in 18 patients with chronic AF, reporting acute termination in 50% and long-term drug-free success in 78%, although following long procedures and redo procedures in 39% [14]. Catheter linear ablation confined to the right atrium was performed in 1994 but was associated with a success rate of less than 10% at 2 years follow-up off antiarrhythmic drugs [15,16]. Recognition of the arrhythmogenic potential of the PVs precipitated a change of emphasis from an attempt to mimic operative procedures to focal ablation of the source of ectopy as an initiating and sustaining mechanism in AF [17].

Many of the important studies published at this time included data not only for paroxysmal but also for persistent and permanent AF and, almost without exception, documented an important difference in outcome between patients with paroxysmal versus chronic AF. Pappone et al., describing their early experience with circumferential PV ablation using an electroanatomic mapping technique, reported freedom from AF in 85% of patients with paroxysmal AF and 68% of those with chronic AF [18]. Using a circumferential mapping catheter-guided approach, Oral et al. reported a much lower freedom from recurrent AF in persistent (22%) versus paroxysmal (70%) AF, despite achieving electrical isolation in 94% of targeted veins [19]. Using a basket catheter to achieve a 100% rate of PVI, Arentz et al. reported freedom from AF in 70% of patients with paroxysmal AF but in only 44% of patients with persistent AF [20], further confirming that extension of the technique of PVI alone to patients with chronic AF was inadequate. A patient age ≥ 50 years and the presence of either persistent or permanent AF were shown to be the only independent predictors of AF recurrence after PVI for symptomatic, drug-refractory AF [21]. When patients with chronic AF underwent 1.7 ± 0.9 ablation procedures with a solitary endpoint of PVI, only 37% were in sinus rhythm and free of antiarrhythmic medication [22].

Nevertheless, others have described excellent outcomes following PVI for persistent AF. Using a double Lasso® technique, Ouyang et al. reported a 95% freedom from arrhythmia after 8 months' follow-up, with 14 of 40 patients requiring a second procedure to treat recurrent atrial tachyarrhythmias associated with recovery of PV–LA conduction [23]. However, with a longer follow-up, these authors reported a success rate off drugs of 47% in those patients with chronic AF lasting more than 1 year prior to ablation, compared to 63% for those with chronic AF of a duration of less than 1 year.

These results are corroborated by the demonstration that the PVs display higher frequency activity in patients with paroxysmal AF compared with persistent AF, and that PVI has a greater impact on the AF cycle length in the former over the latter [24]. It seems clear therefore that AF is mechanistically not uniform and that atrial tissue interventions in addition to addressing the PV–LA junction will be necessary for chronic AF.

Expansion of left atrial targets in chronic atrial fibrillation

A growing appreciation of the inadequacy of PVI as a single ablation strategy for all forms of AF has been accompanied by innovation within existing strategies and development of entirely new ones.

Localized sources

In an isolated, Langendorf-perfused sheep heart model of pacing and acetylcholine-induced AF, Mandapati [25] and Schuessler [26] and coworkers (using an isolated canine atrial preparation) were able to demonstrate the presence of discrete areas of high frequency activity. Using optical mapping techniques, Mandapati et al. showed that the main contributor to the observed dominant frequency was the periodicity of the local rotating spiral wave, with a core perimeter and area of 10.4 ± 2.8 mm and 3.8 ± 2.8 mm^2, respectively [27]. Spectral mapping in humans has shown a discordance of sites of dominant frequency between paroxysmal and persistent AF [28], with atrial sites more prevalent in the latter than the former. High density mapping of AF organized by prior ablation has demonstrated (i) discrete sites driving the atria and harboring varying electrograms; (ii) centrifugal activation with one-to-one conduction from either a discrete point source or an area of complex local conduction or reentry; and (iii) sites of high frequency with variable conduction block to the surrounding tissue and with intermittent or permanent discharges [29]. In a study of 50 consecutive patients with organized AF (i.e. discrete electrograms allowing mapping) occurring after prior ablation, endocardial mapping revealed shorter cycle lengths at sites displaying a frequency gradient than in those with 1 : 1 propagation; mean cycle length was 165 ± 39 ms versus 210 ± 38ms ($P = 0.0015$), and shortest cycle length was 126 ± 21 ms versus 179 ± 39 ms ($P < 0.0001$) [30]. These data provide a rationale for pursuing focal atrial targets unrelated to the PVs in the treatment of chronic AF.

Fractionated potentials

Somewhat countercurrent to established strategies was the demonstration by Nademanee et al. that both chronic and paroxysmal AF could be effectively treated by targeting areas of complex fractionated electrical activity [31] without specifically targeting the LA–PV junction. Targeted electrograms consisted of low voltage signals (0.05–0.25 mV) with highly fractionated potentials or with very short cycle lengths (≤ 120 ms). The most common sites at which fractionated potentials could be recorded were the interatrial septum, the PVs, the left atrial roof, and the proximal coronary sinus. This group also observed that the sites harboring fractionated potentials were anatomically fixed, that is were consistently observed at a given site. The findings reflected those of Jais et al. who demonstrated maximal continuous electrical activity times (expressed as a percentage of a 60 s recording window in each of eight regions distributed throughout both atria) to occur in the septum, roof, and posterior LA [32]. Striking disparities in endocardial activation were observed between adjacent atrial regions and were interpreted as indicators of abnormally conducting, potentially arrhythmogenic tissue.

Fractionated electrograms have been shown to be caused by conduction disturbances including collision, block, pivot points, and slow conduction [33]. More recently, high density contact mapping of complex fractionated atrial endocardial electrograms showed that fractionation was preceded by a shortening of AF cycle length in 84% of sites mapped, consistent with local passive activation [34]. In conjunction with the earlier work showing a broad distribution of continuous electrical activities throughout the left and right atria in paroxysmal AF [35], it is reasonable to deduce that some such electrograms in AF are mechanistically important while others are mere bystanders. In the remaining 16% of patients in the study of Rostock et al., however, local activation during an acceleration of AF cycle length was suggestive of the presence of autonomous local activities that may perpetuate the AF process [36]. Many groups have now modified their ablation strategies for chronic AF to incorporate some element of this technique in spite of the absence of a clear way to determine the "specificity" of these electrograms.

Autonomic targets

The link between the autonomic nervous system and AF has been appreciated for over 85 years [37–39]. In the ablation era there has been renewed interest in cardiac autonomic nervous influences on the trigger–substrate interaction in AF [40–42]. Although there is no firm clinical evidence to date of a role for the autonomic nervous system in chronic AF, the widespread distribution of cardiac autonomic nerves [43] and the early experimental data in animal models of induced AF [44,45] support their clinical relevance.

Results of techniques incorporating novel ablation targets

Ablation of complex atrial electrograms

During ablation targeting fractionated electrograms, Nademanee et al. showed that 53% of 64 chronic AF patients converted to sinus rhythm without pharmacological intervention or electrical cardioversion [46]. A second procedure was necessary in approximately one-third of patients to achieve stable sinus rhythm without drugs in 65% of patients; a further 20% recurred with episodes of paroxysmal AF or atrial tachycardia lasting less than 12 h and not requiring continuous antiarrhythmic therapy (K. Nademannee, personal communication).

In chronic AF, Oral et al. showed that left atrial linear ablation incorporating complex electrograms in the LA roof, septum, anterior wall, mitral isthmus, and atrial aspect of the mitral annulus gave similar results to a PVI strategy in terms of restoration and maintenance of sinus rhythm (60% versus 68% off drugs, respectively) [47]. In this randomized study, all patients ($n = 80$) were pretreated with amiodarone for 6 weeks prior to the procedure, and ibutilide and/or DC cardioversion were necessary to restore sinus rhythm in 78% of patients after completion of the ablation schema.

More recently, Oral et al. reported that only modest short-term efficacy is achievable with radiofrequency ablation of chronic AF guided by complex fractionated atrial electrograms with > 40% patients requiring a second ablation procedure [6]. In 100 patients with chronic AF, complex fractionated atrial electrograms at the PV ostial and antral areas, various regions of the LA, and the coronary sinus were targeted. After the index procedure and mean follow-up of 14 ± 7 months, 33% of patients were in sinus rhythm without antiarrhythmic drugs, 38% had AF, 17% had both AF and atrial flutter, 9% had persistent atrial flutter, and 3% had paroxysmal AF on antiarrhythmic drugs. In the 44% of patients who underwent a second ablation procedure, PV tachycardia was found in all patients in both previously targeted and non-targeted PVs. At a mean follow-up of 13 ± 7 months after the last ablation procedure, 57% of patients were in sinus rhythm without antiarrhythmic drugs, 32% had persistent AF, 6% had paroxysmal AF, and 5% had atrial flutter.

Pulmonary vein isolation plus linear ablation

Incorporation of linear lesions into ablation schema for chronic AF results in improved outcomes. In a well-designed, prospective study of patients with persistent AF, Willems et al. achieved sinus rhythm in 69% of patients (off drugs) who underwent PVI plus ablation at the roof and mitral isthmus, in comparison with only 20% of patients who underwent PVI alone [48]. In patients with chronic AF,

Hsu et al. have demonstrated a 70% success rate (off drugs) in long-term restoration of sinus rhythm following PVI and linear block at the roof and mitral isthmus [49]. Kottkamp et al. showed that circumferential PV ablation and adjunctive roof and mitral isthmus ablation (without demonstration of conduction block) significantly reduced the AF burden at 12 months' follow-up among 20 patients with persistent AF as measured by 7-day Holter, with complete freedom from AF off antiarrhythmic drugs demonstrated in only 22% of these patients [50]. In terms of freedom from AF, the incremental benefit of mitral isthmus ablation in addition to PVI is greater for persistent AF than for paroxysmal AF [51]. At long-term follow-up, 36% of patients without adjunctive mitral isthmus ablation (56% of whom continued antiarrhythmic drugs) and 74% of patients with a mitral line (50% of whom continued antiarrhythmic drugs) were in sinus rhythm.

Wide encircling pulmonary vein ablation

In addition to encircling lesions around each PV, Pappone et al. created ablation lines connecting both the superior and inferior PVs and a mitral isthmus line to reduce the incidence of post-ablation atrial flutter [52–54]. The authors proposed that the following are all contributory to the success of their technique: (i) PVI; (ii) elimination of anatomic anchors for rotors; (iii) ablation at sites of non-PV triggers; (iv) interruption of interatrial communication; (v) atrial debulking; and (vi) PV vagal denervation. Although this is difficult to validate, sinus rhythm can be achieved and maintained following circumferential ablation in 83% of patients with chronic AF. Using the same method, Oral et al. reported a success rate of 68% at 9 months' follow-up off drugs [47], Bertaglia et al. [55] a success rate of 70% at 20 months (64% still taking antiarrhythmics), and Beukema et al. [56] a success rate of 77% at 15 months (44% on antiarrhythmics).

Natale et al. used intracardiac echo to define the proximal edge of the PV antrum and advocated isolation of the veins at this level, guided by a Lasso catheter to confirm wide antral electrical disconnection [57]. It is likely that this approach also includes many of the targets listed above.

Using the double Lasso technique with continuous circular lesions around ipsilateral PVs, sinus rhythm was restored by ablation in 12 of 40 chronic AF patients with freedom from AF in 95% of patients at 8 ± 2 months [23]. However, as stated earlier, the longer term follow-up results are less encouraging with 63% of patients with chronic AF lasting < 1 year and 47% of patients with chronic AF lasting > 1 year in sinus rhythm off antiarrhythmic medication more than 1 year post-ablation.

Although differences exist between the many techniques that are used to treat chronic AF, the immediate and short-term success rates appear to be quite similar, at approximately 60–75% restoration and maintenance of sinus rhythm at 1 year' follow-up (Table 12.1). We can conclude from this similarity of outcome that these different approaches following a predetermined lesion set (i.e. PVI, linear ablation, defragmentation) independently have an impact on AF. No single technique can effectively treat all targets and thereby achieve the best outcome. An ablation strategy incorporating all of the above-mentioned targets and including less frequently targeted structures such as the left atrial appendage (LAA) and the coronary sinus was shown to improve outcomes in ablation of chronic AF.

Stepwise ablation approach for chronic atrial fibrillation

The stepwise ablation approach targets all structures potentially contributing to the initiation and maintenance of AF, and its efficiency is indicated by achieving termination of chronic AF in the majority of patients (Figure 12.1). This approach combined PVI, electrogram-based ablation of the biatrial substrate, and linear ablation [58]. Structures outside the LA (right atrium, superior vena cava) are targeted based on electrogram morphology and frequency. Each region is targeted in sequence and the impact of ablation upon the "global" fibrillatory process is assessed by measurement of the AF cycle length (AFCL) at sites remote from the ablation site, i.e. the right atrium and LA appendage. Ablation is typically accompanied by a progressive increase in the AFCL prior to conversion of AF to sinus rhythm or to atrial tachycardia, which is then mapped and ablated. This flexible

Table 12.1 Success defined as freedom from AF, irrespective of the concomitant use of antiarrhythmic drugs.

Study	*Patients*	*CAF (no. of patients)*	*CAF as % of total study population*	*Follow-up (months)*	*Technique*	*PVI (confirmed)*	*Linear lesions*	*Complex potentials*	*Success in CAF group*	*Drug status (% taking AADs)*
Cox et al. 1995 [8]	123	55	45	180	Maze I-III	Yes (N)	Yes	No	95%	N/S
Sueda et al. 1996 [134]	11	11	100	11	Surgical	No	Yes	No	91%	0%
Pappone et al. 2000 [135]	26	12	46	9 ± 3	CPVA	No	No	No	83%	25%
Fassini et al. 2005 [51]	187	62	33	12	PVI	Yes	MI	No	74 ± 9	50%
Willems et al. 2006 [48]	62	62	100	14–17	PVI	Yes	Roof, MI	No	45% (63% in linear ablation group)	0%
Haissaguerre et al. 2000 [136]	15	15	100	11 ± 8	PVI	Yes	No	No	60%	N/S
Haisaguerre et al. 2005 [58,59]	60	60	100	11 ± 6	PVI	Yes	Yes	Yes	95%	0%
Oral et al. 2005 [47]	80	80	100	9 ± 4	CPVA	No	Yes	Yes	68%	0%
Oral et al. 2006 [54]	146	146	100	12	CPVA	No	PLA, Roof, MI	No	74%	0%
Oral et al. 2002 [19]	70	12	17	5	PVI	Yes	No	No	22%	N/S
Arentz et al. 2003 [20]	55	18	33	12	PVI	Yes	No	No	44%	0%
Lim et al. 2006 [22]	51	51	100	17 ± 9	PVI				45%	17%
Ouyang et al. 2005 [23]	40	40	100	8 ± 2	PVI	Yes	No	No	95%	N/S
Nademanee et al. 2004 [31]	121	64	53	12	CFAE ablation	No	No	Yes	91%	N/S
Kottkamp et al. 2004 [50]	100	20	20	12	CPVA	No	MI	No	22%	33%
Kanagaratnam et al. 2001 [137]	71	71	100	29 ± 8	PVI	Yes (31%)	No	No	21%	0%
Calo et al. 2006 [68]	80	80	100	14 ± 5	CPVA	No	MI	No	72% (85% biatrial group)	N/S
Hsu et al. 2004 [49]	106	116	91	12 ± 7	PVI	Yes	MI, Roof	No	81% overall	0%
Beukema et al. 2005 [56]	105	53	51	15 ± 5	CPVA	No	MI	No	77%	44%
Bertaglia et al. 2006 [55]	74	74	100	20 ± 6	CPVA	No	MI	No	70%	64%

AAD, antiarrhythmic drugs; CAF, chronic atrial fibrillation; CFAE, complex fractionated electrograms; CPVA, circumferential pulmonary vein ablation; MI, mitral isthmus; N/S, not stated in manuscript; PLA, posterior left atrium; PVI, pulmonary vein isolation.

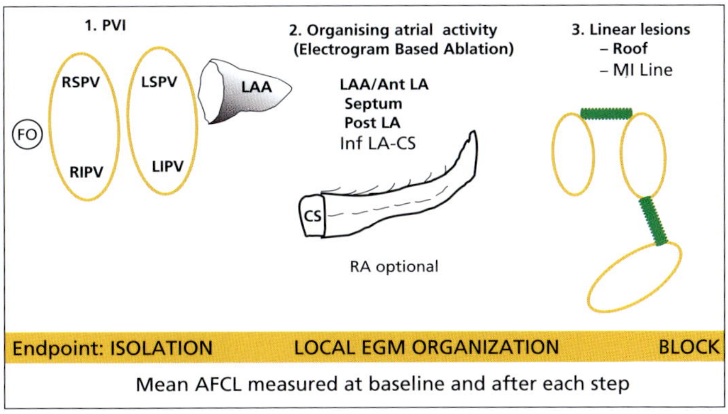

Figure 12.1 Diagram illustrating the catheter ablation strategy for chronic AF guided by measurements of AF cycle length at the right and left appendages. The ablation steps consist of PV isolation (PVI), electrogram-based ablation, and linear ablation. AFCL, atrial fibrillatory cycle length; CS, coronary sinus; EGM, electrogram; FO, foramen ovale; LA, left atrium; LAA, left atrial appendage; LIPV, left inferior pulmonary vein; LSPV, left superior pulmonary vein; MI, mitral isthmus; RA, right atrium; RIPV, right inferior pulmonary vein; RSPV, right superior pulmonary vein.

technique has resulted in an unprecedented level of acute termination of chronic AF by catheter ablation [58,59].

Patient selection

Patients with chronic AF are considered if they are symptomatic and have failed treatment with more than one antiarrhythmic drug, electrical cardioversion, or both. Of note, ablation is offered to patients with AF, echocardiographic evidence of left ventricular dysfunction, New York Heart Association heart failure symptoms of grade II or more, and the absence of an alternative explanation for their cardiac dysfunction [60–62]. The heightened risk of myocardial perforation and thromboembolic complications in very elderly patients and the lower probability of a successful outcome when the LA is markedly dilated, are factors to be considered but are not strict exclusion criterion in our practice.

Evaluation of the effectiveness of ablation: atrial fibrillation cycle length

One of the principal drawbacks of current ablation for chronic AF is the absence of an intraprocedural, real-time measure of effectiveness. Experimental mapping studies have shown that the AFCL is correlated with local refractory periods [63], shortens after initiation of AF [64], and is prolonged with antiarrhythmic drugs [65]. It is reasonable then to consider prolongation of AFCL during catheter ablation at a specific site or area as reflecting an impact upon the underlying AF mechanism and ultimately contributing to a successful outcome. AFCL is generally measured in the LAA and right atrial appendage (RAA) as the average of at least 30 cycle lengths [66]. These structures generally display discrete and unambiguous electrograms for measurement. The AFCL is assessed at each "step" in the ablation process (Figure 12.2). This is a

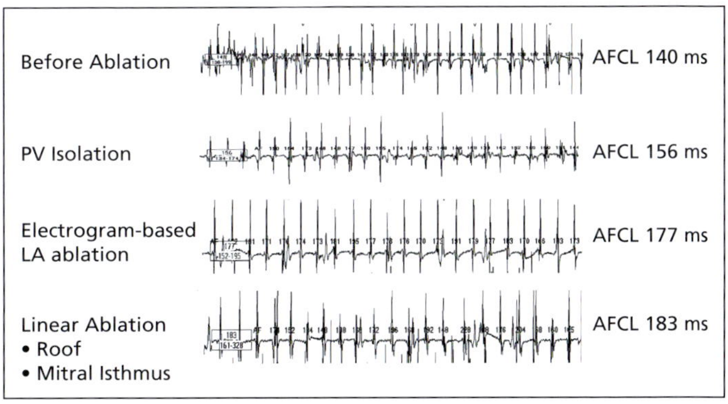

Figure 12.2 Measurements of left appendage atrial fibrillatory cycle length (AFCL) showing progressive prolongation during ablation in the left atrium (LA). When a critical cycle of 180–200 ms is achieved, mapping/ablation is then performed in the right atrium. PV, pulmonary vein.

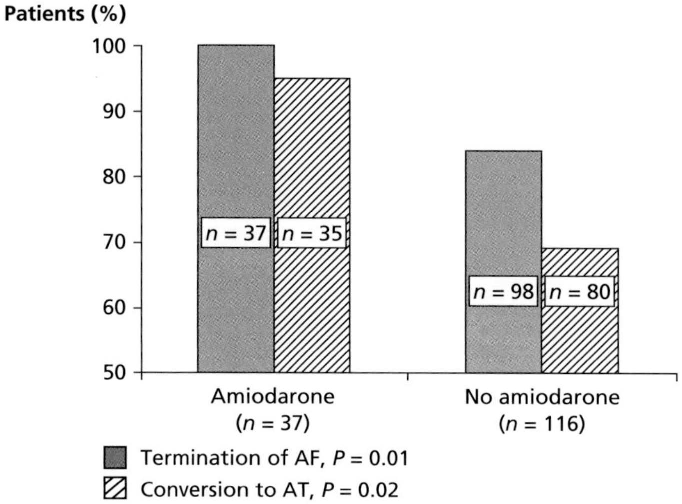

Figure 12.3 Impact of amiodarone in patients with chronic atrial fibrillation (AF) of less than 5 years' duration. The use of amiodarone is associated with increased AF termination and conversion to atrial tachycardia (AT).

relatively stable measurement, with < 5 ms spontaneous variation between two consecutive 30 s measurements in the majority of patients, even with chaotic electrograms in the rest of the atrium and coronary sinus.

A progressive increase in AFCL followed PVI in patients in whom AF was terminated by catheter ablation [67]. Furthermore, with increasing left atrial ablation, a gradual prolongation of the AFCL is seen [68] with the largest increments occurring after ablation of the PV–LA junction, the inferior LA–coronary sinus interface, and the LAA [58,59]; however any anatomic site can be involved in an individual patient. We also have identified a critical threshold of AFCL, generally in the region of 200 ms, where AF terminates to sinus rhythm or to organized atrial tachycardia. The baseline AFCL (prior to any ablation) is significantly longer in patients in whom AF terminates during ablation (156 ± 23 ms, $n = 52$) than in those patients in whom AF persists ($< 130 \pm 14$ ms, $n = 8$) [69]. Furthermore, the facility with which AF can be terminated by ablation, as indicated by the procedure duration, varies inversely with the baseline AFCL. Therefore, a long baseline AFCL indicates that the route to sinus rhythm is shorter than with a short baseline AFCL (< 135 ms), which has been shown to be a strong predictor of failure of ablation therapy to terminate AF [58]. Baseline AFCLs seen in patients with chronic AF on amiodarone are also greater than those not taking the drug, corresponding with a higher rate of termination of AF by ablation [70] (Figure 12.3). These observations reinforce the notion that AFCL provides a meaningful measure of the fibrillatory process.

Technique of stepwise ablation

Pulmonary vein isolation

Pulmonary vein isolation is currently performed as the initial ablation step in all patients with chronic AF in our laboratory [71,72]. All PVs are isolated routinely, guided by a circumferential mapping catheter positioned near the venous ostium. Temperature is limited to 48°C with a target tissue temperature of 42°C achieved by a manual titration of the irrigation rate of between 5 and 20 ml/min (0.9% saline via Cool Flow®, Biosense Webster). Veins are isolated individually or as ipsilateral pairs in accordance with the venous anatomy and operator preference. The Lasso catheter is then withdrawn from the transseptal sheath and positioned within the RAA via the 7 Fr sheath for the remainder of the procedure to monitor the right atrial AFCL. The mapping catheter is returned to the LA via the transseptal sheath. The first ablation step is completed by simultaneous measurement of the AFCL in the LAA and RAA.

Electrogram-based ablation

Ablation targeting left atrial sites of complex electrical activity

Nademanee et al. reported that chronic AF could be terminated in approximately 50% of patients by exclusively targeting sites of complex and fractionated electrical activity [73]. These complex fractionated electrograms may represent sites of slow conduction, pivot points of reentry circuits, or sites of ganglionated plexuses. In our experience [74] and the study by Oral et al. [75], ablation confined to these electrograms has limited efficacy, but is a crucial component of our ablation strategy for chronic AF.

In the stepwise approach, left atrial electrophysiological targets include those areas displaying continuous electrical activity (Figure 12.4), complex fractionated activity, locally short cycle lengths, and a large (> 70 ms) temporal gradient between the activities recorded on the proximal and distal bipoles of the ablation catheter (potentially representing a local circuit or rotor) [58] (Figure 12.5). At the procedural onset, most electrograms recorded in the LA are either continuous or show complex patterns of fractionation, particularly if the AFCL is short. With increasing ablation of the LA, there is gradual prolongation of the AFCL and organization of atrial activities that permits identification of discrete electrograms and their activation sequences (see above), which can then be mapped and targeted for ablation. All parts of the LA are targeted: the interatrial septum around the foramen ovale, the posterior LA, the anterior LA, and the base of the LAA. In particular, ablation at the base of the LAA and the inferior LA–coronary sinus interface (Figures 12.6 and 12.7), which are not part of the standard ablation schemas previously described by other groups, have an important impact on the AFCL recorded in the LAA [58,76].

Forty consecutive patients undergoing catheter ablation were studied to determine electrogram characteristics of favorable ablation sites, defined as those associated with AF termination or an increase in AFCL of ≥ 5 ms. Electrograms at these sites were associated with longer durations of continuous electrical activity (78% of occasions implying that continuous activity was recorded for 8 s out of 10 s) versus 55% of times at unsuccessful sites ($P = 0.016$). A temporal gradient of activation indicating a possible localized reentry was observed in 22% of favorable sites versus 10% of unfavorable sites ($P = 0.03$). Comparisons between favorable and unfavorable sites associated with AF

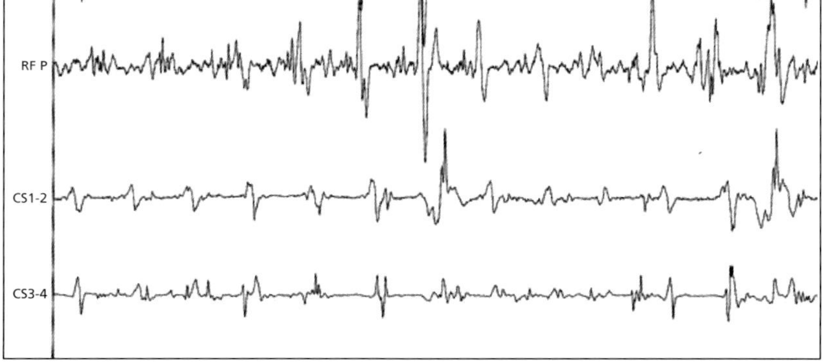

Figure 12.4 Complex fractionated electrograms recorded at the left appendage. The continuous activity is present for 100% of the time window. Ablation at this site resulted in termination of AF.

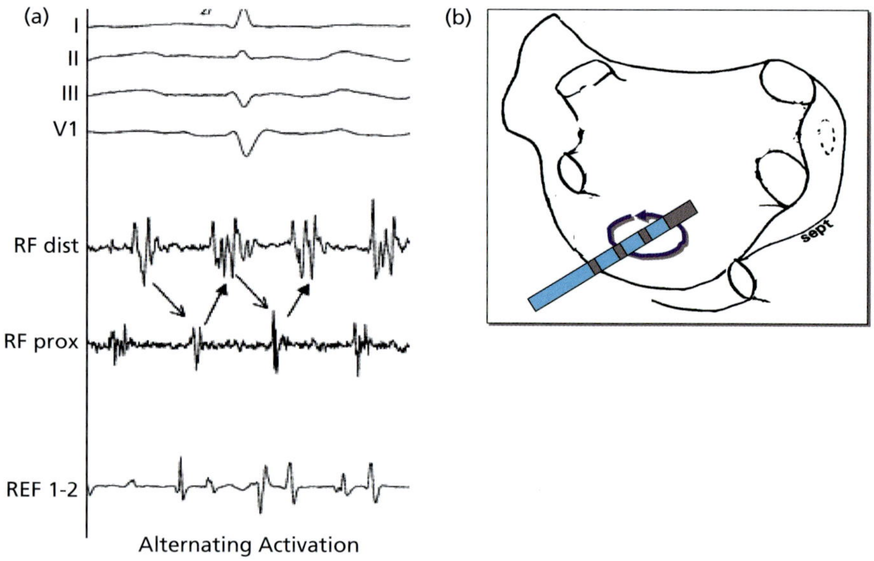

Figure 12.5 Mapping of a discrete source. (a) The local electrogram recording site during organized atrial activity is distal to proximal in the radiofrequency catheter and displays a gradient of local activation (demarcated by arrows in the middle panel). (b) The schematic diagram shows the presence of a "rotating" source mapped at the local electrogram site.

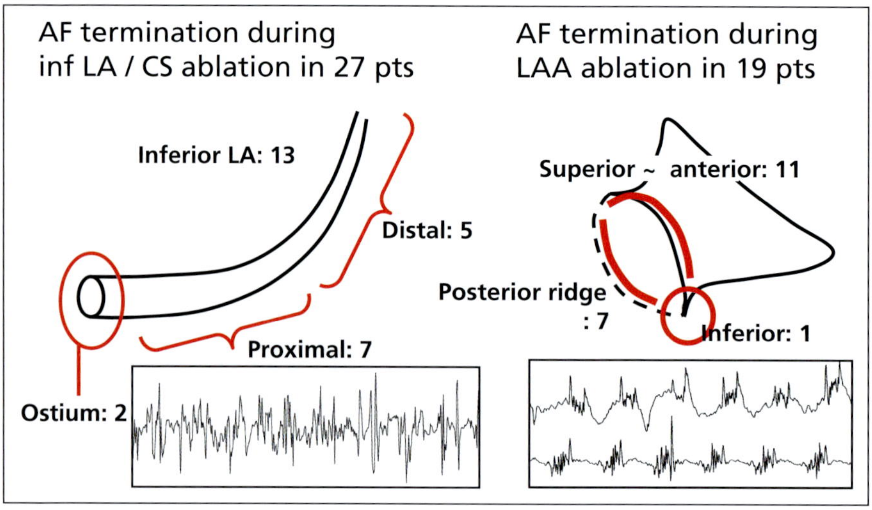

Figure 12.6 The left atrial appendage (LAA) and coronary sinus (CS) represent critical sites for the ablation of chronic atrial fibrillation (AF). Within these structures, electrogram characteristics associated with AF termination display complex fractionation and rapid short cycles. LA, left atrium; pts, patients.

modification or termination did not show significant differences in electrogram voltage (0.18 ± 0.10 mV versus 0.20 ± 0.11 mV; $P > 0.05$), fractionation index (156 ± 64 versus 157 ± 50; $P > 0.05$), and dominant frequency (1.50 ± 3.05 Hz versus 0.97 ± 2.51 Hz; $P > 0.05$).

The coronary sinus and inferior left atrium

Both the coronary sinus (CS) and other thoracic veins have been implicated in arrhythmogenesis [77–82]. The demonstration of the importance of the CS in the termination of chronic AF by catheter ablation implies a broader arrhythmogenic role for

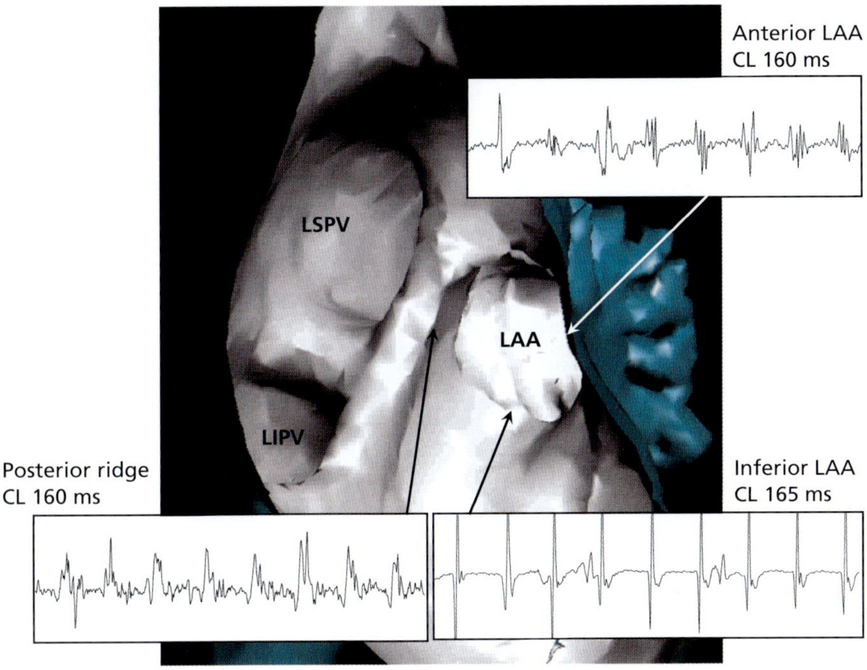

Figure 12.7 Endoscopic view of the left PVs and left atrial appendage (LAA) from a 16-slice cardiac computed tomograph using Philips custom-designed segmentation software. The electrograms recorded at the sites indicated demonstrate the local heterogeneity of electrical activity at the base of the LAA. CL, cycle length; LIPV, left inferior pulmonary vein; LSPV, left superior pulmonary vein.

this structure than just as a source of focal ectopy [58]. The CS is surrounded by a cuff of striated muscle extending up to 4 cm from the vessel ostium. In addition, striated muscular connections ranging from single fascicles to broad myocardial sheets connect the CS to the adjacent LA [83].

In 30 patients undergoing catheter ablation for chronic AF, the CS was targeted if AF persisted after PVI and LA ablation aimed at sites of complex, fractionated electrograms. Ablation within the LA directly abutting the CS (endocardial ablation) significantly prolonged the CS cycle length by 17 ± 5 ms and "organized" the CS activation sequence (from 13% of patients before to 51% after ablation). This strongly suggests interruption of inferior LA wall connections to the CS. Subsequent ablation from within the CS (epicardial) further increased local CS cycle length. Of note, the global AF cycle length measured in the LAA was prolonged significantly both during endocardial and epicardial ablation and was associated with AF termination in 30% of patients with persistent AF.

The mechanisms and sites of arrhythmogenicity from the inferior LA–CS region appear multiple. Endocardial ablation may diminish or terminate interaction or exchange of activity between these two contiguous structures, which may be a mechanism perpetuating AF in these patients (Figure 12.8). In addition, a direct role of the CS musculature is demonstrated by mapping sources of centrifugal or high frequency activity at discrete parts of the venous muscle – from the distal CS (also compatible with the ligament of Marshall [77]) to the CS termination in the right atrium.

From a technical viewpoint, ablation of the inferior LA is achieved by looping the catheter in a "J" (Figure 12.9), pointing towards the interatrial septum and, with the distal electrode parallel to the CS ostium, withdrawing the catheter along a trajectory from 7 o'clock to 4 o'clock in the left anterior oblique (LAO) projection. Electrical artifacts are recorded from the quadripolar catheter within the CS in 68% of cases when this is done. The impact of inferior LA ablation on both local (CS cycle length) and global AF cycle length, the frequency of AF

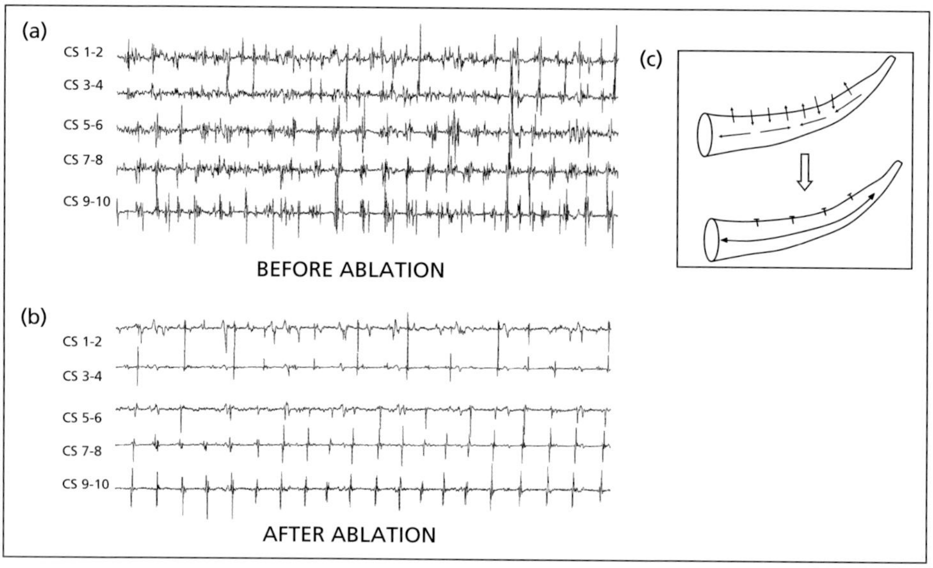

Figure 12.8 Impact of endocardial ablation along the inferior LA on coronary sinus (CS) activation. (a) Before ablation, CS activation is inconsistent and shows a cycle length of 200 ms in CS5-6 and CS7-8. (b) After ablation, CS activation consistently follows a proximal-to-distal sequence with a cycle length of 270 ms. (c) The schema illustrates a putative mechanism to explain this phenomenon.

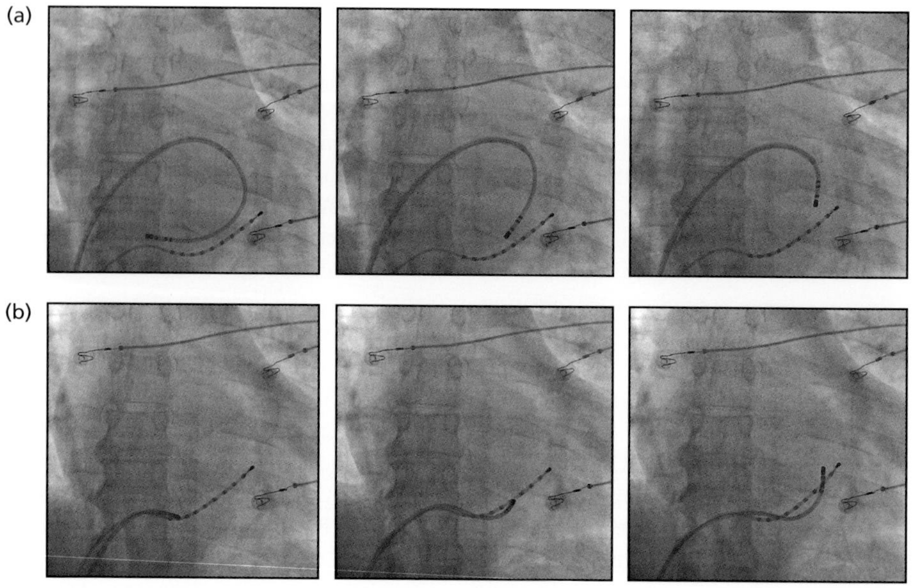

Figure 12.9 Anteroposterior fluoroscopic visualization of the catheter positions during ablation of the inferior LA (a) and CS (b). (a) After looping the catheter into the LA facing the CS ostium (left), the catheter is then gradually withdrawn parallel to the CS along the posterior mitral annulus towards the lateral LA (middle and right images). (b) Corresponding catheter position at the ostial, middle, and distal segments within the CS.

termination during ablation of the inferior LA–CS interface [84], and the CS as a site of origin of atrial tachycardia following termination of AF [85] all support an important role for this structure in perpetuation of AF and a rationale for its inclusion as part of the stepwise ablation approach for chronic AF.

Ablation within the CS is performed by advancing the ablation catheter to the distal CS (approximately 4 o'clock in the LAO projection). Power is limited to an absolute maximum of 25 W and the irrigation rate adjusted manually to achieve the desired power setting. Highest irrigation flow rates are required for ablation in the distal CS. The catheter is withdrawn from along the CS with the tip deflected towards the atrium to minimize the risk of circumflex coronary artery [86] and esophageal injury [87].

Linear ablation

Roof line ablation

This short line generally requires 12 ± 6 min of radiofrequency delivery and 7 ± 2 min of fluoroscopy [88] and can be achieved in 96% of patients. Generally performed during AF, the immediate endpoint is the abolition of local electrograms along a continuous line between the previously isolated left and right superior PVs.

The line is performed as cranially as is permitted by the encircling venous lesions in order to avoid the posterior LA [89]. The preferred catheter orientation during ablation is parallel to the roof, rather than perpendicular, to minimize the likelihood of steam pop and perforation [90]. Confirmation of conduction block at the LA roof is performed following the restoration of sinus rhythm using pacing techniques described [91].

Mitral isthmus ablation

Ablation at the mitral isthmus to achieve bidirectional conduction block may be technically difficult, with a risk of cardiac tamponade [92], and requires ablation within the CS in over two-thirds of patients for completion. In addition, incomplete ablation lesions may be proarrhythmic and are associated with arrhythmia recurrence [93,94]. Consequently, we reserve ablation at the mitral isthmus for those patients in whom AF has not terminated during earlier steps or for those patients with demonstrated perimitral macroreentry following termination of AF.

How to approach an incomplete linear block

Although assessment for linear block can be performed simply, achieving linear block may be difficult. Careful remapping along the ablation line looking for conduction gaps is mandatory. For an incomplete roofline, careful mapping along the line particularly at its junction with the superior PVs should be performed. When no conduction gap is identified, ablation is performed more anteriorly to the previous line.

An incomplete mitral isthmus line should also prompt mapping for conduction gaps from the endocardium aspect. Ablation is required within the distal CS to ablate the epicardial side opposite to the initial mitral line, targeting fractionated or sharp potentials in the distal CS segment enface to the mitral line. The most frequent gap site is the ostium of the lower inferior PV, presumably because of catheter instability at this location [95]. In addition, gaps can be found at the junction between the lower inferior PV and the base of the LAA. In the case of resistant mitral isthmus (usually after 30 min of radiofrequency application), we defer the procedure so as to allow edema regression.

RA ablation targets

Early attempts at catheter ablation for AF focused mainly on the right atrium, with modest success. It seems intuitively obvious, however, that the right atrium should have some role. We have succeeded in terminating AF in 85% of patients with chronic AF by ablation targeting mainly the LA but some patients had termination during right atrial or superior vena cava ablation (Figure 12.10). This concurs with findings reported by Nademanee [96] in which right atrial ablation was required in 15% of patients. Perpetuators of AF, including the right atrium and the superior vena cava, have been identified [97–99]. Although the LA in chronic AF is dominant, spectral analysis during AF shows an important contribution from the right atrium [100]. In addition to LA focal activation with fibrillatory conduction, right atrial focal and reentrant

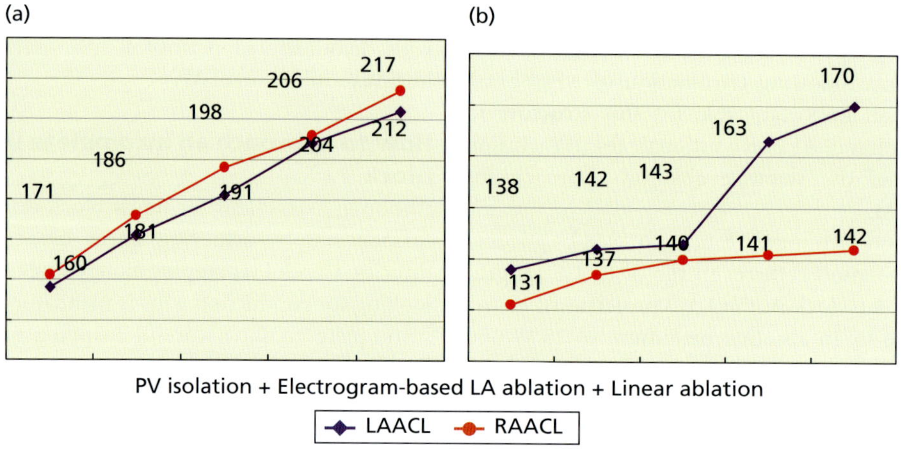

Figure 12.10 The impact on observed AF cycle length after extensive left atrium (LA) ablation. (a) Parallel prolongation of the AF cycle length in the right and left appendages (RAA and LAA, respectively). (b) Disparate prolongation of the LAA and RAA cycle length (LAACL and RAACL, respectively) during ablation; the AF cycle length is shorter in the right appendage compared to the left appendage, suggesting the right atrium may be driving the AF. PV, pulmonary vein.

activity has also been demonstrated during intraoperative high density epicardial mapping of patients with permanent AF [101].

It seems clear that there is a limit or "ceiling" for ablation within the LA beyond which further ablation in that chamber is pointless. The results from 97 consecutive patients undergoing stepwise ablation of chronic AF demonstrate a sigmoidal relationship between the number of ablation steps performed and the success in termination of AF [102]. The relative incremental benefit per stage decreases progressively to a plateau after four stages of ablation. Recognition of when this ceiling is reached during an individual procedure is thus critical.

The left and right atrial appendage cycle lengths measured simultaneously at baseline and following each ablation step during the procedure offer a possible clue to the involvement of structures outside the LA, for example the right atrium. Gradual prolongation of the LAA cycle length by ablation (up to 170 ms) with persisting short AF cycle length in the RAA (140 ms) is suggestive of a potential role for right atrial structures in the perpetuation of AF (Figure 12.11). The electrogram-guided targets for ablation are as for the LA, with the sites of termination – although occurring at any site in the right atrium – predominantly found at the anterior right atrium or at the base of the RAA. Distal-to-proximal activation on the mapping catheter with the distal electrode in the superior vena cava or high frequency activity suggests the presence of an arrhythmogenic source in this vessel. Care must be taken to avoid phrenic nerve and sinus node injury during ablation in this region [103]. Finally, all patients undergo ablation of the cavotricuspid isthmus at the end of the procedure.

The importance of discrete anatomic sites for termination of atrial fibrillation

Discrete sources of rapid activity maintaining AF have been demonstrated in both animals and patients [94,104–107]. Activation mapping should identify sources with 1 : 1 conduction to surrounding tissue, while sources where 1 : 1 conduction to the surrounding atrium is not maintained can be identified by frequency mapping techniques (Figures 12.12 and 12.13).

These discrete sites were dominantly located in any part of the coronary sinus, the base of the LAA, and the interatrial septum. Most of these sources corresponded to localized circuits (rather than focal points) and therefore harbored electrograms covering the entire cycle length in one area, often

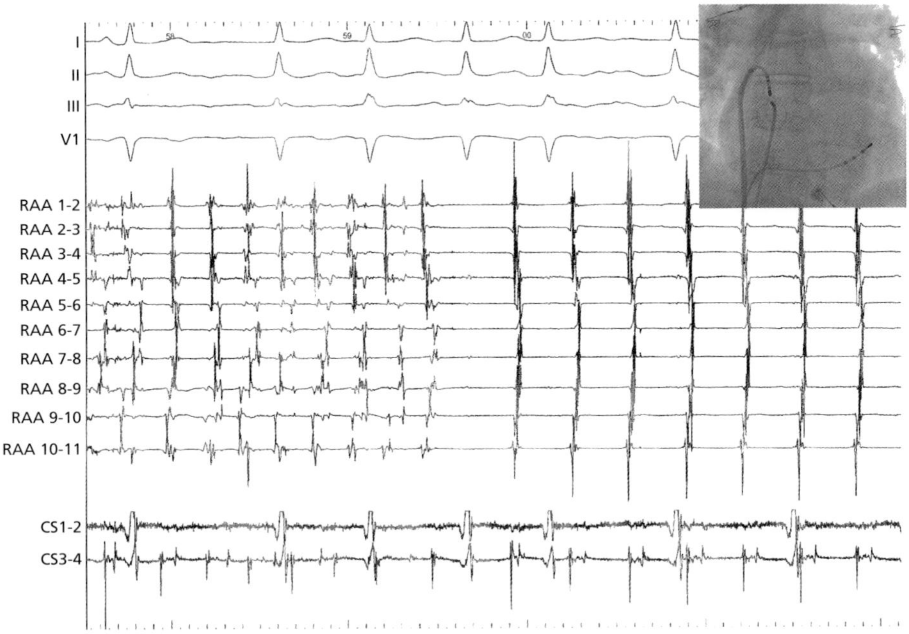

Figure 12.11 Termination of AF by conversion to atrial tachycardia during radiofrequency application at the top of the RAA. The fluoroscopic image shows the ablation site at the RAA.

with long fractionated electrograms indicating a small isthmus. Ablation at sites identified as "sources" prolonged AF cycle length, changed activation sequence, and/or terminated AF [58,108]. It stands to reason that failure to recognize the contribution of these discrete sites to the fibrillatory process will result in failure to terminate AF.

Cumulative benefits of the stepwise approach

Using this approach, there is a progressive increase in AF cycle length resulting in AF termination [58]. The specific sequence in which the structures are targeted does not impact on the overall increase in AF cycle length or procedural success; however, the effect of an individual ablation step is highly dependent on its position within the ablation sequence. For example, for patients with chronic AF, the efficacy of PVI in terminating AF is far greater when it follows ablation of other LA structures, but is almost completely ineffective when performed at the beginning [74]. Although the direct contribution of each step cannot be determined, the stepwise approach progressively arrives at the critical sites for AF termination.

Atrial fibrillation inducibility testing

Inducibility of AF after PVI has been used as an endpoint in paroxysmal AF and is associated with freedom from AF in up to 91% of patients [109,110]. Nonetheless, animal studies have shown that AF is easily reinducible and sustained following AF termination by DC shock, an effect which has been attributed to the remodeling effect of the arrhythmia [111]. Our clinical experience of catheter ablation in chronic AF is in line with this, with patients invariably inducible following termination of AF in spite of good long-term results [59], and this suggests that inducibility is of little use as an endpoint in chronic AF.

Acute procedural outcome

Termination of tachycardia is an obligatory endpoint of ablation performed for atrial, junctional, and ventricular tachycardia. Termination of AF by ablation has been reported in 15–50% of cases of chronic AF but has not yet been validated as a favorable endpoint in terms of risk–benefit ratio. Although intuitively likely that it is better to

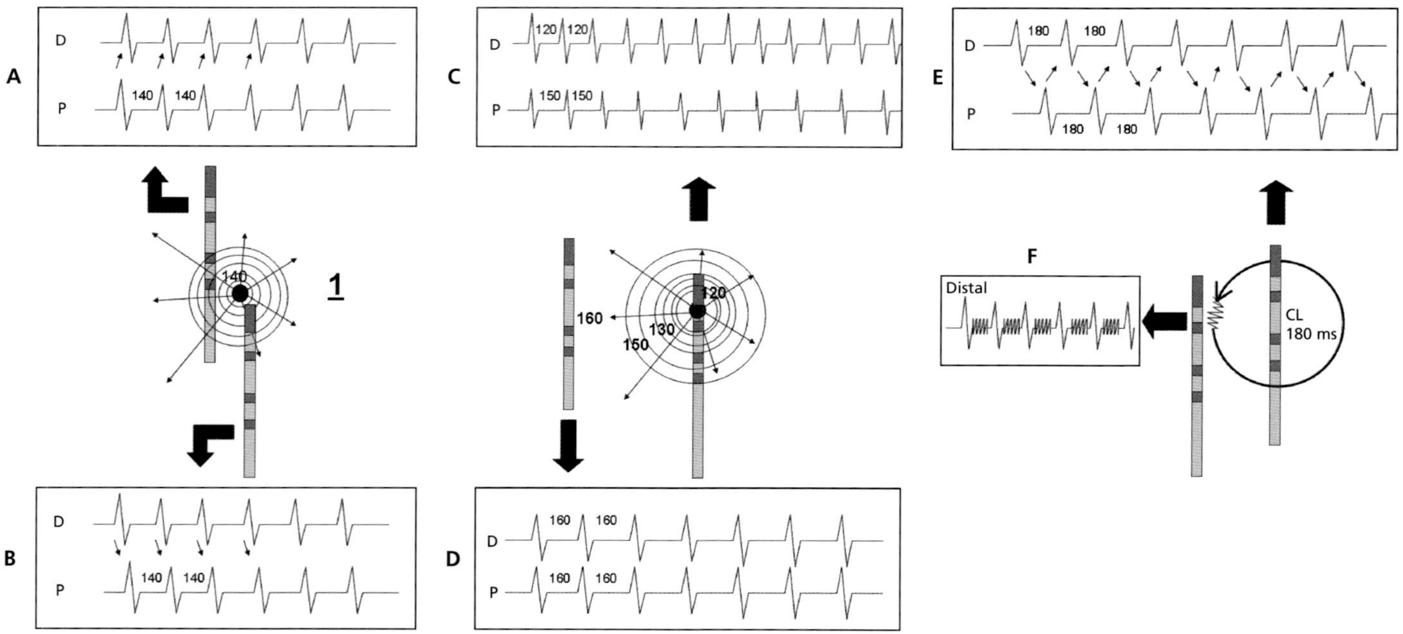

Figure 12.12 Cartoon depiction of electrograms recorded near or at differing hypothetical focal sources. Box A shows a proximal-to-distal activation sequence (arrows) consistent with the catheter position relative to a focal source of cycle length (CL) 140 ms with 1 : 1 activation of the surrounding tissue. Box B shows a distal-to-proximal activation sequence. Box C shows the electrograms recorded with the distal (D) catheter bipole positioned over a high frequency source (shortest cycle length 120 ms) with a frequency gradient to the surrounding tissue, as indicated by the cycle length of 150 ms recorded on the proximal (P) bipole. When the catheter is moved away from the source (Box D), simultaneous activation at the proximal and distal bipoles is seen, with no discernible difference in cycle length. Box E shows a temporal gradient between the proximal and distal bipoles when the catheter is positioned directly over a hypothetical local circuit of cycle length 180 ms. A fractionated signal (Box F) is recorded with the distal bipole at a hypothetical zone of slow conduction within the circuit.

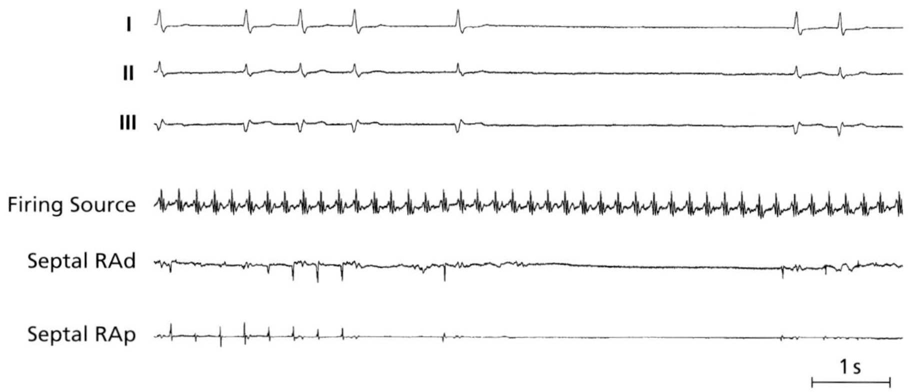

Figure 12.13 Ablation performed within the right atrium (RA) near the sinus node region resulted in the isolation of a local source perpetuating AF. Shown is the local source firing continuously even after termination of AF.

terminate arrhythmia than to resort to electrical or pharmacological cardioversion, the real question is at what electrical and mechanical price? In our experience, termination represents an incontrovertible procedural endpoint as well as impacting significantly upon the mode of arrhythmia recurrence and the final clinical outcome.

We define acute procedural success as termination of AF during radiofrequency application. Of an 178 patient cohort, AF terminated in 149 (84%) patients; 29 patients were deemed "failed" despite having electrical cardioversion to sinus rhythm at the end of the procedure. Direct restoration of sinus rhythm occurs only in a minority of patients. More often, conversion to usually > 1 intermediary atrial tachycardia is observed. It is likely that the presence of de novo tachycardias unmasked by ablation may be the sources responsible for perpetuating AF. Ablation of the initial tachycardia resulted in abrupt tachycardia transition to one which is usually slower (Figures 12.14 and 12.15).

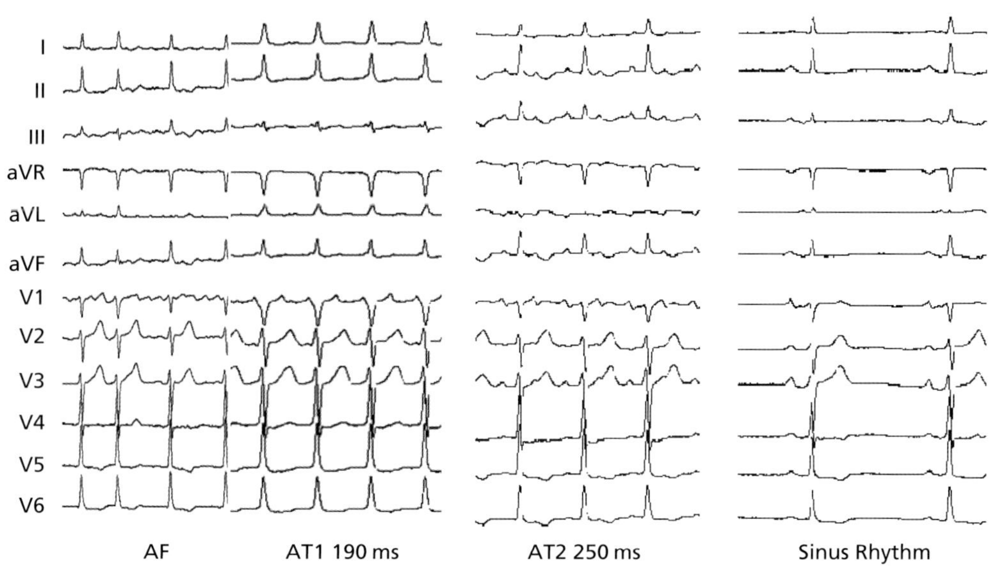

Figure 12.14 In the great majority of patients, termination of atrial fibrillation (AF) during catheter ablation occurs by conversion into more than one atrial tachycardia (AT) prior to the restoration of sinus rhythm, and requiring mapping and ablation.

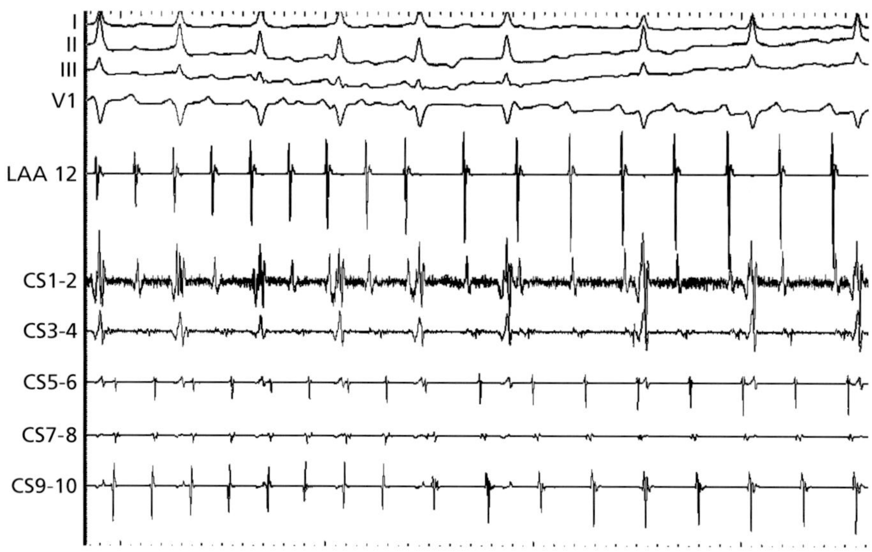

Figure 12.15 Example of the presence of multiple atrial tachycardias (ATs) in patients with persistent and permanent AF. AT1 190 ms (on the left) transitioned to AT2 250 ms (on the right) during radiofrequency application.

Although the use of three-dimensional navigational systems may be helpful, some tachycardias may be unstable. Besides this, using these mapping systems for multiple atrial tachycardias after ablating for 3–4 h can be particularly time-consuming and inpractical. In addition, these systems may introduce unacceptable levels of electrical noise thereby hiding critical low voltage components of local electrograms. We use a simple, yet effective, algorithm which has been extremely valuable in facilitating rapid diagnosis of the type or mechanism of atrial tachycardia and their ablation.

Arrhythmia recurrence post catheter ablation

Although early recurrence of AF carries an independent risk of treatment failure, up to 60% of patients with early recurrence of AF within the first months after ablation will not have any further arrhythmias during long-term follow-up [112–115]. A repeat ablation procedure is therefore deferred for at least 1 month and preferably 3 months following the index procedure. Symptomatic patients with AF and rapid ventricular rates are considered for electrical cardioversion.

New-onset atrial tachycardia has been reported in at least 10% of all arrhythmias observed early post ablation [93,112,116,117]. One study suggested that spontaneous remission of atrial tachycardia may occur in approximately one-third of patients within 6 months of the ablation procedure [116]. The mechanisms underlying post-ablation atrial tachycardias appear to be dependent on the catheter technique used. In patients who underwent segmental PVI, a focal atrial origin due to PV reconduction or outside the PVs at the LA roof or anterior to right PVs have been reported as the dominant mechanisms [93,118,119]. Macroreentrant circuits have been documented with critical isthmuses at various sites – the mitral isthmus, the interatrial septum, the LA roof, and the coronary sinus [116,120,121].

We studied 153 out of 178 patients who had at least 9 months of follow-up to determine the mode of arrhythmia recurrence and longer term clinical outcome. During a mean follow-up of 21 ± 10 months, 58 of 66 patients in whom AF terminated during the index procedure represented with atrial tachycardia, compared to 13 of 21 patients where AF could not be terminated (88% versus 38%, $P = 0.001$). After repeat ablation attempts, sinus rhythm was maintained in 123 out of 129 of patients with AF termination compared to 12 out of 24 of patients without AF termination ($P < 0.001$). In other words, termination of AF is associated with better long-term outcome if sinus rhythm is maintained (Figure 12.16). Patients in whom sinus rhythm is maintained would be expected to have less AF-related complications and,

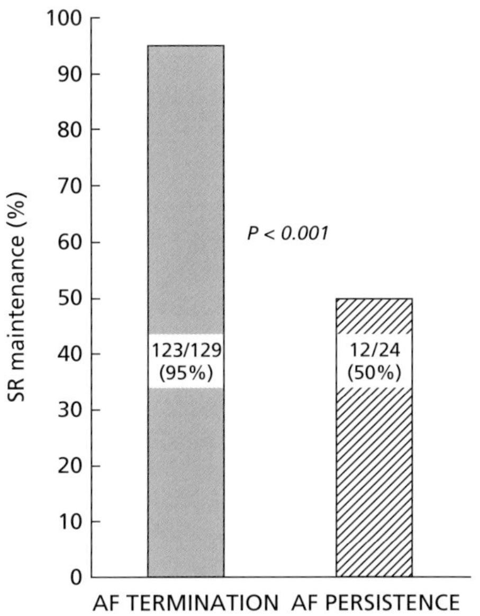

Figure 12.16 Long-term clinical outcome in patients with and without procedural atrial fibrillation (AF) termination showing a significant difference in sinus rhythm (SR) maintenance without antiarrhythmic drugs between the two patient groups.

based on the results of the AFFIRM substudy, would have better prognosis.

During repeat ablation attempts, limited atrial ablation was required for those with atrial tachycardia recurrence compared to the more extensive atrial ablation needed when AF was the primary reason for re-ablation. In our patients, macroreentrant tachycardias comprised approximately half of the left atrial tachycardias and were often related to incomplete linear ablation either at the mitral isthmus or the LA roof. Focal tachycardias were responsible for the rest of tachycardias, most of them being localized circuits [122].

It is striking that patients with successful AF termination during catheter ablation were more likely to have atrial tachycardia recurrence, while those with unsuccessful AF termination re-presented with AF recurrence [123].

Effects of catheter ablation on atrial electrical and mechanical properties

Serial echocardiographic evaluation of left atrial and left ventricular mechanical function confirmed favorable reverse modeling following catheter ablation of chronic AF [124]. Regular follow-up at 1, 3, 6, 9, and 12 months revealed progressive decrease in LA dimensions from 68.4 ± 8.1 mm to 60.7 ± 6.5 mm ($P < 0.05$). Left atrial mechanical function assessed by LA active emptying volume improved from 2.67 ± 1.9 ml/m^2 to 4.7 ± 2.14 ml/m^2 ($P = 0.015$), the LA active emptying fraction improved from 5.5 ± 3.6% to 21.8 ± 11% ($P < 0.05$) and the LA filling fraction increased from 15 ± 7% to 30 ± 5% ($P < 0.05$). Left ventricular remodeling following catheter ablation was demonstrated by significant improvement of the left ventricular ejection fraction from 53 ± 8.5% to 63 ± 7% ($P < 0.05$), improvement of diastolic filling parameters, and decline in the severity of mitral regurgitation.

One of the major issues raised concerning catheter ablation for chronic AF patients is the extent of ablation itself and concerns of negative impact on LA electrical and mechanical function. It is argued that catheter ablation replaces myocardium with scar and prolongs intra-atrial conduction, thereby potentially compromising atrial mechanical performance. In a study of 40 consecutive patients who had stepwise ablation achieving termination of chronic AF, Takahashi et al. performed electroanatomic voltage maps to assess areas of scar and low voltage, which accounted for 31 ± 12% and 32 ± 17% of the total LA surface area, respectively [125] (Figure 12.17). The ablated PV region represented the majority of the scar burden, accounting for 20 ± 4%, approximately two-thirds of the LA surface area [125]. In contrast, ablation in all other atrial regions aiming to achieve local organization and slowing of fibrillation cycle length was associated with a relative preservation of atrial voltages and propagation as well as recovery of atrial mechanical function. The observed LA conduction times were widely spread within the range of 100 to 360 ms, while contraction assessed by the presence of late diastolic mitral flow was 37 ± 15 cm/s, and the mean LA active emptying fraction was 18 ± 11%. Prolongation of LA conduction times due to scar/low voltage tissue in the LA, especially near the Bachmann bundle insertion, was associated with attenuation of atrial contractile performances. In the maze procedure, significant loss in LA contraction occurred in 13–39% of patients.

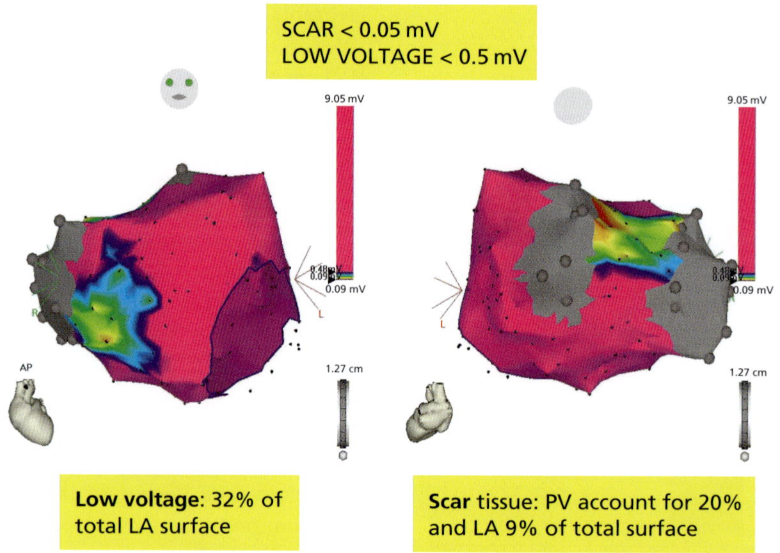

Figure 12.17 Electroanatomic voltage maps showing the impact of extensive left atrium (LA) ablation on LA tissue 3 months' post-ablation and the restoration of sinus rhythm. The pink areas represent healthy tissue. Low voltage regions were defined as < 0.5 mV and represented 32% of the total LA surface, while the presence of scar was defined as a voltage of < 0.05 mV. PV, pulmonary veins.

Factors predictive of procedural AF termination

Observational studies have suggested that paroxysmal AF may become sustained over time [126]. The concept of AF being a progressive disease is supported by marked shortening of the atrial refractory period with electrical maintenance of AF. Progressive increase in AF duration was associated with a marked shortening of atrial refractory period and AF interval and vulnerability to AF.

Success rates of chemical cardioversion have been shown to be much higher for recent AF (< 24 h) than for longer AF [127,128]. Electrical cardioversion studies for patients with longer term AF also supported the influence of chronicity on success or failure of cardioversion [129,130]. Van Gelder et al. investigated the effectiveness of cardioversion for atrial arrhythmias in 246 patients who underwent direct current electrical cardioversion and were followed during a mean of 260 days [129]. Stepwise logistic regression analysis revealed that arrhythmia duration ($P < 0.001$), type of arrhythmia (fibrillation versus flutter; $P < 0.02$), and age ($P < 0.05$) all independently influenced conversion rate [129]. Thus the persistence of AF leads to the development of AF that is more refractory to cardioversion.

In 178 consecutive patients undergoing catheter ablation for chronic AF, AF termination was significantly lower in the 23 patients with chronic AF of more than 5 years' duration (40% versus 84%; $P < 0.001$). It appears that ablation success declines further with increasing chronic AF duration (Figure 12.18), supported by the finding that AF termination occurred in only 13% of patients with chronic AF of more than 10 years' duration. Therefore, catheter ablation for chronic AF should probably be attempted sooner rather than later, and expectations of AF termination by radiofrequency are lower for chronic AF lasting beyond 5 years.

In the vast majority of patients with AF persistent for less than 5 years, multivariate analysis incorporating age, gender, structural heart disease, heart failure, amiodarone use, AF cycle length, and LA size indicate that AF cycle length was the strongest independent predictor of successful AF termination (Figure 12.19).

Future directions for ablation of chronic atrial fibrillation

The currently practiced strategies for ablation of chronic AF have many commonalities and some points of contention. However, all are agreed that

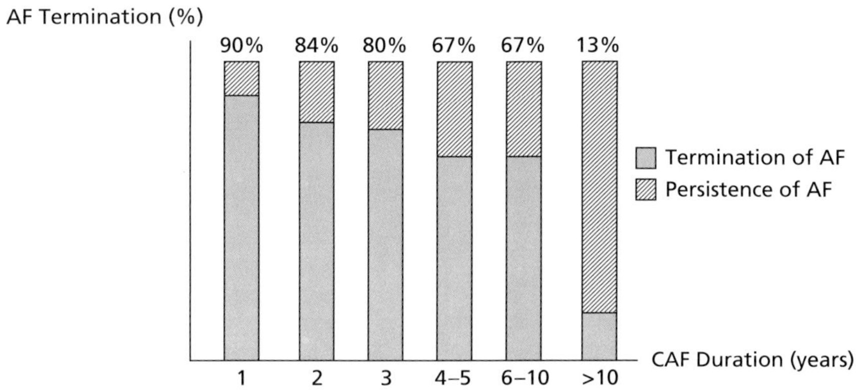

Figure 12.18 Shown is the decline in procedural atrial fibrillation (AF) termination with increasing chronic AF (CAF) duration. High success rates were observed in the initial years, while beyond 10 years results were extremely poor.

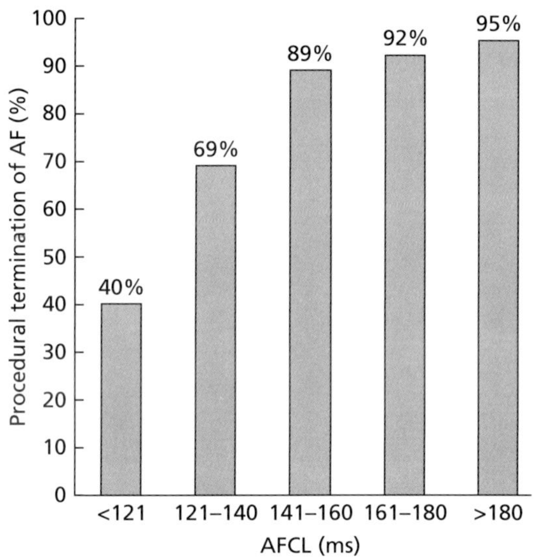

Figure 12.19 Incidence of procedural termination of chronic atrial fibrillation (AF) versus AF cycle length (AFCL) measured in the LAA at the beginning of the procedure. Note that the patients with a short baseline cycle length (< 140 ms) have a low percentage of termination of AF by ablation.

ablation of only those sites critical to initiation and perpetuation of AF, while minimizing collateral damage, is a key goal. PV isolation remains a cornerstone not only because PVs represent important triggers but ablation in their vicinity could potentially give rise to substrates for reentry to promote proarrhythmia even if AF is terminated during the index procedure. The use of conventional catheters to isolate PVs may appear laborious and requires manual dexterity, but it is hoped that balloon-based catheters or equivalents using various energy deliveries will facilitate this step. Such techniques would, however, also pose different problems to the operators given anatomic differences in PVs, sizing issues, and similar potential complications including phrenic nerve injury. The targeting of local sources representing atrial substrates is a relatively new concept. Complex fractionated electrograms indicate areas of slow conduction and/or pivot points where the wavelets propagate around areas of functional block [131]. They are critically dependent on prior cycle length [34] and are found in the boundaries of high frequency excitation [132]. The one challenge is to differentiate electrograms that are critical to AF perpetuation versus those that are not. In the vast majority of patients, linear block is technically challenging to achieve; future improvement in catheter designs and lesion creating tools is desirable. Remote catheter navigation [133] may help to confine lesions to a specific site of interest in addition to increasing the facility with which the procedure can be performed. Novel ablative instruments to provide more controlled and safer ablation will be welcome. Simultaneous global atrial mapping and signal processing may greatly improve the accuracy with which critical sources or drivers can be distinguished within the electrical chaos of the fibrillating atrium.

Conclusion

Catheter ablation for chronic AF has evolved as a result of recognition that both trigger elimination and substrate modification are equally important.

PV isolation alone is insufficient and in these patients additional approaches targeting atrial substrates using individual electrogram-based ablation and linear ablation are necessary to increase success rates. Pending re-ablation for atrial tachycardias, this combined approach may result in the restoration of sinus rhythm in > 90% of patients, associated with great improvement in symptomatic status and general wellbeing. Further refinement in mapping techniques of local sources/drivers and catheter ablation technological advances to improve the creation of contiguous lesions are needed to enhance procedural outcome.

References

1 Fuster V, Ryden LE, Cannom DS, et al. ACC/AHA/ESC 2006 guidelines for the management of patients with atrial fibrillation – executive summary. A report of the American College of Cardiology/American Heart Association Task Force on Practice Guidelines and the European Society of Cardiology Committee for Practice Guidelines (writing committee to revise the 2001 guidelines for the management of patients with atrial fibrillation): developed in collaboration with the European Heart Rhythm Association and the Heart Rhythm Society. *Circulation* 2006;**114**(7):700–52.

2 Krahn AD, Manfreda J, Tate RB, Mathewson FAL, Cuddy TE. The natural history of atrial fibrillation: incidence, risk factors, and prognosis in the manitoba follow-up study. *Am J Med* 1995;**98**(5):476–84.

3 Stewart S, Hart CL, Hole DJ, McMurray JJV. A population-based study of the long-term risks associated with atrial fibrillation: 20-year follow-up of the Renfrew/Paisley study. *Am J Me* 2002;**113**(5):359–64.

4 Cappato R, Calkins H, Chen SA, et al. Worldwide survey on the methods, efficacy, and safety of catheter ablation for human atrial fibrillation. *Circulation* 2005;**111**(9):1100–5.

5 European Heart Rhythm Association and the Heart Rhythm Society, Fuster V, Ryden LE, et al. ACC/AHA/ESC 2006 guidelines for the management of patients with atrial fibrillation – executive summary. A report of the American College of Cardiology, American Heart Association Task Force on Practice Guidelines and the European Society of Cardiology Committee for Practice Guidelines (writing committee to revise the 2001 guidelines for the management of patients with atrial fibrillation). *J Am Coll Cardiol* 2006;**48**(4):854–906.

6 Oral H, Chugh A, Good E, et al. Radiofrequency catheter ablation of chronic atrial fibrillation guided by complex electrograms. *Circulation* 2007;**115**(20):2606–12.

7 Levy S, Maarek M, Coumel P, Guize L, Lekieffre J, Medvedowsky JL, Sebaoun A. Characterization of different subsets of atrial fibrillation in general practice in France: the ALFA Study. *Circulation* 1999;**99**(23):3028–35.

8 Cox JL, Boineau JP, Schuessler RB, Jaquiss RDB, Lappas DG. Modification of the maze procedure for atrial flutter and atrial fibrillation: I. Rationale and surgical results. *J Thoracic Cardiovasc Surg* 1995;**110**(2):473–84.

9 Melo JQ, Santiago T, Gouveia RH, Martins AP. Atrial ablation for the surgical treatment of atrial fibrillation. Principles and limitations. *J Cardiac Surg* 2004;**19**(3):207–10.

10 Sueda T, Imai K, Orihashi K, Okada K, Ban K, Hamamoto M. Midterm results of pulmonary vein isolation for the elimination of chronic atrial fibrillation. *Ann Thoracic Surg* 2005;**79**(2):521–5.

11 Scheinman MM, Morady F, Hess DS, Gonzalez S. Catheter-induced ablation of the atrioventricular junction to control refractory supraventricular arrhythmias. *J Am Med Assoc* 1982;**248**:851–5.

12 Haissaguerre M, Gencel L, Fischer B, Le Metayer P, Poquet F, Marcus FI, Clementy J. Successful catheter ablation of atrial fibrillation. *J Cardiovasc Electrophysiol* 1994;**5**(12):1045–52.

13 Schwartz JF, Pellersels G, Silvers J. A catheter-based curative approach to atrial fibrillation in humans. *Circulation* 1993;**90**:I–335.

14 Packer DL. Linear ablation for atrial fibrillation: the pendulum swings back. In: Zipes DP, Haissaguerre M, eds. *Catheter Ablation of Arrhythmias*, 2nd edn. Futura Publishing, New York, 2002:107–29.

15 Jais P, Shah DC, Takahashi A, Hocini M, Haissaguerre M, Clementy J. Long-term follow-up after right atrial radiofrequency catheter treatment of paroxysmal atrial fibrillation. *Pacing Clin Electrophysiol* 1998;**21**(11):2533–8.

16 Ernst S, Schluter M, Ouyang F, et al. Modification of the substrate for maintenance of idiopathic human atrial fibrillation: efficacy of radiofrequency ablation using nonfluoroscopic catheter guidance. *Circulation* 1999;**100**(20):2085–92.

17 Haissaguerre M, Jais P, Shah DC, et al. Spontaneous initiation of atrial fibrillation by ectopic beats originating in the pulmonary veins. *N Engl J Med* 1998;**339**(10):659–66.

18 Pappone C, Oreto G, Rosanio S, et al. Atrial electroanatomic remodeling after circumferential radiofrequency pulmonary vein ablation: efficacy of an anatomic approach in a large cohort of patients with atrial fibrillation. *Circulation* 2001;**104**(21):2539–44.

19 Oral H, Knight BP, Tada H, et al. Pulmonary vein isolation for paroxysmal and persistent atrial fibrillation. *Circulation* 2002;**105**(9):1077–81.
20 Arentz T, von Rosenthal J, Blum T, et al. Feasibility and safety of pulmonary vein isolation using a new mapping and navigation system in patients with refractory atrial fibrillation. *Circulation* 2003;**108**(20):2484–90.
21 Vasamreddy CR, Lickfett L, Jayam VK, et al. Predictors of recurrence following catheter ablation of atrial fibrillation using an irrigated-tip ablation catheter. *J Cardiovasc Electrophysiol* 2004;**15**(6):692–7.
22 Lim TW, Jassal IS, Ross DL, Thomas SP. Medium-term efficacy of segmental ostial pulmonary vein isolation for the treatment of permanent and persistent atrial fibrillation. *Pacing Clin Electrophysiol* 2006;**29**(4):374–9.
23 Ouyang F, Ernst S, Chun J, et al. Electrophysiological findings during ablation of persistent atrial fibrillation with electroanatomic mapping and double Lasso catheter technique. *Circulation* 2005;**112**(20):3038–48.
24 Sanders P, Nalliah CJ, Dubois R, et al. Frequency mapping of the pulmonary veins in paroxysmal versus permanent atrial fibrillation. *J Cardiovasc Electrophysiol* 2006;**17**(9):965–72.
25 Mandapati R, Skanes A, Chen J, Berenfeld O, Jalife J. Stable microreentrant sources as a mechanism of atrial fibrillation in the isolated sheep heart. *Circulation* 2000; **101**(2):194–9.
26 Schuessler RB, Kawamoto T, Hand DE, Mitsuno M, Bromberg BI, Cox JL, Boineau JP. Simultaneous epicardial and endocardial activation sequence mapping in the isolated canine right atrium. *Circulation* 1993;**88**(1): 250–63.
27 Mandapati R, Skanes A, Chen J, Berenfeld O, Jalife J. Stable microreentrant sources as a mechanism of atrial fibrillation in the isolated sheep heart. *Circulation* 2000; **101**(2):194–9.
28 Sanders P, Berenfeld O, Hocini M, et al. Spectral analysis identifies sites of high-frequency activity maintaining atrial fibrillation in humans. *Circulation* 2005;**112**(6): 789–97.
29 Haissaguerre M, Hocini M, Sanders P, et al. Localized fibrillatory sources maintaining atrial fibrillation. *Heart Rhythm* 2005;**2**(5 Suppl 1):S20.
30 Haissaguerre M, Hocini M, Sanders P, et al. Localized sources maintaining atrial fibrillation organized by prior ablation. *Circulation* 2006;**113**(5):616–25.
31 Nademanee K, McKenzie J, Kosar E, et al. A new approach for catheter ablation of atrial fibrillation: mapping of the electrophysiologic substrate. *J Am Coll Cardiol* 2004;**43**(11):2044–53.
32 Jais P, Haissaguerre M, Shah D, Chouairi S, Clementy J. Regional disparities of endocardial atrial activation in paroxysmal atrial fibrillation. *Pacing Clin Electrophysiol* 1996;**19**(11):1998–2003.
33 Konings KTS, Smeets JLRM, Penn OC, Wellens HJJ, Allessie MA. Configuration of unipolar atrial electrograms during electrically induced atrial fibrillation in humans. *Circulation* 1997;**95**(5):1231–41.
34 Rostock T, Rotter M, Sanders P, et al. High-density activation mapping of fractionated electrograms in the atria of patients with paroxysmal atrial fibrillation. *Heart Rhythm* 2006;**3**(1):27–34.
35 Jais P, Haissaguerre M, Shah D, Chouairi S, Clementy J. Regional disparities of endocardial atrial activation in paroxysmal atrial fibrillation. *Pacing Clin Electrophysiol* 1996;**19**(11):1998–2003.
36 Rostock T, Rotter M, Sanders P, et al. High-density activation mapping of fractionated electrograms in the atria of patients with paroxysmal atrial fibrillation. *Heart Rhythm* 2006;**3**(1):27–34.
37 Lewis T, Drury AN, Bulger HA. Observations upon atrial flutter and fibrillation. VI. Refractory period and rate of propagation in the auricle: their relation to block in the auricular walls and to flutter. *Heart* 1921;**8**: 84–134.
38 Hoff HE, Geddes LA. Cholinergic factor in atrial fibrillation. *J Appl Physiol* 1955;**8**:177–92.
39 Coumel P. Autonomic influences in atrial tachyarrhythmias. *J Cardiovasc Electrophysiol* 1996;**7**(10):999–1007.
40 Scherlag BJ, Yamanashi W, Patel U, Lazzara R, Jackman WM. Autonomically induced conversion of pulmonary vein focal firing into atrial fibrillation. *J Am Coll Cardiol* 2005;**45**(11):1878–86.
41 Schauerte P, Scherlag BJ, Pitha J, Scherlag MA, Reynolds D, Lazzara R, Jackman WM. Catheter ablation of cardiac autonomic nerves for prevention of vagal atrial fibrillation. *Circulation* 2000;**102**(22):2774–80.
42 Takahashi Y, Jais P, Hocini M, et al. Shortening of fibrillatory cycle length in the pulmonary vein during vagal excitation. *J Am Coll Cardiol* 2006;**47**(4):774–80.
43 Tan AY, Li H, Wachsmann-Hogiu S, Chen LS, Chen PS, Fishbein MC. Autonomic innervation and segmental muscular disconnections at the human pulmonary vein–atrial junction: implications for catheter ablation of atrial–pulmonary vein junction. *J Am Coll Cardiol* 2006;**48**(1):132–43.
44 Scherlag BJ, Nakagawa H, Jackman WM, Yamanashi WS, Patterson E, Po S, Lazzara R. Electrical stimulation to identify neural elements on the heart: their role in atrial fibrillation. *J Interv Cardiac Electrophysiol* 2005;**13**: 37–42.
45 Scherlag BJ, Yamanashi W, Patel U, Lazzara R, Jackman WM. Autonomically induced conversion of pulmonary vein focal firing into atrial fibrillation. *J Am Coll Cardiol* 2005;**45**(11):1878–86.

46 Nademanee K, McKenzie J, Kosar E, et al. A new approach for catheter ablation of atrial fibrillation: mapping of the electrophysiologic substrate. *J Am Coll Cardiol* 2004;**43**(11):2044–53.

47 Oral H, Chugh A, Good E, et al. Randomized comparison of encircling and nonencircling left atrial ablation for chronic atrial fibrillation. *Heart Rhythm* 2005;**2**(11): 1165–72.

48 Willems S, Klemm H, Rostock T, et al. Substrate modification combined with pulmonary vein isolation improves outcome of catheter ablation in patients with persistent atrial fibrillation: a prospective randomized comparison. *Eur Heart J* 2006;**27**:2871–8.

49 Hsu LF, Jais P, Sanders P, et al. Catheter ablation for atrial fibrillation in congestive heart failure. *N Engl J Med* 2004;**351**(23):2373–83.

50 Kottkamp H, Tanner H, Kobza R, et al. Time courses and quantitative analysis of atrial fibrillation episode number and duration after circular plus linear left atrial lesions. Trigger elimination or substrate modification: early or delayed cure? *J Am Coll Cardiol* 2004;**44**(4): 869–77.

51 Fassini G, Riva S, Chiodelli R, et al. Left mitral isthmus ablation associated with PV isolation: long-term results of a prospective randomized study. *J Cardiovasc Electrophysiol* 2005;**16**(11):1150–6.

52 Pappone C, Santinelli V. Atrial fibrillation ablation: state of the art. *Am J Cardiol* 2005;**96**(12 Suppl 1): 59–64.

53 Pappone C, Manguso F, Vicedomini G, et al. Prevention of iatrogenic atrial tachycardia after ablation of atrial fibrillation: a prospective randomized study comparing circumferential pulmonary vein ablation with a modified approach. *Circulation* 2004;**110**(19):3036–42.

54 Oral H, Pappone C, Chugh A, et al. Circumferential pulmonary-vein ablation for chronic atrial fibrillation. *N Engl J Med* 2006;**354**(9):934–41.

55 Bertaglia E, Stabile G, Senatore G, et al. Long term outcome of right and left atrial radiofrequency ablation in patients with persistent atrial fibrillation. *Pace* 2006; **29**:153–8.

56 Beukema WP, Elvan A, Sie HT, Misier AR, Wellens HJ. Successful radiofrequency ablation in patients with previous atrial fibrillation results in a significant decrease in left atrial size. *Circulation* 2005;**112**:2089–95.

57 Verma A, Marrouche NF, Natale A. Pulmonary vein antrum isolation: intracardiac echocardiography-guided technique. *J Cardiovasc Electrophysiol* 2004;**15**(11):1335–40.

58 Haissaguerre M, Sanders P, Hocini M, et al. Catheter ablation of long-lasting persistent atrial fibrillation: critical structures for termination. *J Cardiovasc Electrophysiol* 2005;**16**(11):1125–37.

59 Haissaguerre M, Hocini M, Sanders P, et al. Catheter ablation of long-lasting persistent atrial fibrillation: clinical outcome and mechanisms of subsequent arrhythmias. *J Cardiovasc Electrophysiol* 2005;**16**(11): 1138–47.

60 Chen MS, Marrouche NF, Khaykin Y, et al. Pulmonary vein isolation for the treatment of atrial fibrillation in patients with impaired systolic function. *J Am Coll Cardiol* 2004;**43**(6):1004–9.

61 Hsu LF, Jais P, Sanders P, et al. Catheter ablation for atrial fibrillation in congestive heart failure. *N Engl J Med* 2004;**351**(23):2373–83.

62 O'Neill MD, Sanders P, Takahashi Y, et al. Treatment of chronic atrial fibrillation by catheter ablation in patients with heart failure. *Pacing Clin Electrophysiol* 2006;**29**: S8–S9.

63 Kim KB, Rodefeld MD, Schuessler RB, Cox JL, Boineau JP. Relationship between local atrial fibrillation interval and refractory period in the isolated canine atrium. *Circulation* 1996;**94**(11):2961–7.

64 Wijffels MCEF, Kirchhof CJHJ, Dorland R, Allessie MA. Atrial fibrillation begets atrial fibrillation: a study in awake chronically instrumented goats. *Circulation* 1995; **92**(7):1954–68.

65 Wang Z, Page P, Nattel S. Mechanism of flecainide's antiarrhythmic action in experimental atrial fibrillation. *Circ Res* 1992;**71**(2):271–87.

66 Haissaguerre M, Sanders P, Hocini M, et al. Changes in atrial fibrillation cycle length and inducibility during catheter ablation and their relation to outcome. *Circulation* 2004;**109**(24):3007–13.

67 Haissaguerre M, Sanders P, Hocini M, et al. Changes in atrial fibrillation cycle length and inducibility during catheter ablation and their relation to outcome. *Circulation* 2004;**109**(24):3007–13.

68 Calo L, Lamberti F, Loricchio ML, et al. Left atrial ablation versus biatrial ablation for persistent and permanent atrial fibrillation: a prospective and randomized study. *J Am Coll Cardiol* 2006;**47**(12):2504–12.

69 Verma A, Kilicaslan F, Adams JR, et al. Extensive ablation during pulmonary vein antrum isolation has no adverse impact on left atrial function: an echocardiography and cine computed tomography analysis. *J Cardiovasc Electrophysiol* 2006;**17**(7):741–6.

70 Sanders P, Sacher F, Jais P, et al. P4-44: restoration of atrial mechanical function after catheter ablation of AF. Impact of the mode of termination and arrhythmia duration. *Heart Rhythm* 2006;**3**(5 Suppl 1):S232–S233.

71 Hocini M, Sanders P, Jais P, et al. Techniques for curative treatment of atrial fibrillation. *J Cardiovasc Electrophysiol* 2004;**15**(12):1467–71.

72 Sanders P, Hocini M, Jais P, et al. Pulmonary vein isolation for atrial fibrillation. In: Stephen Huang SK, Wood

MA, eds. *Catheter Ablation of Cardiac Arrhythmias.* Saunders Elsevier, Philadelphia, 2006:269–87.

73 Nademanee K, McKenzie J, Kosar E, et al. A new approach for catheter ablation of atrial fibrillation: mapping of the electrophysiologic substrate. *J Am Coll Cardiol* 2004;**43**(11):2044–53.

74 O'Neill MD, Jais P, Takahashi Y, et al. The stepwise ablation approach for chronic atrial fibrillation – evidence for a cumulative effect. *J Interv Cardiac Electrophysiol* 2006;**16**(3):153–167.

75 Oral H, Chugh A, Good E, et al. Radiofrequency catheter ablation of chronic atrial fibrillation guided by complex electrograms. *Circulation* 2007;**115**(20):2606–12.

76 Takahashi Y, Jais P, Hocini M, et al. AB25-3: sites of termination of chronic atrial fibrillation by catheter ablation. *Heart Rhythm* 2006;**3**(5 Suppl 1):S52.

77 Kamunu S, Tan AY, Peter CT, Hwang C, Chen P. Vein of Marshall activity during sustained atrial fibrillation. *J Cardiovasc Electrophysiol* 2006;**17**(8):839–46.

78 Elayi CS, Fahmy TS, Wazni OM, Patel D, Saliba W, Natale A. Left superior vena cava isolation in patients undergoing pulmonary vein antrum isolation: impact on atrial fibrillation recurrence. *Heart Rhythm* 2006; **3**(9):1019–23.

79 Tsai CF, Tai CT, Hsieh MH, et al. Initiation of atrial fibrillation by ectopic beats originating from the superior vena cava: electrophysiological characteristics and results of radiofrequency ablation. *Circulation* 2000; **102**(1):67–74.

80 Lin WS, Tai CT, Hsieh MH, et al. Catheter ablation of paroxysmal atrial fibrillation initiated by non-pulmonary vein ectopy. *Circulation* 2003;**107**(25):3176–83.

81 Oral H, Ozaydin M, Chugh A, et al. Role of the coronary sinus in maintenance of atrial fibrillation. *J Cardiovasc Electrophysiol* 2003;**14**(12):1329–36.

82 Kistler PM, Fynn SP, Haqqani H, et al. Focal atrial tachycardia from the ostium of the coronary sinus: electrocardiographic and electrophysiological characterization and radiofrequency ablation. *J Am Coll Cardiol* 2005;**45**(9):1488–93.

83 Chauvin M, Shah DC, Haissaguerre M, Marcellin L, Brechenmacher C. The anatomic basis of connections between the coronary sinus musculature and the left atrium in humans. *Circulation* 2000;**101**(6):647–52.

84 Takahashi Y, Jais P, Hocini M, et al. AB25-3: Sites of termination of chronic atrial fibrillation by catheter ablation. *Heart Rhythm* 2006;**3**(5 Suppl 1):S52.

85 Hocini M, Takahashi Y, Sanders P, et al. P6-83: multifocal arrhythmogenicity of the coronary sinus in chronic atrial fibrillation. *Heart Rhythm* 2006;**3**(5 Suppl 1):S329.

86 Takahashi Y, Jais P, Hocini M, et al. Acute occlusion of the left circumflex coronary artery during mitral isthmus linear ablation. *J Cardiovasc Electrophysiol* 2005;**16**(10):1104–7.

87 Tsao HM, Wu MH, Chern MS, et al. Anatomic proximity of the esophagus to the coronary sinus: implication for catheter ablation within the coronary sinus. *J Cardiovasc Electrophysiol* 2006;**17**(3):266–9.

88 Hocini M, Jais P, Sanders P, et al. Techniques, evaluation, and consequences of linear block at the left atrial roof in paroxysmal atrial fibrillation: a prospective randomized study. *Circulation* 2005;**112**(24):3688–96.

89 Pappone C, Oral H, Santinelli V, et al. Atrio-esophageal fistula as a complication of percutaneous transcatheter ablation of atrial fibrillation. *Circulation* 2004;**109**(22): 2724–6.

90 Nakagawa H, Wittkampf FHM, Yamanashi WS, et al. Inverse relationship between electrode size and lesion size during radiofrequency ablation with active electrode cooling. *Circulation* 1998;**98**(5):458–65.

91 Hocini M, Jais P, Sanders P, et al. Techniques, evaluation, and consequences of linear block at the left atrial roof in paroxysmal atrial fibrillation: a prospective randomized study. *Circulation* 2005;**112**(24):3688–96.

92 Hsu LF, Jais P, Hocini M, et al. Incidence and prevention of cardiac tamponade complicating ablation for atrial fibrillation. *Pacing Clin Electrophysiol* 2005;**28**(s1): S106–S109.

93 Gerstenfeld EP, Callans DJ, Dixit S, et al. Mechanisms of organized left atrial tachycardias occurring after pulmonary vein isolation. *Circulation* 2004;**110**(11): 1351–7.

94 Chugh A, Oral H, Lemola K, et al. Prevalence, mechanisms, and clinical significance of macroreentrant atrial tachycardia during and following left atrial ablation for atrial fibrillation. *Heart Rhythm* 2005;**2**(5):464–71.

95 Rostock T, O'Neill M, Sanders P, et al. Characterization of conduction recovery across left atrial linear lesions in patients with paroxysmal and persistent atrial fibrillation. *J Cardiovasc Electrophysiol* 2006;**17**(10):1106–11.

96 Nademanee K. Trials and travails of electrogram-guided ablation of chronic atrial fibrillation. *Circulation* 2007; **115**(20):2592–4.

97 Tsai CF, Tai CT, Hsieh MH, et al. Initiation of atrial fibrillation by ectopic beats originating from the superior vena cava: electrophysiological characteristics and results of radiofrequency ablation. *Circulation* 2000; **102**(1):67–74.

98 Elayi CS, Fahmy TS, Wazni OM, Patel D, Saliba W, Natale A. Left superior vena cava isolation in patients undergoing pulmonary vein antrum isolation: impact on atrial fibrillation recurrence. *Heart Rhythm* 2006; **3**(9):1019–23.

99 Saksena S, Skadsberg ND, Rao HB, Filipecki A. Biatrial and three-dimensional mapping of spontaneous atrial

arrhythmias in patients with refractory atrial fibrillation. *J Cardiovasc Electrophysiol* 2005;**16**(5):494–504.

100 Sanders P, Berenfeld O, Hocini M, et al. Spectral analysis identifies sites of high-frequency activity maintaining atrial fibrillation in humans. *Circulation* 2005;**112**(6): 789–97.

101 Nitta T, Ishii Y, Miyagi Y, Ohmori H, Sakamoto S, Tanaka S. Concurrent multiple left atrial focal activations with fibrillatory conduction and right atrial focal or reentrant activation as the mechanism in atrial fibrillation. *J Thoracic Cardiovasc Surg* 2004;**127**(3):770–8.

102 O'Neill MD, Jonsson A, Hocini M, et al. P5-78: sigmoidal relationship between extent of left atrial ablation and termination of chronic atrial fibrillation. *Heart Rhythm* 2006;**3**(5 Suppl 1):S286.

103 Sacher F, Monahan KH, Thomas SP, et al. Phrenic nerve injury after atrial fibrillation catheter ablation: characterization and outcome in a multicenter study. *J Am Coll Cardiol* 2006;**47**(12):2498–503.

104 Sanders P, Berenfeld O, Hocini M, et al. Spectral analysis identifies sites of high-frequency activity maintaining atrial fibrillation in humans. *Circulation* 2005;**112**(6): 789–97.

105 Nitta T, Ishii Y, Miyagi Y, Ohmori H, Sakamoto S, Tanaka S. Concurrent multiple left atrial focal activations with fibrillatory conduction and right atrial focal or reentrant activation as the mechanism in atrial fibrillation. *J Thoracic Cardiovasc Surg* 2004;**127**(3): 770–8.

106 Haissaguerre M, Hocini M, Sanders P, et al. Localized sources maintaining atrial fibrillation organized by prior ablation. *Circulation* 2006;**113**(5):616–25.

107 Mandapati R, Skanes A, Chen J, Berenfeld O, Jalife J. Stable microreentrant sources as a mechanism of atrial fibrillation in the isolated sheep heart. *Circulation* 2000;**101**(2):194–9.

108 Haissaguerre M, Hocini M, Sanders P, et al. Localized sources maintaining atrial fibrillation organized by prior ablation. *Circulation* 2006;**113**(5):616–25.

109 Oral H, Chugh A, Lemola K, et al. Noninducibility of atrial fibrillation as an end point of left atrial circum ferential ablation for paroxysmal atrial fibrillation: a randomized study. *Circulation* 2004;**110**(18):2797–801.

110 Jais P, Hocini M, Sanders P, et al. Long-term evaluation of atrial fibrillation ablation guided by noninducibility. *Heart Rhythm* 2006;**3**(2):140–5.

111 Allessie M, Ausma J, Schotten U. Electrical, contractile and structural remodeling during atrial fibrillation. *Cardiovasc Res* 2002;**54**(2):230–46.

112 Oral H, Knight BP, Ozaydin M, et al. Clinical significance of early recurrences of atrial fibrillation after pulmonary vein isolation. *J Am Coll Cardiol* 2002; **40**(1):100–4.

113 Bertaglia E, Stabile G, Senatore G, et al. Predictive value of early atrial tachyarrhythmias recurrence after circumferential anatomical pulmonary vein ablation. *Pacing Clin Electrophysiol* 2005;**28**(5):366–71.

114 Vasamreddy CR, Lickfett L, Jayam VK, et al. Predictors of recurrence following catheter ablation of atrial fibrillation using an irrigated-tip ablation catheter. *J Cardiovasc Electrophysiol* 2004;**15**(6):692–7.

115 O'Donnell D, Furniss SS, Dunuwille A, Bourke JP. Delayed cure despite early recurrence after pulmonary vein isolation for atrial fibrillation. *Am J Cardiol* 2003;**91**(1):83–5.

116 Chugh A, Oral H, Lemola K, et al. Prevalence, mechanisms, and clinical significance of macroreentrant atrial tachycardia during and following left atrial ablation for atrial fibrillation. *Heart Rhythm* 2005;**2**(5):464–71.

117 Villacastin J, Perez-Castellano N, Moreno J, Gonzalez R. Left atrial flutter after radiofrequency catheter ablation of focal atrial fibrillation. *J Cardiovasc Electrophysiol* 2003;**14**(4):417–21.

118 Ouyang F, Antz M, Ernst S, et al. Recovered pulmonary vein conduction as a dominant factor for recurrent atrial tachyarrhythmias after complete circular isolation of the pulmonary veins: lessons from double Lasso technique. *Circulation* 2005;**111**(2):127–35.

119 Oral H, Knight BP, Morady F. Left atrial flutter after segmental ostial radiofrequency catheter ablation for pulmonary vein isolation. *Pacing Clin Electrophysiol* 2003;**26**(6):1417–19.

120 Jais P, Sanders PRAS, Hsu LF, et al. Flutter localized to the anterior left atrium after catheter ablation of atrial fibrillation. *J Cardiovasc Electrophysiol* 2006;**17**(3):279–85.

121 Chugh A, Oral H, Good E, et al. Catheter ablation of atypical atrial flutter and atrial tachycardia within the coronary sinus after left atrial ablation for atrial fibrillation. *J Am Coll Cardiol* 2005;**46**(1):83–91.

122 O'Neill MD, Lim KT, Jais P, et al. Chronic AF termination by catheter ablation is associated with a better clinical outcome. *Heart Rhythm* 2007;**4**(5S):S67 (abstract).

123 Haissaguerre M, Sanders P, Takahashi Y, et al. AB41-2: relationship between mode of arrhythmia recurrence and the achievement of chronic AF termination by ablation. *Heart Rhythm* 2006;**3**(5 Suppl 1):S84.

124 Reant P, Lafitte S, Jais P, et al. Reverse remodeling of the left cardiac chambers after catheter ablation after 1 year in a series of patients with isolated atrial fibrillation. *Circulation* 2005;**112**(19):2896–903.

125 Takahashi Y, O'Neill MD, Hocini M, et al. Effects of stepwise ablation of chronic atrial fibrillation on atrial electrical and mechanical properties. *J Am Coll Cardiol* 2007;**49**(12):1306–14.

126 Kopecky SL, Gersh BJ, McGoon MD, Whisnant JP, Holmes DR, Jr., Ilstrup DM, Frye RL. The natural history of lone atrial fibrillation. A population-based study over three decades. *N Engl J Med* 1987;**317**(11):669–74.

127 Crijns HJ, van Wijk LM, van Gilst WH, Kingma JH, van G, I, Lie KI. Acute conversion of atrial fibrillation to sinus rhythm: clinical efficacy of flecainide acetate. Comparison of two regimens. *Eur Heart J* 1988;**9**(6): 634–8.

128 Suttorp MJ, Kingma JH, Lie AH, Mast EG. Intravenous flecainide versus verapamil for acute conversion of paroxysmal atrial fibrillation or flutter to sinus rhythm. *Am J Cardiol* 1989;**63**(11):693–6.

129 van Gelder, I, Crijns HJ, van Gilst WH, Verwer R, Lie KI. Prediction of uneventful cardioversion and maintenance of sinus rhythm from direct-current electrical cardioversion of chronic atrial fibrillation and flutter. *Am J Cardiol* 1991;**68**(1):41–6.

130 Resnekov L, McDonald L. Appraisal of electroconversion in treatment of cardiac dysrhythmias. *Br Heart J* 1968;**30**(6):786–811.

131 Konings KTS, Smeets JLRM, Penn OC, Wellens HJJ, Allessie MA. Configuration of unipolar atrial electrograms during electrically induced atrial fibrillation in humans. *Circulation* 1997;**95**(5):1231–41.

132 Kalifa J, Tanaka K, Zaitsev AV, et al. Mechanisms of wave fractionation at boundaries of high-frequency excitation in the posterior left atrium of the isolated sheep heart during atrial fibrillation. *Circulation* 2006;**113**(5):626–33.

133 Pappone C, Vicedomini G, Manguso F, et al. Robotic magnetic navigation for atrial fibrillation ablation. *J Am Coll Cardiol* 2006;**47**(7):1390–400.

134 Sueda T, Nagata H, Shikata H, et al. Simple left atrial procedure for chronic atrial fibrillation associated with mitral valve disease. *Ann Thoracic Surg* 1996;**6**:1796–800.

135 Pappone C, Rosanio S, Oreto G, et al. Circumferential radiofrequency ablation of pumonary vein ostia: a new anatomic approach for curing atrial fibrillation. *Circulation* 2000;**21**:2619–28.

136 Haissaguerre M, Jais P, Shah D, et al. Catheter ablation of chronic atrial fibrillation targeting the reinitiating triggers. *J Cardiovasc Electrophsiol* 2000;**1**:2–10.

137 Kanagaratnam L, Tomassoni G, Schweikert R, et al. Empirical pulmonary vein isolation in patients with chronic atrial fibrillation using a three-dimensional nonfluoroscopic mapping system: long-term follow-up. *Pacing Clin Electrophysiol* 2001;**12**:1774–9.

PART 3

Special challenges in atrial fibrillation

13

CHAPTER 13

Diagnostic algorithm of atrial tachycardia following atrial fibrillation ablation: importance of localized reentries

Pierre Jaïs, Sébastien Knecht, Seiichiro Matsuo, Mark D. O'Neill, Rajesh Subbiah, Leonardo Arantès, Kang Teng Lim, Nicolas Derval, Frédéric Sacher, Antoine Deplagne, Pierre Bordachar, Mélèze Hocini, Jacques Clémenty, & Michel Haïssaguerre

Introduction

In recent years, catheter ablation for atrial fibrillation (AF) has emerged as an important therapeutic option for patients with not only paroxysmal AF [1–4] but persistent and longstanding persistent AF [5–11]. Pulmonary vein (PV) isolation alone has been associated with a high success rate in patients with paroxysmal AF [3,12,13] but is insufficient for patients with persistent and longstanding persistent AF. For these conditions, different approaches have been proposed including PV antrum isolation [14], ablation at rapid or fractionated sites [9,15], and linear lesions [7,8,16]. We have previously described a stepwise strategy combining these approaches, which is associated with a high rate of conversion of AF and long-term clinical efficacy [5,6]. However, in more than 70% of patients, AF first converted to atrial tachycardia (AT) instead of a direct restoration of sinus rhythm [5]. In addition, there are often multiple different ATs, which add significant complexity and constitute the last but frequently difficult step in ablation for persistent or longstanding AF (Figure 13.1).

Contact mapping using three-dimensional navigational systems with sequential single electrode recordings are useful in the context of stable AT but may excessively prolong the procedure or be challenging to interpret because of non-sustained or multiple morphology ATs. This chapter reviews the main clinical mechanisms of these ATs and our diagnostic approach to allow rapid and effective mapping of these arrhythmias.

Definitions

According to an arrhythmia expert group, ATs can be categorized as macroreentrant or focal, based on their electrophysiological properties [17]. Macroreentry AT was defined as a circuit with a diameter greater than 2 cm, generally circling around a large central obstacle, while focal AT was

Catheter Ablation of Atrial Fibrillation Edited by Etienne Aliot, Michel Haïssaguerre and Warren M. Jackman
© 2008 Blackwell Publishing, ISBN: 978-1-4501-6349-1.

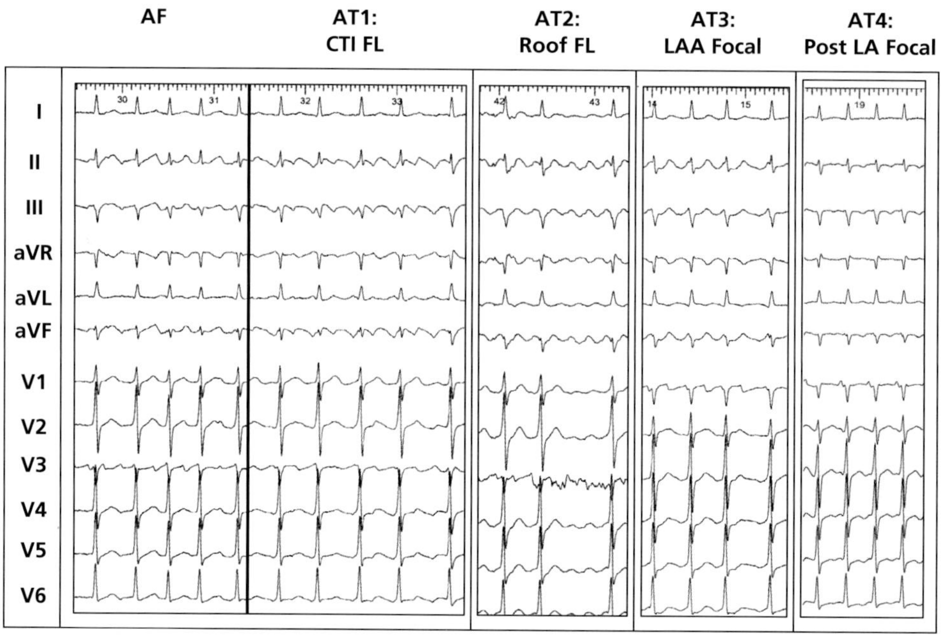

Figure 13.1 A typical example of the sequence of arrhythmias observed during ablation for chronic atrial fibrillation (AF). The first panel shows the initial AF, while after conversion four different atrial tachycardias (AT1 to AT4) are observed. AT1 is a cavotricuspid isthmus (CTI) dependent flutter; AT2 is a roof-dependent flutter; and AT3 and AT4 are focal from the left atrial appendage (LAA) and posterior left atrium (LA), respectively.

defined as atrial activity originating from a focus and spreading out centrifugally. However, in the context of AF ablation, we have reported a distinct mechanism of AT where centrifugal activation emanates not from a focal point but instead from a small area (about 2 cm in diameter), which contains the entire cycle length of the AT [18]. High density mapping, programmed stimulation, and entrainment confirmed the reentrant mechanism of the arrhythmia, named "localized reentry". Such localized reentries have also been shown to participate in the process of AF [15]. Therefore, we use the following definitions:

- *Macroreentry* (Figure 13.2a) uses a circuit involving more than three atrial segments where the entire (or at least more than 75%) circuit is mapped. In practice, macroreentry ATs in the context of AF ablation are essentially perimitral, roof dependent, or peritricuspid circuits. Entrainment maneuvers show a post pacing interval (PPI) not exceeding the tachycardia cycle length (TCL) by more than 20 ms in the three involved atrial segments. The term of "flutter" commonly refers to macroreentry.
- *Localized reentry* (Figure 13.2b) uses a circuit (usually smaller than 2 cm) involving one or two adjacent segments with the entire (or at least more than 75%) cycle length present within those segments. Centrifugal activation from the localized circuit to other segments of the chamber is observed. There is a good PPI close to the site only.
- *Focal point atrial tachycardia* (Figure 13.2c) is defined as a tachycardia originating from one atrial segment with centrifugal activation. It is commonly associated with less than 75% of the cycle length in the involved chamber. The PPI increases with the distance from the focal source.

Focal point tachycardia and localized reentry both display centrifugal activation. For both, resetting and entrainment maneuvers show a PPI not exceeding the cycle length by more than 20 ms in the atrial segment harboring the tachycardia [19,20]. When mapped within the entire chamber,

Figure 13.2 (*opposite*) Diagnostic characteristics of (a) macroreentries, (b) localized reentries, and (c) focal tachycardias. Values in the figures refer to PPI-TCL during pacing maneuvers. CS, coronary sinus; LAA, left atrial appendage; Peri M, perimitral; RFD, radiofrequency, distal.

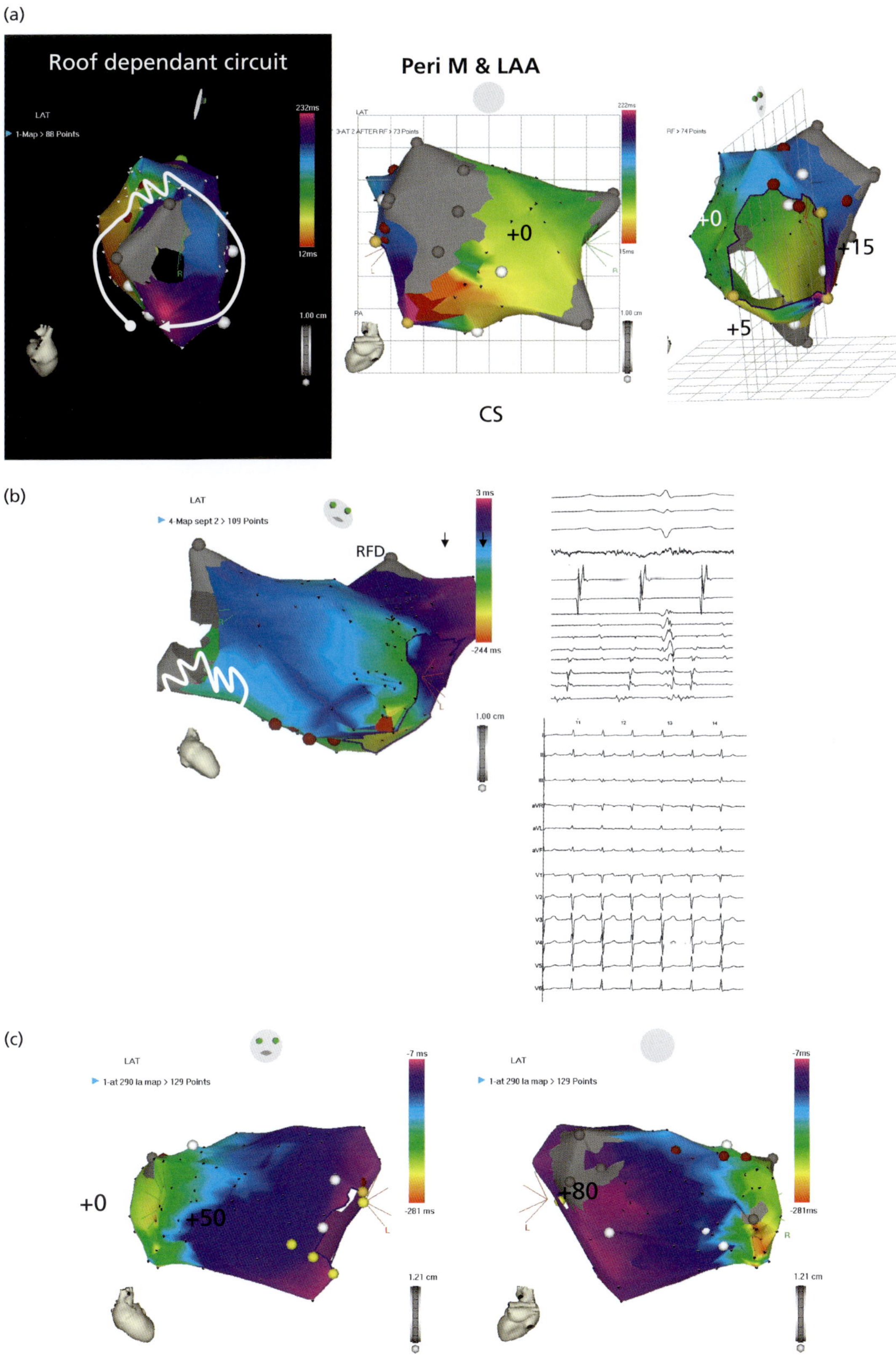
(a)
Roof dependant circuit
LAT
1-Map > 88 Points
232ms
12ms
1.00 cm
Peri M & LAA
+0
222ms
15ms
1.00 cm
+0
+15
+5
CS
(b)
LAT
4-Map sept 2 > 109 Points
3 ms
-244 ms
RFD
1.00 cm
(c)
LAT
1-at 290 la map > 129 Points
-7 ms
-281 ms
+0
+50
1.21 cm
LAT
1-at 290 la map > 129 Points
-7ms
-281ms
+80
1.21 cm

both appear as focal ATs with progressively earlier activity converging to the origin. But when mapped at the origin, the focal point AT converges on a single point, while in localized reentry the entire circuit will be recorded, often with long fractionated electrograms indicating slow conduction.

Mechanisms

Mechanisms of AT after prior AF ablation vary with ablation approach. While focal origins from reconnected PVs are usual after ostial PV isolation [21,22], macro and localized reentries are more frequent after linear, wide area circumferential, or antral ablation approaches [23–25].

Focal atrial tachycardia

Focal mechanisms of AT classically include three main types: triggered activity, abnormal automaticity, and microreentry [26].

1 *Triggered activity* is used to define impulse initiation in cardiac muscles fibers that is dependent on after-depolarizations, which are oscillations in membrane potential that follow the upstroke of an action potential. Early after-depolarizations (EADs) occur in phase 2 or 3 of the action potential, while delayed after-depolarizations (DADs) occur when repolarization is complete or nearly complete. If an after-depolarization reaches a threshold potential sufficient to generate an inward current, it results in a "triggered" new action potential. Thus, triggered activity must be linked to a prior action potential. Even though triggered activity has been demonstrated in vitro in isolated cardiac tissue and cells, it is difficult to highlight in vivo. Chen et al. [26] have proposed the following criteria for triggered activity: initiation is cycle length dependent; AT can be terminated with overdrive pacing (without entrainment) or by programmed stimulation with a single premature impulse; and after-depolarizations are observed on the monophasic action potential. However, there are exceptions, as artifacts can produce deflections similar to after-depolarizations on the monophasic action potential recording and pacing maneuvers can correspond to reentry. The only clear distinguishing features of triggered activity from reentry are inability to entrain and the dependence of initiation on a critical cycle length.

2 *Enhanced automaticity* is due to enhanced phase 4 excitability in both abnormal (abnormal automaticity) and normal cells. It is the property of a fiber to initiate an impulse spontaneously without the need for prior stimulation. Normally, atrial myocardial cells do not exhibit spontaneous diastolic depolarizations. However, when the resting membrane potential of atrial myocardial cells is reduced, for example by pathological processes such as prolonged ischemia, spontaneous diastolic depolarizations may occur, leading to abnormal or depolarization-induced automaticity. ATs due to enhanced automaticity are not predictably initiated or terminated by electrical stimulation. They are catecholamine-dependent, and so can be initiated by isoproterenol, and terminated by beta-blockers. Monophasic action potential recordings show an increased phase 4 diastolic slope just prior to the onset of AT in the area near the exit site [26].

3 *Reentry* was defined by Chen et al. [26] using the entrainment criteria described by Waldo, and termination with adenosine, dipyridamole, and verapamil.

Practically, it is often laborious to differentiate these three classical mechanisms of focal tachycardia in the laboratory. Adenosine does not help clarify the situation as it has inconsistent and overlapping results [26–28]. In general, automatic ATs can be transiently suppressed but not terminated by adenosine, while triggered activity and microreentry can be terminated (macroreentry being insensitive to adenosine) [29].

In addition to these uncertainties, Sanders et al. described, with high density mapping, ATs displaying centrifugal activation wavefronts from a discrete origin but with the entire tachycardia cycle length within the localized region at the origin of the AT [18]. Half of these patients had arrhythmias induced by programmed stimulation, and a reentrant mechanism was confirmed by entrainment. They postulated that these observations were consistent with localized reentry.

Other authors have also reported evidence for microreentry in patients with repaired congenital heart disease. Recently, Markowitz et al. identified "focal reentry adenosine insensitive tachycardia" as a de novo mechanism in patients with coexisting AF but without prior ablation [30]. Thus, there seems to be a spectrum between micro and localized reentry.

Macroreentrant tachycardia

Macroreentry is reentrant activation around a large central obstacle, greater than 2 cm [17]. This obstacle can be fixed, functional, or a combination of both. There is no single point of origin of activation, and the atrial myocardium surrounding the circuit is activated from various parts of the circuit. Thus, reentrant activation can be recorded continuously throughout the atrial cycle length and the point of earliest activity can not be determined.

Macroreentry occurs in any region of the atria that supports the substrate for reentry. As in cavotricuspid isthmus-dependent flutter, this substrate consists of an isthmus that represents a critical zone of slow conduction facilitating reentry. Reentry also requiries boundaries of zones of electrical silence, which for typical flutter are the crista terminalis posteriorly and the tricuspid annulus anteriorly. In the context of prior AF ablation, these boundaries are mainly constituted in the left atrium (LA) by the mitral annulus, the PVs, and regions of conduction abnormalities or electrical silence occurring spontaneously or due to radiofrequency applications. These boundaries may occur in the right [31], left [32,33], or both atria. However, the vast majority of them are perimitral or roof dependent, encircling either the right or left PVs. Thus the targets for ablation are the area between the left inferior PV and the mitral annulus (the mitral isthmus line) and the area between the superior PVs (the roof line), respectively.

Differentiation

The differentiation of macroreentrants from focal ATs is essential for subsequent effective ablation. Macroreentrant circuits are generally easy to map but may be difficult to ablate (with complete block), while focal ATs may be difficult to localize but are easy to ablate. In our experience, localized reentry is the most frequent AT mechanism, comprising 37% of all ATs and 71% of focal ATs.

Electrocardiogram morphology

In the context of prior AF ablation, electrocardiogram (ECG) characteristics of AT are not distinctive and rarely useful in differentiating mechanisms of AT or localizing focal AT. Atrial conduction properties vary according to the patients because of wider electrophysiological and structural alterations of the tissue, resulting in longer atrial conduction times (sometimes reaching more than 200 ms). Significant atrial damage has been demonstrated by scar outside the PV region in 9% of patients and low voltage of the LA tissue in 32% of patients [34]. Interpretation can also be inaccurate due to block on previously performed linear lesions. Finally, the exit block of a focal AT can be located far from the origin because of prior ablation.

Typical counter-clockwise right atrial macroreentry flutter often displays the classic "sawtooth" pattern in inferior leads, with positive deflections in V1, but may show atypical morphologies after LA ablation.

LA macroreentries can result in discrete P waves and isoelectric baseline or of typical or atypical cavotricuspid isthmus-dependent macroreentry with a predominantly positive flutter wave morphology in lead V1. Algorithms validated to determine PV origin of focal AT [21,35] can rarely be applied in the context of extensive prior left atrial ablation.

Cycle length variability

A dynamic and intermittent arrhythmia pattern with interruptions followed by reinitiations is probably the most convincing pattern favoring a focal mechanism. In addition, cycle length (CL) variability accurately distinguished focal from macroreentrant AT. In a cohort of 72 patients (21 paroxysmal and 51 long-lasting AF) with 128 ATs, we found that a variability of $> 15\%$ of the AT CL was highly suggestive of a focal origin, whereas there was no discriminating value if the AT CL variability was $< 15\%$. The mean CL of macroreentrant arrhythmias was not significantly different to focal arrhythmias: 271 ± 79 ms and 306 ± 102 ms, respectively.

This criterion of AT variability can be assessed on the surface ECG, and is helpful in guiding mapping strategies. Pitfalls can result from atrial ectopy that either terminates or reinitiates macroreentrant arrhythmia, circuits passing through multiple gaps [36], or multiple loop reentries [37].

Percentage of the cycle length

Focal tachycardia displays a discrete origin, spreading out centrifugally. Conventional mapping consequently focuses on the site of earliest atrial

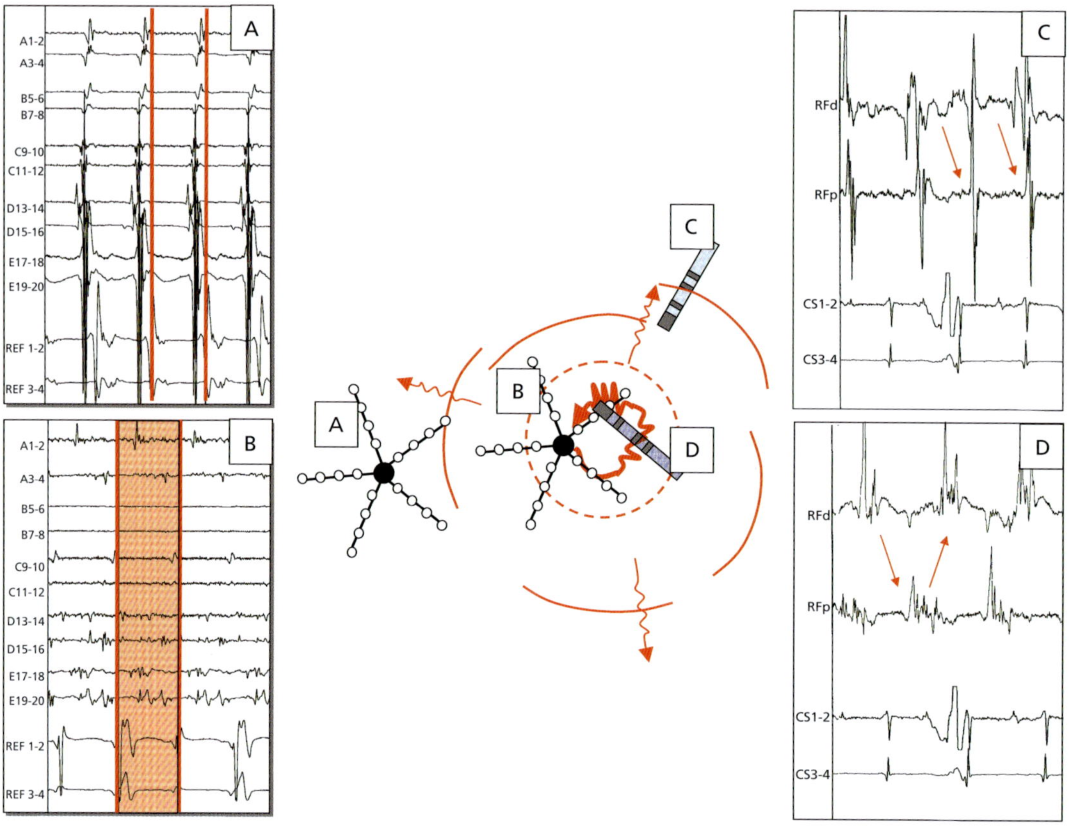

Figure 13.3 An example of localized reentry with mapping using a Pentaray® multispine catheter in panels A and B, while conventional mapping with the rove catheter is shown in panels C and D. The activation sequence recorded by the Pentaray in A allows localization of the catheter to the source where fractionated potentials spanning the entire CL are recorded (B). The same applies to mapping with the rove catheter in C, albeit with a lower mapping resolution. The tracing in D is typical of the activation gradient observed in localized reentries.

activation for automaticity and triggered activity, while activation throughout the CL has to be detected in the context of localized reentry. If only a small part of the CL can be mapped in the region of origin, it rules out a reentry mechanism. If local activity spans all or most of the AT CL (> 70%), it suggests a reentrant mechanism (Figure 13.3). However, slow conduction around a focus in the context of prior ablation is possible and can make the diagnosis difficult. Very low amplitude signals (< 0.04 mV) are common for localized reentry and lack of amplification or noise can make mapping challenging or sometimes impossible.

Entrainment

Entrainment remains the cornerstone of the diagnosis of reentry [20]. Pacing maneuvers revealing a PPI not exceeding the tachycardia CL (TCL) by more than 20 ms in three different atrial segments confirm the diagnosis of macroreentry.

A recent article from Mohamed et al. highlighted the role of atrial overdrive pacing maneuvers to localize the origin and identify the mechanism of focal AT [19]. In seven patients, they demonstrated a direct relationship between the PPI-TCL and proximity to the tachycardia focus. PPI-TCL was systematically less than 20 ms at successful ablation sites. They postulated that "entrainment" (or resetting) maneuvers could also help determine the area of interest. However, it seems that most of their patients had reentrant tachycardias, with only one patient having probable automaticity.

The aim of overdrive pacing in the context of focal arrhythmia is not to entrain but to reset tachycardia. As described above, automaticity and triggered activity have a broad range of responses to overdrive maneuvers. Automaticity often demonstrates high variability of the CL, spontaneous termination, or a period of silence in response to pacing maneuvers. Therefore, inconsistent resetting may be observed in a truly focal mechanism depending on its recovery time. However, in the case of localized reentry, which is the most common in the context of prior AF ablation, entrainment and PPI are accurate methods to localize the arrhythmia.

Localization of atrial tachycardias

PV reconduction is the main cause of AT in the context of prior segmental PV isolation [21]. Therefore, PV isolation should be systematically checked as the first step in the AT mapping process. As the majority of so-called ATs are localized reentries, these ATs are often related to areas targeted during AF ablation. In our experience, the most common sites for localized reentries are the PV–LA junctions, the left interatrial septum, and the entrance of the left atrial appendage (LAA). Other sites include the anterior LA, inferior LA/coronary sinus, and the right atrium. Occasionally, in a single patient, two different localized reentries coexist in the same region.

Influence of prior radiofrequency applications on atrial tachycardia mechanisms

This correlation between AT localization and prior ablation begs the question as to whether these localized reentries are caused by prior radiofrequency application. Non-radiofrequency-related LA scar, which may be idiopathic or related to underlying structural heart disease, could result in local zones of slow conduction predisposing to reentrant circuits. A recent study showed evidence of "small reentrant circuits" in non-ablated patients. Furthermore, some authors described that lesions occurring because of radiofrequency ablation do not give rise to arrhythmogenicity [38]. However, in the context of electrogram-based ablation, the relation between locations of radiofrequency deliveries and reentrant circuits is more than coincidental. Injury or edema of the atrial tissue provoked by radiofrequency applications could provide the substrate for arrhythmia [39] by creating an anchoring point potentially able to maintain reentry. Therefore mechanism of AT after AF ablation may be different from that of spontaneous AT.

Technical aspects of atrial tachycardia mapping and ablation

Mapping and ablation of atrial tachycardia

The first step is to ensure complete isolation of all four PVs and to deliver further ablation if required. After confirming isolation of the PVs, the regularity of the AT is then assessed. Variations in CL of more than 15% would suggest the presence of a focal AT and less than 15% would be compatible with either a focal or reentrant mechanism.

Three-dimensional navigation systems

Three-dimensional navigation systems are not routinely used during AT mapping and ablation in the context of AF ablation. A three-dimensional navigation system was used for the purposes of illustration after the achievement of a complete understanding of the arrhythmia. There was a consensus on tachycardia mechanisms with and without three-dimensional mapping strategies in all patients.

Macroreentrant arrhythmia

In the presence of a regular cycle length, macroreentry either around the tricuspid annulus or mitral annulus or around the right PVs (roof-dependent circuit) is assessed. Linear lesions either at the cavotricuspid isthmus, mitral isthmus, or left atrial roof are subsequently created depending on the reentrant circuit participating in the AT. Incomplete lines are reablated either by identifying the "gaps" from previous ablation or by the creation of additional lines where appropriate. The electrogram-based mapping of the annulus-related circuit is performed by moving the rove catheter around the annulus, looking for consistent atrial activation sequence covering the entire cycle length. The decapolar catheter placed in the coronary sinus is also useful to assess the activation sequence of the inferior LA. Consistent activation, either proximal to distal or distal to proximal is typically observed in the presence of a perimitral circuit. Following this, the activation of the anterior

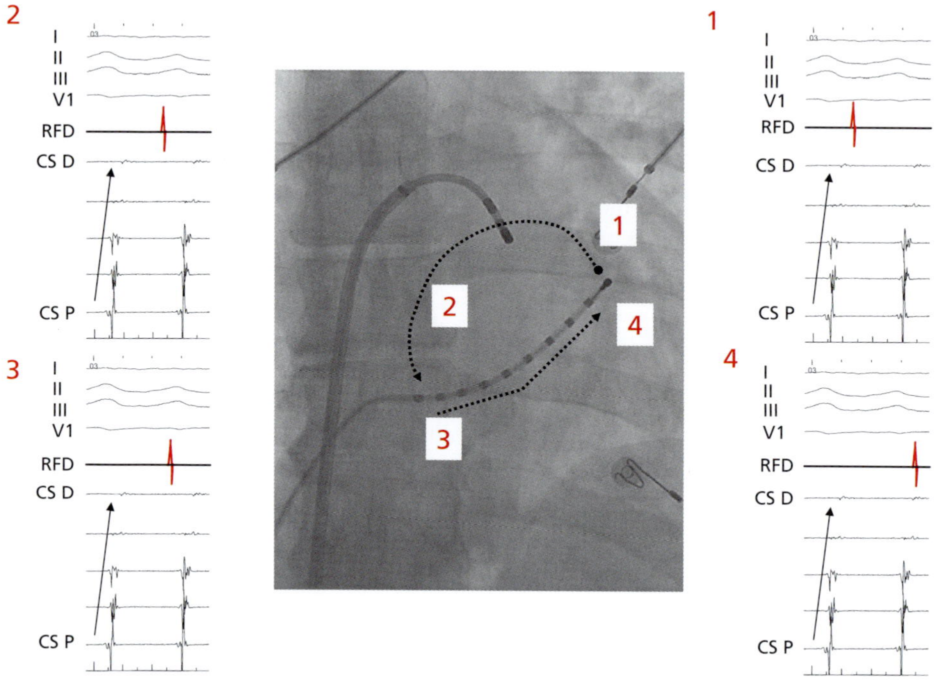

Figure 13.4 The concept of conventional mapping for assessing perimitral flutters. The first step is to check that the coronary sinus (CS) activation is consistent, showing either proximal (P) to distal (D) (as shown here) or distal to proximal. In this example, CS activation is compatible with a counter-clockwise perimitral circuit. Then the rove catheter is used to assess the activation on the anterior LA. Panels 1 and 2 show the expected timing of the potentials at the anterior LA; panels 3 and 4 at the posterior LA. Note that this maneuver confirms a counter-clockwise perimitral activation, but this can also be observed with a focal source and complete mitral isthmus block. Therefore final proof requires entrainment and good return cycles during pacing maneuvers at three or four segments around the annulus. RF, radiofrequency.

LA can be assessed using the rove catheter as shown in Figure 13.4.

The mapping of a roof-dependent circuit is performed by recording the activation front of the anterior and posterior LA. In the presence of a roof-dependent circuit, atrial activation is ascending in one direction and descending in the other, while in the presence of a perimitral circuit, both activation wavefronts are ascending from the mitral annulus to the roof (Figures 13.5 and 13.6). Entrainment maneuvers may then be used to confirm the diagnosis.

Non-macroreentrant arrhythmia

In the absence of macroreentry, we look for local reentry or focal atrial tachycardia (see Figure 13.2b, c), which may be located anywhere in the atria. Entrainment and resetting maneuvers with analysis of the PPI are then used to progressively approach the site of origin. If the PPI exceeds the CL by more than 50 ms, pacing is performed at another segment of the atrium. This is repeated until a PPI lower or equal to 20 ms is recorded. Then fractionated long duration potentials spanning the entire TCL are looked for in case of localized reentry (Figures 13.3, 13.7, and 13.8). In the presence of a focal tachycardia, the earliest bipolar activity associated with a QS pattern and a rapid initial slope in the unipolar recording (when interpretable) is targeted.

While localized reentry displays low voltage continuous activation, focal tachycardia propagating from a defined source is typically characterized by higher voltage electrograms. These mapping strategies have been used to build the algorithm detailed in Figure 13.9. An example of the use of the algorithm is shown in Figure 13.10.

More complex atrial tachycardias

In a small percentage of cases, focal versus macroreentry AT can not be determined using the algorithm approach because of widespread altered

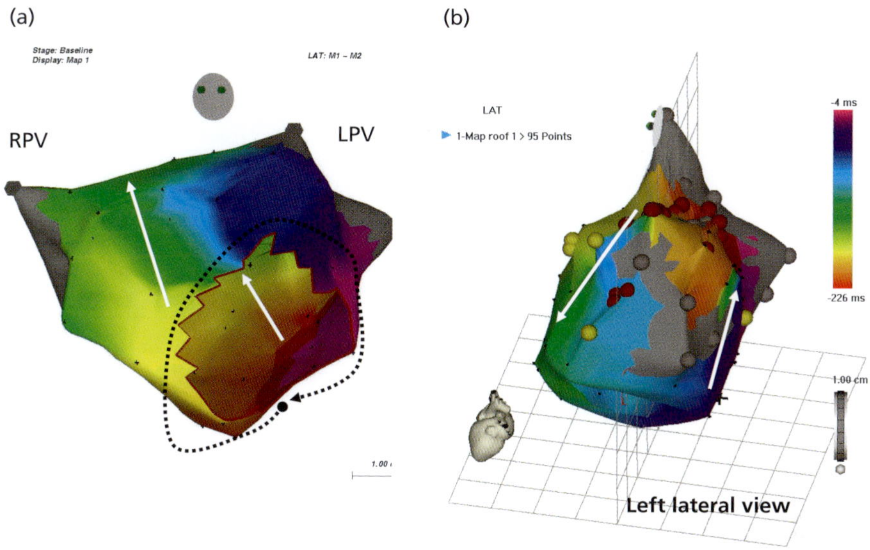

Figure 13.5 The concept of conventional mapping for assessing roof-dependent flutters. (a) A perimitral circuit. The activation of the anterior and posterior LA are both upward, from the mitral annulus to the roof. (b) A roof-dependent circuit is associated with opposite activations of the anterior and posterior LA. LPV, left pulmonary vein; RPV, right pulmonary vein.

electrograms or scars creating large activation gradients or more complex arrhythmias.

A challenging situation is encountered when a focal arrhythmia is located in the vicinity of a complete ablation line. The activation front will propagate around the atrium, simulating the activation observed during macroreentry. An example is shown in Figure 13.11 where a focus located above a complete mitral isthmus line produces an activation front consistent with that of a perimitral circuit. This is in fact similar to what happens during pacing maneuvers to check for completeness of linear block. In this situation, three methods can be used to facilitate the identification and ablation of the AT:

1 Entrainment maneuvers performed during the arrhythmia will suggest a focal origin by demonstrating long return CLs around the mitral annulus except at sites adjacent to the focus. The same applies for foci located close to a complete ablation line at the LA roof.

2 An area of early activity will display local activity spanning the entire AT CL in the case of localized reentry.

The variant of perimitral circuits with a gap located between the LAA and the left PVs is challenging to diagnose. The slow conduction recorded at the posterior ridge of the LAA can be misleading and interpreted as being local reentry. The diagnosis is ascertained using entrainment maneuvers demonstrating a perfect PPI around the mitral annulus (Figure 13.12).

Fusion between two macroreentrant circuits (dual-loop reentry [37]) is also possible after prior AF ablation. In this case, ablation of one loop will result in transition to the other. This can be observed in the presence of a perimitral and roof-dependent circuit and can be suspected when the PPI-TCL does not exceed 50 ms around the mitral annulus and at the posterior LA.

Another complex situation was observed in one patient with dual perimitral flutters with two alternating CLs. Macroreentrant tachycardia was circulating around the mitral annulus via two different conduction gaps on the mitral isthmus [36]. The most difficult situation, however, is observed in the setting of multiple focal ATs firing sequentially and not stable enough to be mapped.

Algorithm and ablation results

Using the approach described above (the algorithm in Figure 13.9), a total of 128 ATs were prospectively mapped and successfully ablated in 72 patients (1.7 ± 0.8 per patient).

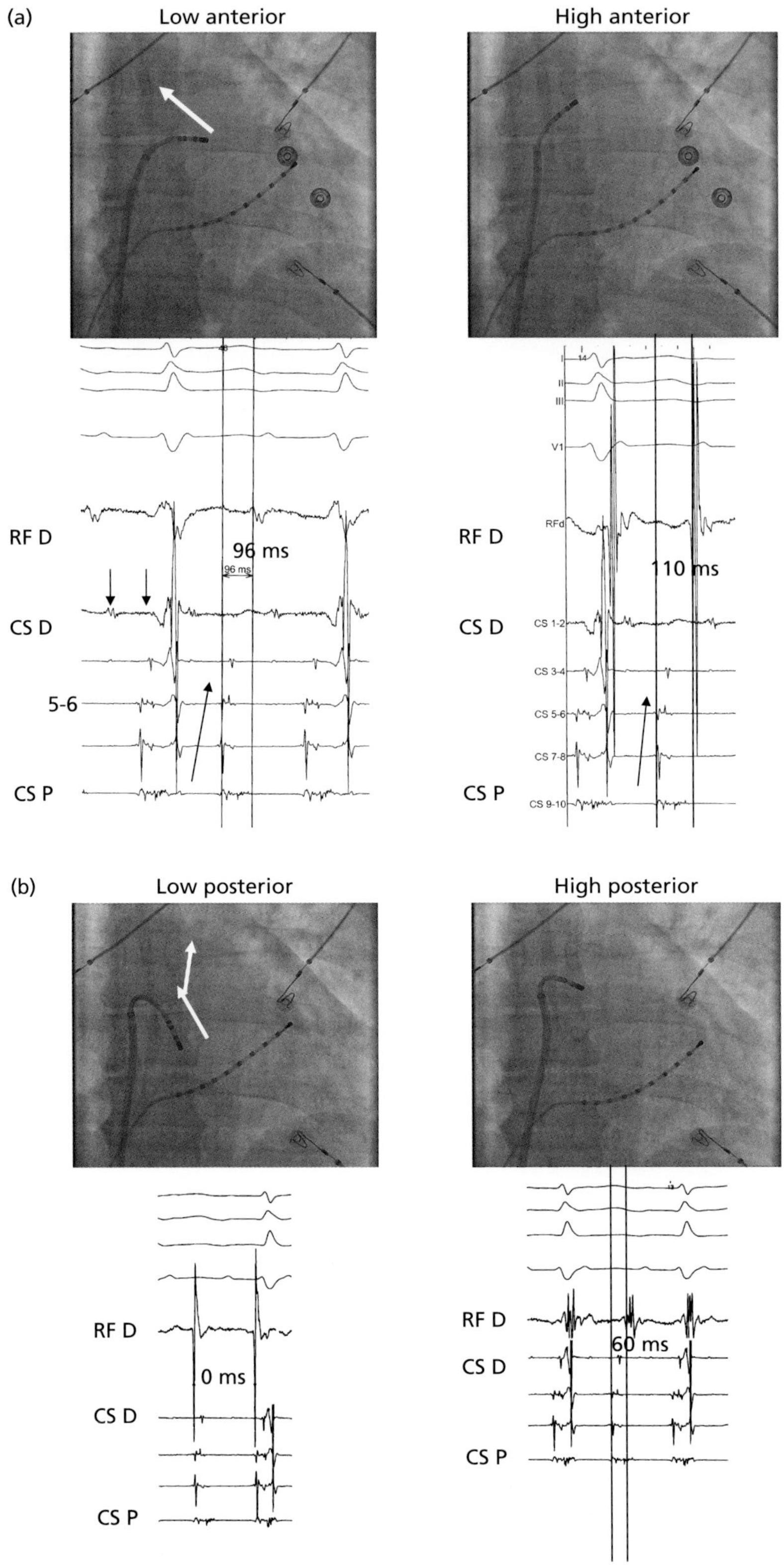
(a)
Low anterior
High anterior
RF D
96 ms
96 ms
CS D
5-6
CS P
I
II
III
V1
RFd
RF D
110 ms
CS D
CS 1-2
CS 3-4
CS 5-6
CS 7-8
CS P
CS 9-10
(b)
Low posterior
High posterior
RF D
0 ms
CS D
CS P
RF D
CS D
60 ms
CS P

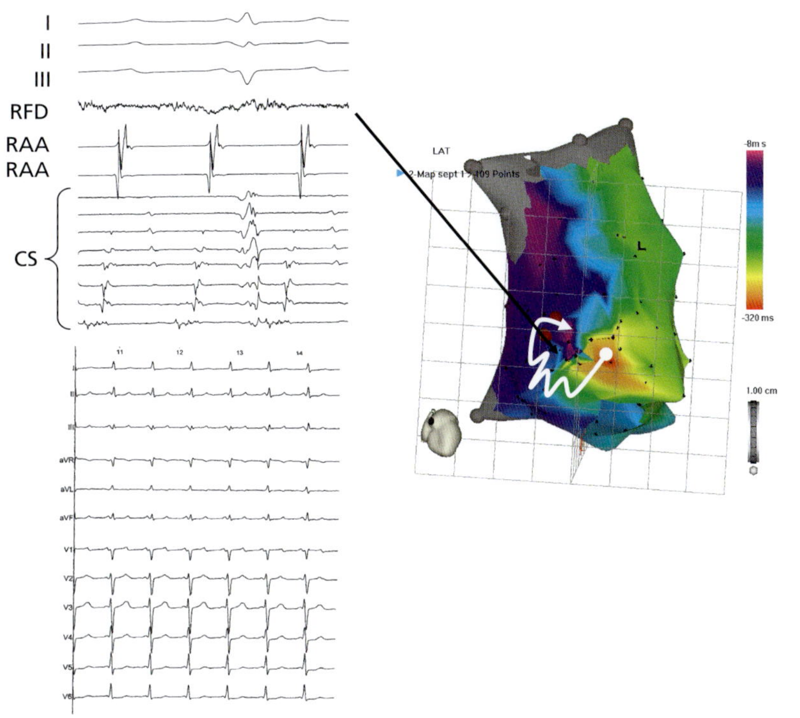

Figure 13.7 Recording showing, in the same patient, a local reentrant circuit located in the inferior left septum (drawn in white). The ablation site is shown in the middle panel. A highly fractionated long duration signal is recorded. The amplitude does not exceed 0.02 mV. This type of activity at the successful ablation site is typical of local reentrant circuits. CS, coronary sinus; RAA, right atrial appendage; RFD, radiofrequency, distal.

Methods

Patient population

A total of 128 ATs were mapped and ablated in 72 patients undergoing catheter ablation, aged 60 ± 9 years, comprising of 10 female and 62 male patients. The indication for catheter ablation was paroxysmal AF in 21 patients, and persistent/permanent AF in 51. Atrial tachycardia occurred during the index ablation procedure in 21 patients or during a repeated ablation procedure in 51 patients. Hypertension was present in 10 patients, idiopathic dilated cardiomyopathy in eight patients, hypertrophic cardiomyopathy in six patients, mitral valve disease in one patient, and ischemia in two patients.

Definitions

For the purpose of this study, the LA was anatomically divided into anterior, posterior, lateral, and septal segments, in addition to the PVs and LAA. For diagnostic characteristics of different ATs, see above and Figure 13.2.

Figure 13.6 (*opposite*) (a) Conventional mapping of the anterior aspect of the LA during atrial tachycardia. A reference is chosen in the coronary sinus (5-6 in this example). The low anterior LA is activated 96 ms after the reference as compared to 110 ms at the high anterior LA. This means that the activation goes from the mitral annulus to the roof on the anterior aspect. (b) A similar maneuver is performed for the posterior LA. The low posterior LA is activated on time with the coronary sinus (CS) reference. The high posterior LA is activated 60 ms after, demonstrating again an activation front propagating from the mitral annulus to the roof. The upward activation of both anterior and posterior left atrial segments rules out a circuit dependent on the roof and may be consistent with a perimitral circuit if macroreentry has been demonstrated earlier. D, distal; P, proximal; RF, radiofrequency.

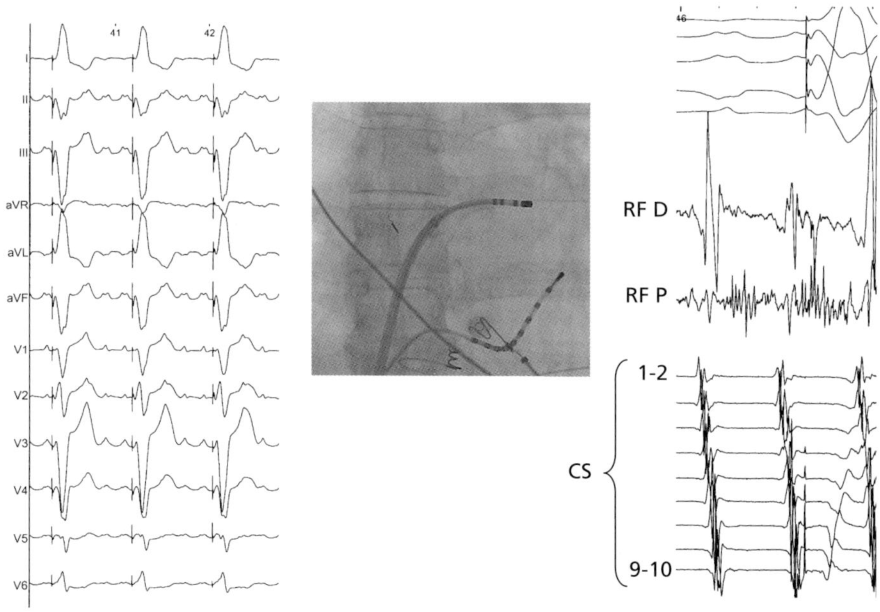

Figure 13.8 This tachycardia was observed in the context of an ablation performed for persistent AF. The ablation catheter is at the entrance of the LAA and the proximal bipole records a highly fractionated long duration activity typical of the slow conduction area of this local reentrant circuit. The coronary sinus (CS) is activated from distal (D) to proximal (P) as expected. This suggests the absence of complete block at the mitral isthmus line. In contrast, proximal-to-distal activation of the CS would have been expected in the presence of a complete mitral isthmus line. RF, radiofrequency.

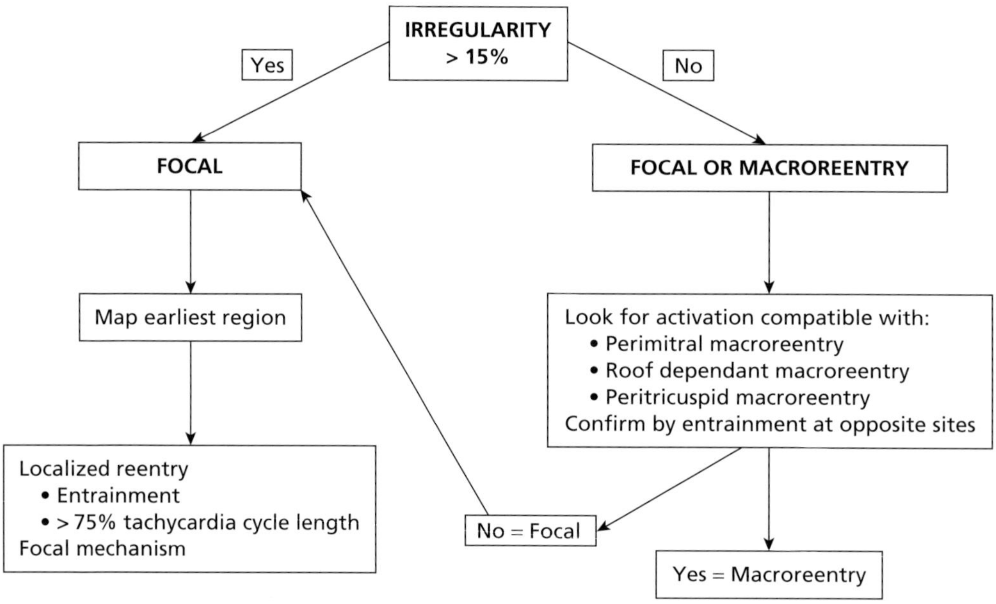

Figure 13.9 The diagnostic algorithm used for this study.

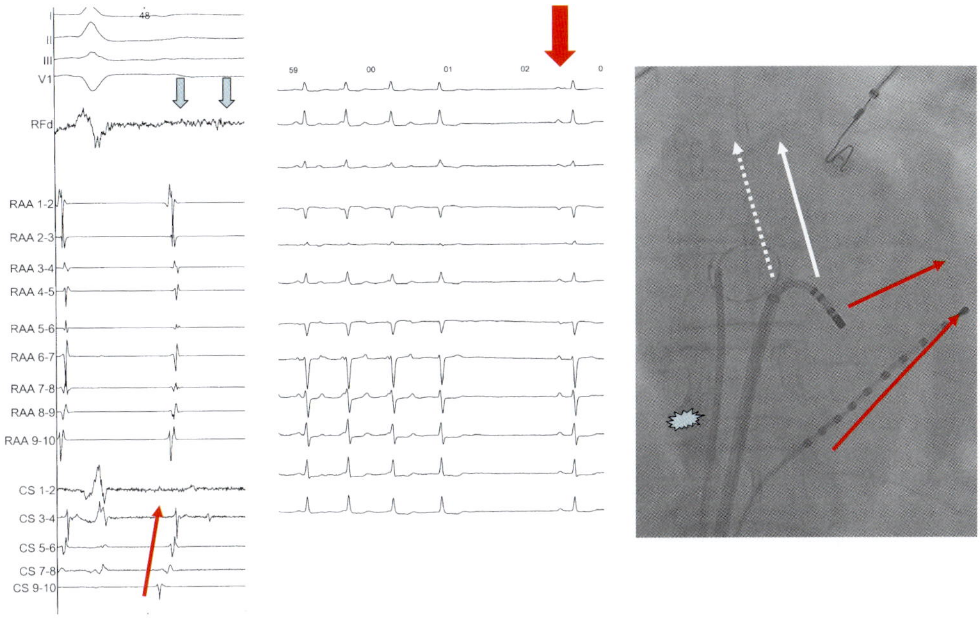

Figure 13.10 Diagnostic mapping strategy to identify a local reentrant circuit in the left septum. The first step is to look for activation compatible with a perimitral or roof-dependent circuit. The coronary sinus (CS) shows a proximal-to-distal activation, and the anterior LA a septolateral activation, eliminating a perimitral circuit. The anterior and posterior LAs are activated from the mitral to the roof, eliminating a roof-dependent circuit. A non-macroreentrant arrhythmia is then looked for. Given the previously collected mapping data, the septum (the right veins have been proven to be disconnected earlier) is the area to look for as anterior, inferior, and posterior LAs are activated from the septum. Mapping this region showed long duration fractionated potentials of very low amplitude (wider blue arrows) and that ablation terminated the tachycardia (wide red arrow, middle panel). Other arrows show the directions of the activation sequence. RAA, right atrial appendage; RFd, radiofrequency, distal.

Results

Macroreentrant arrhythmia

There were 60 macroreentrant arrhythmias out of the 128 mapped (47%). This included 35 (27%) typical perimitral circuits ablated at the mitral isthmus, with complete block achieved in 33 (95%). A variant was observed in four patients (3%) in whom a complete ablation line connecting the mitral annulus to the LAA ostium terminated the tachycardia. The slow conduction was posterior to the LAA and anterior to the left PVs, at the LAA ridge (see Figure 13.12). This was the site of successful ablation and resulted in complete block at the mitral isthmus in all four patients.

Circuits rotating around right PVs propagating through the roof were observed in 18 patients (14%) and successfully ablated using a linear lesion connecting both superior PVs at the most superior part of the LA. Complete block was achieved in 17 patients.

Peritricuspid isthmus tachycardia was observed in three patients (2%) and was successfully ablated in all using the classical cavotricuspid isthmus ablation line. Complete block was observed in all patients. Of note, the 12-lead morphology was atypical in all three patients despite a counter-clockwise propagation, with a proximal-to-distal activation sequence in the coronary sinus.

The coronary sinus activation recorded using a decapolar catheter in cases of perimitral circuits demonstrated a distal-to-proximal activation sequence in 50% of patients and a proximal-to-distal sequence in the other 50%. In the presence of macroreentry propagating over the roof, the coronary sinus activation in patients was proximal to distal in 30% and distal to proximal in 30%, while in 40% neither the proximal nor the distal bipole were the earliest.

Assessment of anterior and posterior LA activation aiming to identify or exclude a roof-dependent circuit was not possible in two patients because of

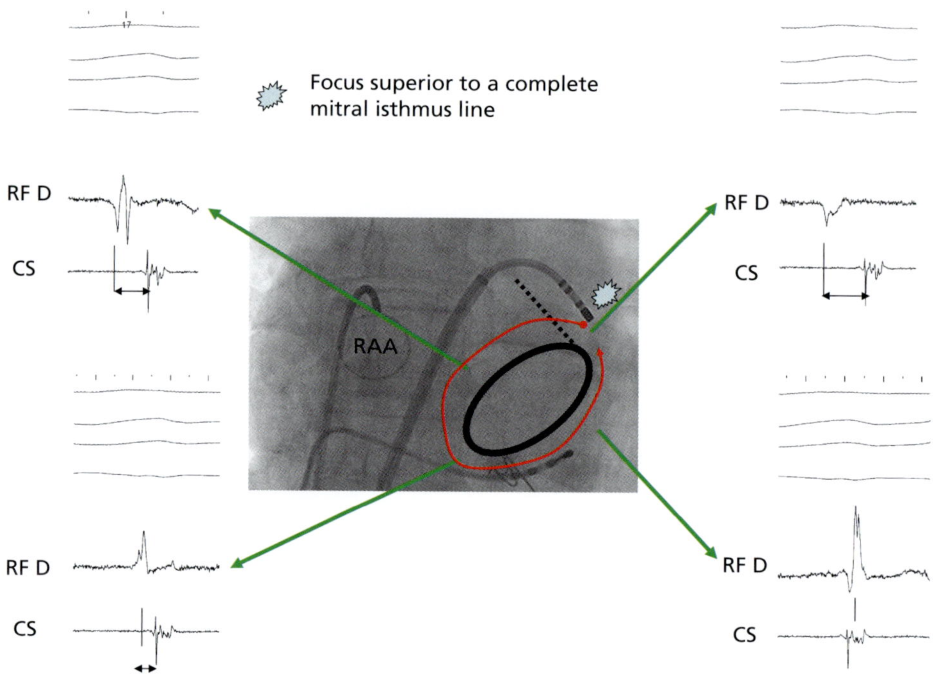

Figure 13.11 This figure illustrates a classical pitfall where a focus adjacent to an ablation line with complete block produces an activation compatible with a reentrant perimitral circuit. The activation recorded with the rove catheter around the mitral annulus is shown. However, this can be suspected by pacing maneuvers demonstrating a long return cycle in the atrial segments not harboring the focus: the septum and the inferior LA in this case. CS, coronary sinus; D, distal; RAA, right atrial appendage; RF, radiofrequency.

the absence of recordable potentials in the posterior LA.

In 70 out of the 72 patients (97%), the arrhythmias were successfully mapped and ablated using this approach. In two patients, the arrhythmia could not be identified but macroreentry was excluded by mapping and pacing maneuvers. The tachycardias were either pace terminated or electrically cardioverted.

The most common macroreentrant circuit was related to reentry around the mitral annulus in this study. Despite being technically challenging, complete linear block was achieved in 29 of 31 cases (94%). In a minority of cases, three of 29 (9%), linear block was observed only after ablating the posterior ridge, where slow conduction perpetuated the perimitral circuit. Linear roof block occurred in 11 of 12 cases (92%), highlighting also the technically challenging aspects of linear ablation.

Non-macroreentrant arrhythmia

Sixty-six (52%) non-macroreentrant arrhythmias were identified and ablated. They were located anywhere in both atria, but significantly clustered in the LA (Figure 13.13). The left septum, the entrance of the LAA, and the PVs were the most frequent sites. After eliminating macroreentry, activation mapping and pacing maneuvers to identify the shortest PPI were found to be highly effective in localizing the site of origin. An example of the diagnostic strategy is shown in Figure 13.10. The vast majority of non-macroreentrant arrhythmias were local reentries in 47 of 66 patients (71%), while in 19 of 66 (29%) a focal origin appeared to be more likely. Local reentrant tachycardias characteristically displayed low amplitude signals and continuous activity spanning a significant portion (> 70%) of the TCL. Preferential locations for these local reentrant circuits were the PV–LA junction (10 patients), the left septum (10), and the entrance of the LAA (10). They were also observed at the anterior LA (8), inferior LA/coronary sinus (7), and in the right atrium: one in the superior vena cava and one in the right lateral free wall. A mean CL of 290 ± 92 ms was observed, with a range of 200 to 650 ms.

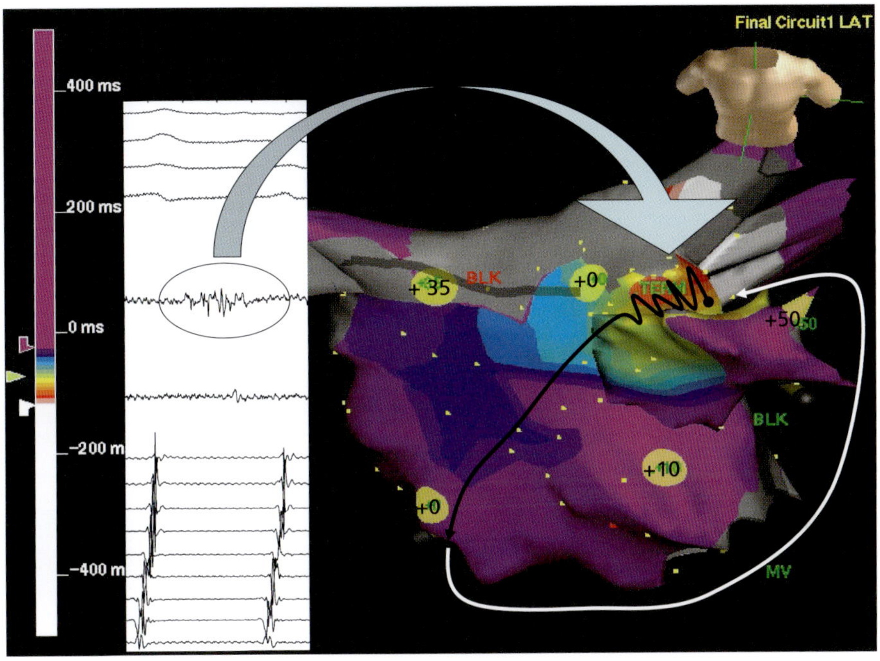

Figure 13.12 A variant of perimitral circuits with a gap located between the LAA and the left PVs. The slow conduction recorded at the posterior ridge of the LAA can be misleading and interpreted as being a local reentry. The diagnosis is ascertained using entrainment maneuvers demonstrating a perfect PPI around the mitral annulus. Values in the figure refer to PPI-TCL.

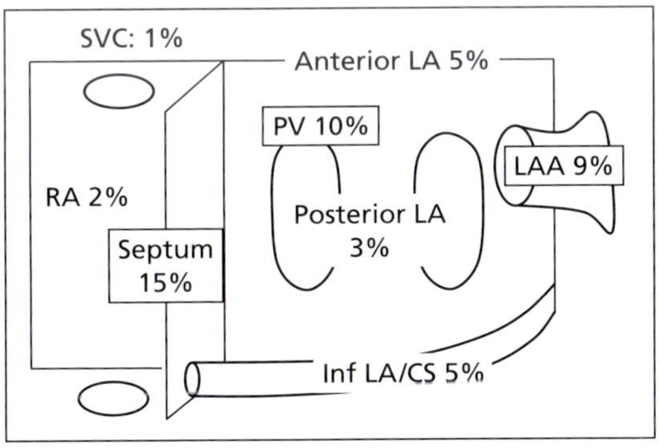

Figure 13.13 Summary of the locations of non-macroreentrant tachycardias observed in the study. The left atrial appendage (LAA), pulmonary veins (PV), and septum are the most prominent sites. LA, left atrium; RA, right atrium; SVC, superior vena cava.

Pitfalls and tricks

During focal arrhythmia, the atrial chamber is not being depolarized during the entire CL, in contrast to reentries. However, this may be observed by chance if bystander slow conduction or a prior linear lesion has produced enough delay to cover the entire CL.

Macroreentries are easy to map but may be difficult to ablate as they require complete ablation lines. This is particularly true of the mitral isthmus line, which frequently (70%) requires ablation from within the coronary sinus. Non-macroreentrant arrhythmias are more difficult to localize but their ablation is usually straightforward. This is principally true of the local reentrant circuits where the slow conduction area is particularly sensitive to radiofrequency delivery (see Figures 13.3, 13.7, and 13.8).

The mapping phase being complete, ablation is then performed at the identified target. It is crucial, however, to remain vigilant to identify any change in CL and/or activation, which indicates that the ablation has modified the arrhythmia, possibly producing a transition to another tachycardia requiring reassessment. The transition may be obvious, as shown in Figure 13.14, or subtle, as shown in Figure 13.15. The extreme can be observed when the successful ablation of the tachycardia is not associated with any change in CL or activation in the coronary sinus reference catheter. This justifies repeating entrainment maneuvers in

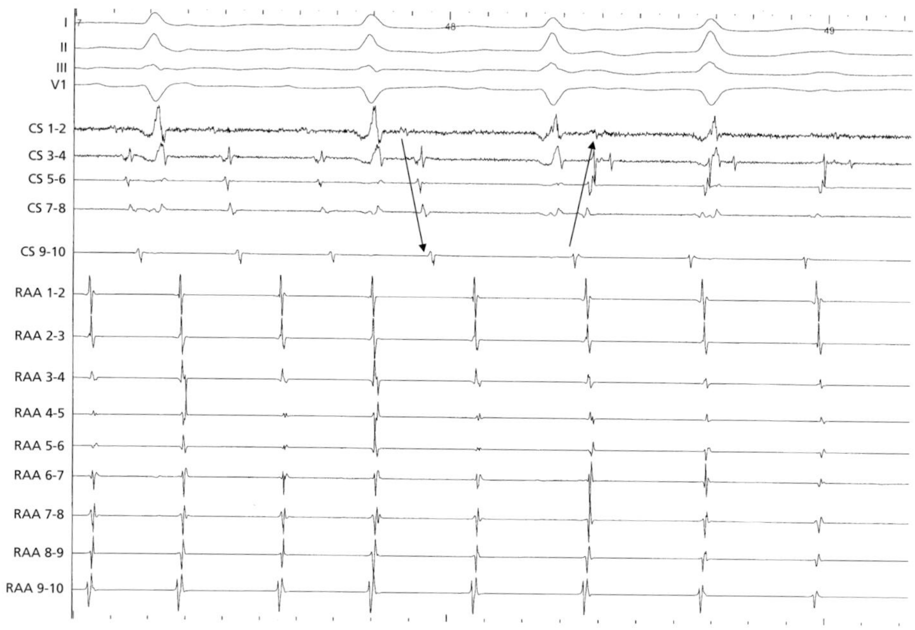

Figure 13.14 This figure shows the transition from a perimitral circuit to a septal focus. The activation recorded from the Lasso® catheter placed in the right atrial appendage (RAA) does not change appreciably, but the activation recorded by the decapolar diagnostic catheter in the coronary sinus (CS) shows a dramatic change due to catheter-induced block at the mitral isthmus. Note the following reversed CS activation from proximal to distal, compatible with a focus in the septum, that was finally ablated in this patient.

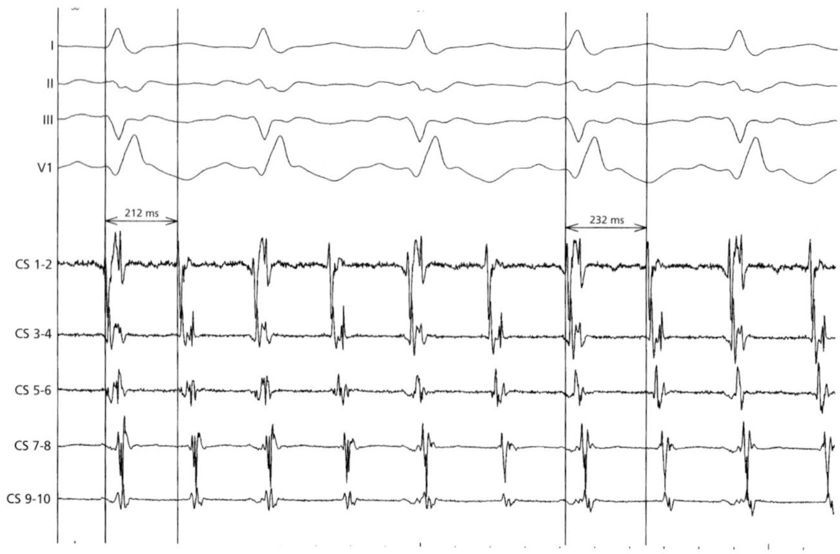

Figure 13.15 In this patient the transition from a perimitral circuit to a roof-dependent one during ablation at the mitral isthmus is difficult to identify and could be missed, leading to further unnecessary radiofrequency applications at the already blocked isthmus. Surprisingly, no significant change in the coronary sinus (CS) activation is observed. The only difference is a prolongation in the tachycardia CL by 20 ms.

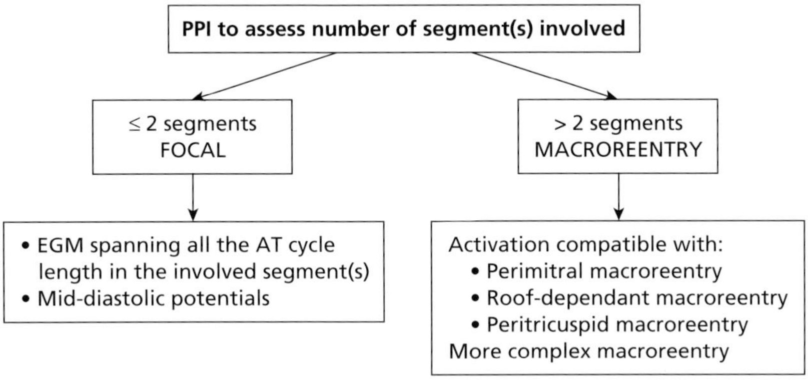

Figure 13.16 The algorithm used in difficult cases of extensive scar or ablation. AT, atrial tachycardia; EGM, electrogram; PPI, post pacing interval.

the presence of a resistant tachycardia to be sure that it has not changed to another one.

The most significant limitation of this approach is observed in patients in whom very few potentials are recordable because of previous ablations and/or spontaneous tissue alterations. This limits the utility of both activation mapping and entrainment maneuvers in areas of possible scar. The same may apply to coronary sinus activity rendering the coronary sinus catheter useless in some patients in whom the reference has to be placed elsewhere. For more difficult cases a second algorithm is proposed (Figure 13.16).

Conclusion

In the vast majority of patients ablated for long-standing persistent AF, sinus rhythm is restored only after mapping and ablation of multiple ATs, adding to the complexity of the procedure. Mapping and ablation of AT has become an indispensable step in the process of AF ablation and makes the difference between procedural success and failure. Given the context of emerging electrogram-based ablation, electrophysiologists will inevitably be confronted by an incoming tide of iatrogenic AT arising late after AF ablation.

Atrial tachycardia in the context of prior AF ablation displays different characteristics from classical AT. The main difference resides in the importance of localized reentry due to spontaneous or ablated tissue alterations creating an anchoring point. The described practical algorithm allows simple and accurate differentiation of macroreentrant and non-macroreentrant AT, which facilitates subsequent successful ablation. Difficult cases due to prior extensive ablation or scar can also be resolved using PPI maneuvers and searching for localized reentries expressing the entire AT CL in a circumscribed region.

Acknowledgments

Sébastien Knecht is supported by the Belgian "Funds for cardiac surgery" and Mark O'Neill is supported by the British Heart Foundation.

References

1 Haissaguerre M, Jais P, Shah DC, et al. Spontaneous initiation of atrial fibrillation by ectopic beats originating in the pulmonary veins. *N Engl J Med* 1998;**339**(10):659–66.

2 Pappone C, Rosanio S, Oreto G, et al. Circumferential radiofrequency ablation of pulmonary vein ostia: a new anatomic approach for curing atrial fibrillation. *Circulation* 2000;**102**(21):2619–28.

3 Ouyang F, Bansch D, Ernst S, et al. Complete isolation of left atrium surrounding the pulmonary veins: new insights from the double-Lasso technique in paroxysmal atrial fibrillation. *Circulation* 2004;**110**(15):2090–6.

4 Chen SA, Hsie MH, Tai CT, et al. Initiation of atrial fibrillation by ectopic beats originating from the pulmonary veins: electrophysiological characteristics, pharmacological responses, and effects of radiofrequency ablation. *Circulation* 1999;**100**(18):1879–86.

5 Haissaguerre M, Sanders P, Hocini M, et al. Catheter ablation of long-lasting persistent atrial fibrillation: critical structures for termination. *J Cardiovasc Electrophysiol* 2005;**16**(11):1125–37.

6 Haissaguerre M, Hocini M, Sanders P, et al. Catheter ablation of long-lasting persistent atrial fibrillation: clinical outcome and mechanisms of subsequent arrhythmias. *J Cardiovasc Electrophysiol* 2005;**16**(11):1138–47.
7 Hsu LF, Jais P, Sanders P, et al. Catheter ablation for atrial fibrillation in congestive heart failure. *N Engl J Med* 2004;**351**(23):2373–83.
8 Oral H, Pappone C, Chugh A, et al. Circumferential pulmonary-vein ablation for chronic atrial fibrillation. *N Engl J Med* 2006;**354**(9):934–41.
9 Nademanee K, McKenzie J, Kosar E, et al. A new approach for catheter ablation of atrial fibrillation: mapping of the electrophysiologic substrate. *J Am Coll Cardiol* 2004;**43**(11):2044–53.
10 Ouyang F, Ernst S, Chun J, et al. Electrophysiological findings during ablation of persistent atrial fibrillation with electroanatomic mapping and double Lasso catheter technique. *Circulation* 2005;**112**(20):3038–48.
11 Verma A, Marrouche NF, Natale A. Pulmonary vein antrum isolation: intracardiac echocardiography-guided technique. *J Cardiovasc Electrophysiol* 2004;**15**(11):1335–40.
12 Haissaguerre M, Shah DC, Jais P, et al. Electrophysiological breakthroughs from the left atrium to the pulmonary veins. *Circulation* 2000;**102**(20):2463–5.
13 Jais P, Hocini M, Sanders P, et al. Long-term evaluation of atrial fibrillation ablation guided by noninducibility. *Heart Rhythm* 2006;**3**(2):140–5.
14 Verma A, Kilicaslan F, Adams JR, et al. Extensive ablation during pulmonary vein antrum isolation has no adverse impact on left atrial function: an echocardiography and cine computed tomography analysis. *J Cardiovasc Electrophysiol* 2006;**17**(7):741–6.
15 Haissaguerre M, Hocini M, Sanders P, et al. Localized sources maintaining atrial fibrillation organized by prior ablation. *Circulation* 2006;**113**(5):616–25.
16 Sanders P, Hocini M, Jais P, et al. Complete isolation of the pulmonary veins and posterior left atrium in chronic atrial fibrillation. Long-term clinical outcome. *Eur Heart J* 2007;**28**:1862–71.
17 Saoudi N, Cosio F, Waldo A, et al. A classification of atrial flutter and regular atrial tachycardia according to electrophysiological mechanisms and anatomical bases. A statement from a Joint Expert Group from the Working Group of Arrhythmias of the European Society of Cardiology and the North American Society of Pacing and Electrophysiology. *Eur Heart J* 2001;**22**(14):1162–82.
18 Sanders P, Hocini M, Jais P, et al. Characterization of focal atrial tachycardia using high-density mapping. *J Am Coll Cardiol* 2005;**46**(11):2088–99.
19 Mohamed U, Skanes AC, Gula LJ, et al. A novel pacing maneuver to localize focal atrial tachycardia. *J Cardiovasc Electrophysiol* 2007;**18**(1):1–6.
20 Waldo AL, MacLean WA, Karp RB, Kouchoukos NT, James TN. Entrainment and interruption of atrial flutter with atrial pacing: studies in man following open heart surgery. *Circulation* 1977;**56**(5):737–45.
21 Gerstenfeld EP, Callans DJ, Dixit S, et al. Mechanisms of organized left atrial tachycardias occurring after pulmonary vein isolation. *Circulation* 2004;**110**(11):1351–7.
22 Ouyang F, Antz M, Ernst S, et al. Recovered pulmonary vein conduction as a dominant factor for recurrent atrial tachyarrhythmias after complete circular isolation of the pulmonary veins: lessons from double Lasso technique. *Circulation* 2005;**111**(2):127–35.
23 Mesas CE, Pappone C, Lang CCE, et al. Left atrial tachycardia after circumferential pulmonary vein ablation for atrial fibrillation: electroanatomic characterization and treatment. *J Am Coll Cardiol* 2004;**44**(5):1071–9.
24 Pappone C, Manguso F, Vicedomini G, et al. Prevention of iatrogenic atrial tachycardia after ablation of atrial fibrillation: a prospective randomized study comparing circumferential pulmonary vein ablation with a modified approach. *Circulation* 2004;**110**(19):3036–42.
25 Deisenhofer I, Estner H, Zrenner B, et al. Left atrial tachycardia after circumferential pulmonary vein ablation for atrial fibrillation: incidence, electrophysiological characteristics, and results of radiofrequency ablation. *Europace* 2006;**8**(8):573–82.
26 Chen SA, Chiang CE, Yang CJ, et al. Sustained atrial tachycardia in adult patients. Electrophysiological characteristics, pharmacological response, possible mechanisms, and effects of radiofrequency ablation. *Circulation* 1994;**90**(3):1262–78.
27 Engelstein ED, Lippman N, Stein KM, Lerman BB. Mechanism-specific effects of adenosine on atrial tachycardia. *Circulation* 1994;**89**(6):2645–54.
28 Kall JG, Kopp D, Olshansky B, Kinder C, O'Connor M, Cadman CS, Wilber D. Adenosine-sensitive atrial tachycardia. *Pacing Clin Electrophysiol* 1995;**18**(2):300–6.
29 Markowitz SM, Stein KM, Mittal S, Slotwtner DJ, Lerman BB. Differential effects of adenosine on focal and macroreentrant atrial tachycardia. *J Cardiovasc Electrophysiol* 1999;**10**(4):489–502.
30 Markowitz SM, Nemirovksy D, Stein KM, et al. Adenosine-insensitive focal atrial tachycardia: evidence for de novo micro-re-entry in the human atrium. *J Am Coll Cardiol* 2007;**49**(12):1324–33.
31 Kall JG, Rubenstein DS, Kopp DE, et al. Atypical atrial flutter originating in the right atrial free wall. *Circulation* 2000;**101**(3):270–9.
32 Jais P, Shah DC, Haissaguerre M, et al. Mapping and ablation of left atrial flutters. *Circulation* 2000;**101**(25):2928–34.

33 Ouyang F, Ernst S, Vogtmann T, et al. Characterization of reentrant circuits in left atrial macroreentrant tachycardia: critical isthmus block can prevent atrial tachycardia recurrence. *Circulation* 2002;**105**(16):1934–42.

34 Takahashi Y, O'Neill MD, Hocini M, et al. Effects of stepwise ablation of chronic atrial fibrillation on atrial electrical and mechanical properties. *J Am Coll Cardiol* 2007;**49**(12):1306–14.

35 Kistler PM, Roberts-Thomson KC, Haqqani HM, et al. P-wave morphology in focal atrial tachycardia: development of an algorithm to predict the anatomic site of origin. *J Am Coll Cardiol* 2006;**48**(5):1010–17.

36 O'Neill MD, Hocini M, Matsuo S, Haissaguerre M. Twin perimitral atrial flutters with alternating cycle lengths. *J Cardiovasc Electrophysiol* 2007;**18**(4):455–6.

37 Shah D, Jais P, Takahashi A, Hocini M, Peng JT, Clementy J, Haissaguerre M. Dual-loop intra-atrial reentry in humans. *Circulation* 2000;**101**(6):631–9.

38 Chiang CE, Chen SA, Wang DC, et al. Arrhythmogenicity of catheter ablation in supraventricular tachycardia. *Am Heart J* 1993;**125**:388–95.

39 Wood MA, Fuller IA. Acute and chronic electrophysiologic changes surrounding radiofrequency lesions. *J Cardiovasc Electrophysiol* 2002;**13**(1):56–61.

14

CHAPTER 14

Catheter ablation of atrial fibrillation in patients with heart failure

Ibrahim Abu Romeh, Mohammed Nasir Khan, & Andrea Natale

Introduction

Atrial fibrillation (AF) is the most common arrhythmia requiring medical treatment, with a lifetime risk for development of AF of approximately 25% in the general population and significant associated morbidity, mortality, and health care expenditure. Heart failure (HF) is among the greatest contributors to morbidity, mortality, and medical expenditure in modern society – currently afflicting nearly 5 million Americans. These two cardiac disorders are intertwined, for each can result in the other [1–3], and when combined, AF and HF together carry a substantially worse prognosis than either alone. There is an increase in AF prevalence in patients afflicted with more advanced HF. AF is present in 40–50% of patients in New York Heart Association (NYHA) functional class IV compared with 10% of patients with class II symptoms. After a 38-year follow-up of subjects from the Framingham study, HF was associated with an approximately 5-fold increase in the risk of developing AF [4]. In further analysis from the Framingham study, Wang et al. showed that patients with HF who develop AF, as well as AF patients who develop HF, have increased mortality [5].

The adverse hemodynamic consequences of AF, including chronically elevated heart rates, elevated cardiac filling pressures, irregular ventricular intervals, lack of effective atrial contraction, and atrioventricular (AV) synchrony, can impair ventricular function and contribute to symptoms of HF. Similarly, elevated cardiac filling pressures, dysregulation of intracellular calcium, and autonomic and neuroendocrine dysfunction associated with HF can markedly increase the risk for the development of AF. Strategies including both medical therapy and interventional procedures have proven effective at preventing and treating AF and HF. In this review, we discuss the treatment options for AF in the HF population.

Atrial fibrillation and heart failure: mechanisms

In the laboratory, the relationship between HF and AF has been validated in multiple experimental models. Persistent marked elevation of the ventricular rate, as during poorly controlled AF, can be mimicked experimentally by rapid pacing. This can lead to ventricular dysfunction and HF. Similarly, the inducibility of AF in animal models can be increased either by HF or by isolated increases in biatrial pressures. Interestingly, although AF inducibility can be increased either by HF (induced by rapid ventricular pacing) or by rapid atrial pacing, the electrophysiological mechanisms appear

Catheter Ablation of Atrial Fibrillation Edited by Etienne Aliot, Michel Haïssaguerre and Warren M. Jackman
 ISBN: 978-1-4501-6349-1.

to be different in these situations. Rapid atrial pacing induces substantially greater decreases in atrial refractory periods, compared with HF. In contrast, HF causes greater atrial interstitial fibrosis than does rapid atrial pacing, leading to heterogeneity of atrial conduction and regions of slow electrical conduction. Clinical AF is likely related to a combination of these factors, so both mechanisms deserve consideration.

Atrial fibrillation and congestive heart failure: treatment

Rate control versus rhythm control

Despite new insights into the pathophysiological triggers of AF and the development of novel ablative techniques and antiarrhythmic drugs, the management of this chronic rhythm disturbance remains problematic. During the past few years, five randomized trials investigating the two treatment strategies have been completed: PIAF (Pharmacological Intervention in Atrial Fibrillation), STAF (Strategies of Treatment of Atrial Fibrillation), RACE (RAte Control versus Electrical conversion), AFFIRM (Atrial Fibrillation Follow-up of Rhythm Management), and HOT CAFE (How to Treat Chronic Atrial Fibrillation) [6–10]. Results from these studies indicate that in a selected group of patients, a strategy of rate control in AF patients can be at least as effective as pharmacological efforts to control rhythm with respect to several specific outcomes. However, there are limitations to keep in mind with these trials. For one, patients who, in the mind of the enrolling physician, were not candidates for either arm of the study could be excluded from enrollment. This potentially eliminated very symptomatic patients from being enrolled in the rate control arm. Additionally, these trials compared rate control versus rhythm control using pharmacological strategies. Pharmacological studies have achieved, at best, only 50% conversion to sinus rhythm and this benefit may be offset by proarrhythmic effects of the antiarrhythmic medications. In patients with HF, the issue of rate versus rhythm control is still unsettled. In a predefined analysis of the RACE study, 261 patients were in NYHA classes II and III. Rate control was not inferior to rhythm control. However, the authors concluded that if sinus rhythm can be maintained, outcomes may be improved.

In a recently reported substudy of the AFFIRM trial, restoration and maintenance of sinus rhythm were associated with a 47% reduction in the risk of death as compared with that of patients who were in AF, whereas the use of antiarrhythmic drugs and the presence of HF significantly increased the risk of death by 49% and 57%, respectively, thereby reversing the benefit of restoration of normal sinus rhythm [11]. The maintenance of sinus rhythm without antiarrhythmic drugs may thus be of critical importance and can now be achieved through curative ablation with the use of catheter or surgical techniques.

In patients with heart failure at entry, a mortality trend in the AFFIRM study favored the rhythm control arm. The issue of survivorship and rhythm control in AF in congestive HF is undergoing further testing. The AF-CHF (Atrial Fibrillation and Congestive Heart Failure) study is currently investigating this issue in a large number of patients [12].

Antiarrrhythmic drugs

Among patients with HF, maintaining sinus rhythm with the use of antiarrhythmic drugs is challenging, owing to the limited efficacy and potentially deleterious effects of the drugs. Patients with HF are particularly prone to the ventricular proarrhythmic effects of antiarrhythmic drugs. Randomized trials have demonstrated the safety of amiodarone and dofetilide (given separately) in patients with HF, and these are the recommended drugs for the maintenance of sinus rhythm in the HF population [13,14].

Non-pharmacological options

Five non-pharmacological approaches have been evaluated to prevent recurrent AF: (i) radiofrequency catheter ablation of the AV node; (ii) radiofrequency catheter ablation of triggers and substrates for AF; (iii) surgery for the maze procedure; (iv) pacing; and (v) implantable atrial defibrillators. The last three options are beyond the scope of this chapter. Ablative and surgical procedures are directed at disrupting the conduction of electrical activity between the tissues that contain arrhythmogenic triggers, most commonly the pulmonary veins and the atrial myocardium, and at modifying the atrial substrate(s) responsible for the maintenance of AF.

Atrioventricular node ablation

It is estimated that 12% of patients with AF and a normal or near normal ejection fraction (EF) are refractory to medical therapy. Radiofrequency catheter ablation of the AV node to produce complete heart block followed by permanent pacemaker implantation with right ventricular pacing (ablation and pacing therapy) is a recognized treatment to alleviate symptoms in medically refractory patients. In a meta-analysis of 21 studies by Wood et al., 1181 patients with medically refractory atrial tachyarrhythmias, mostly AF, underwent AV ablation followed by permanent pacemaker implantation [15]. The outcome analysis included 642 patients in 15 studies. Only 11 studies had documented mean baseline EF. The average duration of follow-up ranged from 3 months to 2.3 years. In two studies with a total of 36 patients, the mean EF was less than 40% at baseline; the mean EF was unchanged by ablation and pacing therapy in five of 11 studies. The ablate and pace strategy improved rate control, quality of life, functional status, EF, and exercise capacity and reduced the number of hospital admissions. Of note, left ventricular function was particularly improved in patients with baseline impairment in two trials. This was attributed to enhanced diastolic filling times, improved cardiac mechanics, withdrawal of negative inotropic drugs, and reversal of tachycardia-induced cardiomyopathy. This meta-analysis included primarily small, uncontrolled studies. Most of the patients had normal EF with only two studies having a mean EF of < 40%.

Although this strategy provides effective rate control and regularization of ventricular rhythm, it does not restore atrial contraction or AV or interventricular synchrony. In addition, right ventricular pacing has been associated with cardiac dyssynchrony. The PAVE (Post AV Node Ablation Evaluation) trial compared chronic biventricular pacing to right ventricular pacing in patients undergoing ablation of the AV node for treatment of AF with rapid ventricular rate. The mean EF was 0.45 and 0.47 in both groups [15]. Biventricular pacing provided a significant improvement in EF and the 6 min hallway walk test compared to right ventricular pacing. Patients with an EF of < 0.45 or class II/III NYHA symptoms had a greater improvement in the 6 min walk distance compared to patients with normal systolic function or class I symptoms.

Atrial fibrillation ablation

The observation that AF can be initiated by ectopic beats originating in the pulmonary veins guided the development of catheter-based strategies to eliminate these foci [15]. The initial attempts to selectively identify and ablate these pulmonary vein foci directly were frequently complicated by AF recurrence and pulmonary vein stenosis. Subsequently, all four pulmonary veins were isolated without incorporating the ostia. There continued to be risk of pulmonary vein stenosis. This risk has been reduced by the technique of electrical isolation of the pulmonary veins by contiguous ablation lesions around the pulmonary vein ostia [16,17]. This technique avoids ablating near the pulmonary vein, yet isolates both the pulmonary veins and the antrum. Another strategy has been the creation of large circumferential lesions around the pulmonary veins using electroanatomic mapping without the requirement for electrical isolation of the veins [18,19].

Several studies have shown the efficacy of AF ablation for restoration of normal sinus rhythm. In a controlled, non-randomized study in predominantly normal EF patients, there was 80% efficacy in restoration to sinus rhythm using a circumferential ablation technique. Additionally, there was a 54% reduction in mortality and a 55% reduction in cardiovascular-related morbidity as compared to matched control patients who were treated with antiarrhythmic medications [18]. A randomized controlled trial comparing pulmonary vein antrum isolation (PVAI) versus antiarrhythmic medications as first-line treatment showed 87% efficacy in the restoration of sinus rhythm in patients with primarily normal EF. Patients undergoing PVAI also had a 45% reduction in hospitalizations and an improved quality of life [20]. Thus, in patients with a normal EF with predominantly paroxysmal AF, there is a plethora of ablation data that point toward high efficacy (greater than 80%) for sinus rhythm restoration with minimal side effects

(1–2% risk of major adverse events including pulmonary vein stenosis, cardiac tamponade, atrio-esophogeal fistula, and stroke).

Ablation in low ejection fraction

Atrial fibrillation ablation can be technically more challenging in patients with impaired left ventricular function, as these patients have elevated filling pressures and larger pulmonary vein ostia. This results in a larger area that potentially needs to be ablated. Many of the early trials on AF ablation focused on patients with a normal EF or those without congestive HF. However, as shown above, AF, congestive HF, and low EF are often intertwined. Recently, several studies have focused on this population.

Hsu et al. studied 58 patients with HF from any cause who underwent catheter ablation for AF that was resistant to at least two antiarrhythmic drugs [21] (Table 14.1). All patients had a left ventricular EF of less than 45% and NYHA class II or higher. A group of 58 matched patients without HF who underwent the same procedure served as controls. Seventy eight percent of patients with HF and 84% of controls were free of AF at 12 months. In the HF group, EF increased by an average of 21%, left ventricular end-diastolic and end-systolic diameters decreased by 7 and 9 mm, respectively. Catheter ablation in this study involved PVAI with one or more linear lesions, which included a roofline between the left and right superior veins and a mitral isthmus line between the mitral annulus and left inferior pulmonary vein.

Another study examining this population looked specifically at patients with low EFs. In a retrospective series of AF patients undergoing pulmonary vein isolation, Chen et al. studied 377 patients, comparing 94 patients with EFs < 40% versus those with EFs ≥ 40% [22]. All patients had symptomatic AFs refractory to medical treatment and were adequately rate controlled. The ablation procedure consisted of PVAI with ablation of the cavotricuspid isthmus at the discretion of the physician. Similar to Hsu et al., there was an AF-free rate of 73% at 14 months in the low EF group as compared to an AF-free rate of 87% in the normal EF group. In contrast, EFs in the low EF group improved non-significantly from 36% before ablation to 41% after ablation. However, 60% of the patients showed an improvement in EF after pulmonary vein isolation, and in these responders the average increase in EF was 7%. One difference that may account for the discrepancy in improvement in EF may be the proportion of patients with permanent or persistent AF. In Chen et al.'s study, 57% of patients had permanent or persistent AF as compared to 91% in the study by Hsu et al. Another factor may be the requirement for rate control in the study by Chen et al., which may have effectively limited the number of patients with tachycardia-mediated cardiomyopathy.

A third study retrospectively examined patients undergoing ablation and compared 40 patients with EFs of < 40% to 65 patients with EFs of ≥ 40% [23]. The ablation procedure consisted of a hybrid procedure wherein electroanatomic mapping-guided ablation was supplemented with demonstration of PVAI, mitral isthmus line, and cavotricuspid isthmus line in most patients. At 14 months, there was a 62% rate of freedom from AF and antiarrhythmic medications in the low EF group with a concomitant increase in EF from 33% to 47%. In

Table 14.1 Studies of patients with low ejection fractions (EFs) undergoing atrial fibrillation (AF) ablation.

	Patients (no.)	*Mean EF (%)*	*LA size (cm)*	*Freedom from AF* (%)*
Hsu et al. [21]	58	35	5	69
Chen et al. [22]	94	36	4.7	73
Tondo et al. [23]	40	33	4.8	62
Gentlesk et al. [27]	53	43	NA	90†

NA, not available.

* Freedom from AF without the use of antiarrhythmic medications.

† No AF with or without antiarrhythmic medications or > 90% reduction in AF burden.

addition, there was significant improvement in exercise capacity and quality of life scores.

Critical structures for ablation

All three trials taken together demonstrate not only the feasibility of catheter ablation in patients with HF and low EF, but also show an efficacy rate between 62% and 73% that rivals efficacy rates in patients with normal EF. In addition, the complication rate in this population was similar to the population with normal EF. What is different, especially in patients with persistent or permanent AF, is the need to ablate critical structures in addition to the pulmonary vein ostia. Haïssaguerre et al. elegantly described other critical structures for AF sustainment [24,25]. They designed a stepwise approach of ablation of persistent or permanent AF that includes: (i) pulmonary vein isolation; (ii) isolation of the superior vena cave; (iv) isolation of the coronary sinus; (iv) atrial ablation at sites of complex fractionated electrograms in the anterior, roof, posterior, and septal portions of the left atrium; and (v) linear ablation of the cavotricuspid isthmus, roofline connecting the superior pulmonary veins, and mitral isthmus line. Isolation of the coronary sinus involves first approaching from the endocardial inferior aspect of the left atrium and then proceeding into the coronary sinus if isolation is not complete.

The end goal of the ablation procedure was prolongation of the AF cycle length and conversion of AF directly to sinus rhythm or from AF to focal atrial tachycardia or to reentrant atypical atrial flutter. Ablation of the atrial tachycardia or atrial flutter would then lead to sinus rhythm. Each step allows for the organization of the rhythm. This approach, incorporating many of the techniques used to ablate AF, is exhaustive, requiring an average of 264 min of fluoroscopy time. However, the results may be well worth the effort. Haïssaguerre et al. report an 87% acute termination of AF and 95% long-term conversion to sinus rhythm with improvement in exercise capacity. The structures found to be the most important in both acute conversion of AF and in sites of atrial tachycardia or atrial flutter occurrence were the pulmonary vein–left atrium junction, coronary sinus, and anterior left atrium near the left atrial appendage. The authors hypothesize that these structures may be important in that they interface with the left atrium with wide diameters and may lead to heterogeneous fiber orientation which may be conducive for AF rotors. Regardless of the mechanism, it appears evident that pulmonary vein isolation by itself is not enough in patients with persistent or permanent AF, especially those with low EFs.

Ablation versus atrioventricular node ablation in low ejection fraction

Before the advent of catheter ablation for AF in a low EF populations, the only option for patients with symptomatic, refractory AF was AV node ablation with subsequent pacemaker implantation. The PAVE trial showed improvements in exercise capacity and quality of life scores when biventricular pacing was substituted for right ventricular pacing in patients undergoing AV node ablation for AF [26]. The question remains as to whether patients with refractory AF and low EFs would derive greater benefit from AV node ablation with biventricular pacing or from AF ablation.

Recently, the PABA-CHF (PVAI vs AV Node Ablation with Biventricular Pacing for Treatment of AF in Patients with Congestive Heart Failure) study, a multicenter randomized controlled trial, was presented in which patients with symptomatic, drug-resistant AF with EFs of ≥ 40% and NYHA class I–III were randomized to either AF ablation with PVAI or AV node ablation with a biventricular implantable cardioverter-defibrillator (ICD). The triple endpoint consisted of the quality of life score as measured by the Minnesota Living with Heart Failure questionnaire, the EF, and the 6 min walk score. All of the endpoints significantly favored the PVAI group with EFs improving from 27% to 34% in the PVAI group and no measurable change in EFs in the AV node ablation group. In addition, there was improvement in left atrial size in the PVAI group. The PVAI group achieved 79% freedom from AF and antiarrhythmic medications at the 6-month follow-up. Even more interestingly, the AV node ablation group had continued progression of AF severity as defined by paroxysmal, persistent, and permanent AF. There were no major complications and minor complications were equivalent between the two strategies. The overall results of this randomized controlled trial indicate that PVAI as compared to AV node ablation with biventricular ICD provides improved functional and objective parameters for heart failure severity and should be considered as a superior option for patients with AF and low EFs.

Conclusion

Catheter ablation for AF in patients with HF has been validated in several clinical trials. While ablation techniques and targets for ablation are still a work in progress, ablation of AF in HF patients is not only a viable option at experienced centers, but may also provide advantages over other treatment modalities such as AV node ablation.

References

1 Van den Berg MP, Tuinenburg AE, Crijns HJ, Van Gelder IC, Gosselink AT, Lie KI. Heart failure and atrial fibrillation: current concepts and controversies. *Heart* 1997; 77(4):309–13.

2 Stevenson WG, Stevenson LW. Atrial fibrillation in heart failure. *N Engl J Med* 1999;**341**(12):910–11.

3 Shinagawa K, Shi YF, Tardif JC, Leung TK, Nattel S. Dynamic nature of atrial fibrillation substrate during development and reversal of heart failure in dogs. *Circulation* 2002;**105**(22):2672–8.

4 Kannel WB, Wolf PA, Benjamin EJ, Levy D. Prevalence, incidence, prognosis, and predisposing conditions for atrial fibrillation: population-based estimates. *Am J Cardiol* 1998;**82**(8A):2N–9N.

5 Wang TJ, Larson MG, Levy D, et al. Temporal relations of atrial fibrillation and congestive heart failure and their joint influence on mortality: the Framingham Heart Study. *Circulation* 2003;**107**(23):2920–5.

6 Van Gelder IC, Hagens VE, Bosker HA, et al. A comparison of rate control and rhythm control in patients with recurrent persistent atrial fibrillation. *N Engl J Med* 2002;**347**(23):1834–40.

7 Wyse DG, Waldo AL, DiMarco JP, et al. A comparison of rate control and rhythm control in patients with atrial fibrillation. *N Engl J Med* 2002;**347**(23):1825–33.

8 Hohnloser SH, Kuck KH, Lilienthal J. Rhythm or rate control in atrial fibrillation-- Pharmacological Intervention in Atrial Fibrillation (PIAF): a randomised trial. *Lancet* 2000;**356**(9244):1789–94.

9 Carlsson J, Miketic S, Windeler J, et al. Randomized trial of rate-control versus rhythm-control in persistent atrial fibrillation: the Strategies of Treatment of Atrial Fibrillation (STAF) study. *J Am Coll Cardiol* 2003;**41**(10): 1690–6.

10 Opolski G, Torbicki A, Kosior DA, et al. Rate control vs rhythm control in patients with nonvalvular persistent atrial fibrillation: the results of the Polish How to Treat Chronic Atrial Fibrillation (HOT CAFE) Study. *Chest* 2004;**126**(2):476–86.

11 Corley SD, Epstein AE, DiMarco JP, et al. Relationships between sinus rhythm, treatment, and survival in the Atrial Fibrillation Follow-Up Investigation of Rhythm Management (AFFIRM) Study. *Circulation* 2004;**109** (12):1509–13.

12 Roy D. Rationale for the Atrial Fibrillation and Congestive Heart Failure (AF-CHF) trial. *Cardiac Electrophysiol Rev* 2003;7(3):208–10.

13 Chun SH, Sager PT, Stevenson WG, Nademanee K, Middlekauff HR, Singh BN. Long-term efficacy of amiodarone for the maintenance of normal sinus rhythm in patients with refractory atrial fibrillation or flutter. *Am J Cardiol* 1995;**76**(1):47–50.

14 Torp-Pedersen C, Moller M, Bloch-Thomsen PE, et al. Dofetilide in patients with congestive heart failure and left ventricular dysfunction. Danish Investigations of Arrhythmia and Mortality on Dofetilide Study Group. *N Engl J Med* 1999;**341**(12):857–65.

15 Wood MA, Brown-Mahoney C, Kay GN, Ellenbogen KA. Clinical outcomes after ablation and pacing therapy for atrial fibrillation: a meta-analysis. *Circulation* 2000;**101** (10):1138–44.

16 Haissaguerre M, Jais P, Shah DC, et al. Electrophysiological end point for catheter ablation of atrial fibrillation initiated from multiple pulmonary venous foci. *Circulation* 2000;**101**(12):1409–17.

17 Marrouche NF, Dresing T, Cole C, et al. Circular mapping and ablation of the pulmonary vein for treatment of atrial fibrillation: impact of different catheter technologies. *J Am Coll Cardiol* 2002;**40**(3):464–74.

18 Pappone C, Rosanio S, Augello G, et al. Mortality, morbidity, and quality of life after circumferential pulmonary vein ablation for atrial fibrillation: outcomes from a controlled nonrandomized long-term study. *J Am Coll Cardiol* 2003;**42**(2):185–97.

19 Oral H, Pappone C, Chugh A, et al. Circumferential pulmonary-vein ablation for chronic atrial fibrillation. *N Engl J Med* 2006;**354**(9):934–41.

20 Wazni OM, Marrouche NF, Martin DO, et al. Radiofrequency ablation vs antiarrhythmic drugs as first-line treatment of symptomatic atrial fibrillation: a randomized trial. *J Am Med Assoc* 2005;**293**(21):2634–40.

21 Hsu LF, Jais P, Sanders P, et al. Catheter ablation for atrial fibrillation in congestive heart failure. *N Engl J Med* 2004;**351**(23):2373–83.

22 Chen MS, Marrouche NF, Khaykin Y, et al. Pulmonary vein isolation for the treatment of atrial fibrillation in patients with impaired systolic function. *J Am Coll Cardiol* 2004;**43**(6):1004–9.

23 Tondo C, Mantica M, Russo G, et al. Pulmonary vein vestibule ablation for the control of atrial fibrillation in patients with impaired left ventricular function. *Pacing Clin Electrophysiol* 2006;**29**(9):962–70.

24 Haissaguerre M, Hocini M, Sanders P, et al. Catheter ablation of long-lasting persistent atrial fibrillation: clinical outcome and mechanisms of subsequent arrhythmias. *J Cardiovasc Electrophysiol* 2005;**16**(11):1138–47.

25 Haissaguerre M, Sanders P, Hocini M, et al. Catheter ablation of long-lasting persistent atrial fibrillation: critical structures for termination. *J Cardiovasc Electrophysiol* 2005;**16**(11):1125–37.

26 Doshi RN, Daoud EG, Fellows C, et al. Left ventricular-based cardiac stimulation post AV nodal ablation evaluation (the PAVE study). *J Cardiovasc Electrophysiol* 2005; **16**(11):1160–5.

27 Gentlesk PSW, Zodo ES, McKernan ML, et al. Ablation of atrial fibrillation in patients with decreased ejection fraction: outcome and evidence for reversible cardiomyopathy. *Heart Rhythm* 2004;**1**(1):S171–S172.

CHAPTER 15

Morbidity and mortality of ablation versus drugs

Carlo Pappone, & Vincenzo Santinelli

Introduction

Atrial fibrillation (AF) is associated with an increased morbidity and mortality risk. However, despite important advances in its treatment, AF remains an independent predictor of both morbidity and mortality. Morbidity is related to frequent hospitalizations due to debilitating symptoms, heart failure (HF), stroke, and systemic thromboembolism. Although AF is considered a non-life-threatening arrhythmia, it is associated with a 1.5–1.9-fold excess mortality after adjustment for preexisting cardiovascular conditions [1]. The rise in hospital admission rates for AF among elderly patients worldwide is striking and its cost to society is exponentially increasing with the aging of the population as well as the rising prevalence of risk factors. In order to face this emerging socioeconomic challenge, there is a need for a deeper understanding of AF pathophysiology. Since AF is a highly pleomorphic and dynamic condition progressing from a first episode to long-lasting persistent or permanent AF, morbidity and mortality risks may be different for each clinical form and may increase over time during AF progression. Better characterization of the predictors, natural history, and clinical course of AF should ultimately support improvements in prevention and clinical decision-making. Unfortunately, at present there are no prospective studies in the literature on progression times and associated risks to elucidate this issue. In an ongoing prospective study from 2001 to 2006 (unpublished observations) we have observed that: (i) about half of untreated patients with a first episode of paroxysmal AF had no further recurrences during follow-up; (ii) compared to patients with AF only, those with associated diseases were more likely to rapidly progress to permanent AF despite antiarrhythmic drug therapy including amiodarone; and (ii) age and HF were independent predictors of progression to permanent AF. Taken together, these findings emphasize the need for an effective and safe strategy that is able to eliminate AF in all its clinical forms, possibly by an early timing of intervention to avoid its rapid progression to the permanent form which, particularly in patients with concomitant diseases and HF, is associated with the highest morbidity and mortality. We believe that every patient admitted to hospital with a stroke and AF represents an opportunity that was lost to prevent a stroke.

The need for sinus rhythm maintenance in patients with atrial fibrillation

Currently, two basic strategies are used to treat patients with AF: (i) maintain sinus rhythm (rhythm control); and (ii) let the patient remain in AF but control the ventricular response (rate control). We believe that the best strategy is long-term sinus rhythm maintenance in the absence of antiarrhythmic drug therapy (ADT) since it represents the physiological condition. Many advantages are associated with rhythm control, which include

Catheter Ablation of Atrial Fibrillation Edited by Etienne Aliot, Michel Haïssaguerre and Warren M. Jackman
© 2008 Blackwell Publishing, ISBN: 978-1-4501-6349-1.

improved cardiac function, better quality of life, prevention of thromboembolic events, and possible increased life expectancy. The advantages of the rate control strategy include the avoidance of ADT, which is frequently necessary to maintain sinus rhythm and is associated with risks of serious complications [2], and a reduced need for repeated direct current cardioversions for recurrences of AF. Evidence indicates an improved outcome if sinus rhythm is maintained long term [3]. An analysis of on-treatment outcomes in the AFFIRM (Atrial Fibrillation Follow-up of Rhythm Management) study has shown that the presence of sinus rhythm is associated with reduced mortality (47% reduction) [4].

Pharmacological or transcutaneous radiofrequency ablation therapy for rhythm control?

If sinus rhythm maintenance is the strategy to be pursued, the next step is to decide which approach to adopt. At present, the two main alternatives for rhythm control are ADT and/or catheter ablation. The potential advantages and disadvantages of each strategy should be explained to patients before it is agreed which one should be adopted. Regardless of the approach, the need for anticoagulation is based on stroke risk and not on whether sinus rhythm is maintained. Unfortunately, ADT available for rhythm control has poor efficacy and significant drawbacks. A study showed that deleterious effects of ADT (mortality increase of 49%) may have offset the benefits of sinus rhythm (which was associated with a 53% reduction in mortality) [5]. Thus, sinus rhythm maintenance is inherently beneficial but the toxic effects and poor efficacy of presently available antiarrhythmic drugs may negate this benefit. These findings led to a search for new drugs that have different ion channel effects, or that work by a different mechanism of action, but there is still a need for proof of efficacy/safety from adequately powered, controlled, and randomized trials.

Fueled by dissatisfaction with ADT and following the development of catheter-based technologies, catheter AF ablation has matured from an investigational technique to an effective alternative to ADT [6–17], as recently stated by the current ACC/AHA/ESC (American College of Cardiology/American Heart Association/European Society of Cardiology) management guidelines [1]. The most effective ablative procedure for patients with paroxysmal, persistent, and permanent AF is circumferential pulmonary vein ablation (CPVA) as currently performed by Pappone et al. [9], which is effective in up to 90% of patients with AF. CPVA focuses on pulmonary vein trigger elimination, electrophysiological substrate modification, and transient vagal denervation – which are all crucial in perpetuating AF (Figure 15.1).

Efficacy: trials comparing atrial fibrillation ablation strategy versus antiarrhythmic drug therapy

At present, there are five milestone trials that compared AF catheter ablation strategy with long-term ADT among patients with AF [9–13] (Table 15.1).

1 The first trial by Pappone et al. [9] in 2003 was a long-term (median follow-up, 900 days), nonrandomized study that demonstrated the striking superiority of AF ablation strategy over ADT in 1171 patients with paroxysmal and chronic AF. The ablation group had more patients with longer arrhythmia duration (5.5 years vs 3.6 years). Freedom from AF was significantly higher (78% vs 37% in the ablated and medical groups, respectively). In addition, ablated patients had fewer hospitalizations than patients treated medically.

2 The second trial by Wazni et al. [10] in 2005 was a randomized study that compared AF ablation as first-line strategy to long-term ADT among 70 patients with initial episodes of paroxysmal AF. Pulmonary vein isolation was superior to initial ADT at 1-year follow-up (87% vs 37%, respectively).

3 The third trial by Stabile et al. [11] in 2006 was a randomized study that confirmed the superiority of AF ablation strategy when combined with ADT over ADT alone (56% vs 9%, respectively) in preventing AF recurrences among 137 patients with paroxysmal or persistent AF in whom ADT had already failed.

4 The fourth trial by Oral et al. [12] in 2006 was the first multicenter, randomized study among 146 patients with chronic AF that demonstrated that sinus rhythm was maintained long term in the majority of ablated patients independently of the

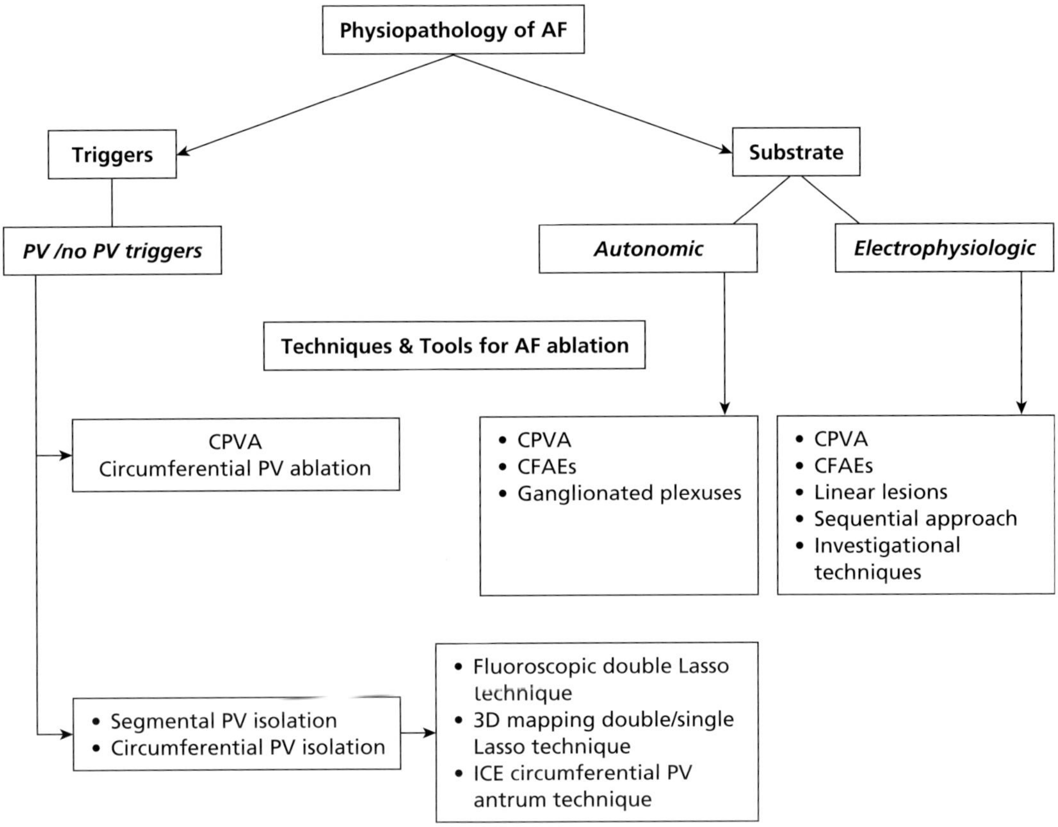

Figure 15.1 Schematic representation of the physiopathology of atrial fibrillation (AF) and ablation strategies. CFAE, complex fractionated atrial electrograms; CPVA, circumferential pulmonary vein ablation; ICE, intracardiac echocardiography; PV, pulmonary vein.

Table 15.1 Characteristics and results of trials comparing atrial fibrillation (AF) ablation strategy versus antiarrhythmic drug therapy (ADT).

Study	*Randomization*	*Type of AF*	*Patients*	*Age (years)*	*Technique*	*Outcome: ablation vs ADT*	*Follow-up*
Pappone et al. 2003 [9]	No	PAF, CAF	1171	65	CPVA	78% vs 37%	900 days
Wazni et al. 2005 [10]	Yes	PAF	70	54	PVI	87% vs 37%	365 days
Stabile et al. 2006 [11]	Yes	PAF, PersAF	137	62	CPVA	56% vs 9%	365 days
Pappone et al. 2006 [12]	Yes	PAF	198	56	CPVA	86% vs 22%	365 days
Oral et al. 2006 [12]	Yes	CAF	146	57	CPVA	74% vs 4%	365 days

CAF, chronic atrial fibrillation; CPVA, circumferential pulmonary vein ablation; PAF, paroxysmal atrial fibrillation; PersAF, persistent atrial fibrillation; PVI, pulmonary vein isolation.

effects of ADT, cardioversion, or both. The maintenance of sinus rhythm was associated with a significant decrease in both the severity of symptoms and the left atrial diameter while no left atrial remodeling was observed in the group of patients assigned to ADT.

5 The last trial, by Pappone et al. [13] in 2006, was a randomized study among 198 patients with

paroxysmal AF, which also demonstrated a striking superiority of ablation over long-term ADT with three widely used antiarrhythmic drugs, amiodarone, flecainide, and sotalol, at maximum tolerable doses. Ablation was much more effective than amiodarone (86% vs 35%, respectively) in preventing AF recurrences in the absence of serious complications. Asymptomatic post-ablation AF recurrences were recorded in about 3% of patients who also experienced symptomatic recurrences and in 27% of the ADT group.

The results of all these five trials demonstrate that AF ablation strategy is more effective than ADT in selected patients in whom maintenance of sinus rhythm is desired.

Morbidity: atrial fibrillation ablation strategy versus antiarrhythmic drug therapy

Morbidity is a concern that needs to be taken into consideration when comparing ablation strategy to ADT since type, time, and number of complications are different. Long-term ADT is frequently associated with significant morbidities that often require ADT discontinuation. Amiodarone is the most effective antiarrhythmic drug, but its long-term administration is frequently associated with the most dangerous side effects. ADT not only produces side effects but may also increase patient mortality according to the well-known results of the CAST (Cardiac Arrhythmia Suppression Trial) and SWORD (Survival With Oral D-sotalol) trials. Proarrhythmic effects leading to hemodynamic instability may be frequently observed in patients with heart diseases, particularly after flecainide or propafenone administration. The Stroke Prevention in Atrial Fibrillation Investigators also reported that in patients given ADT for AF, both cardiac mortality and arrhythmic death were significantly increased, particularly in patients with HF [18]. Analysis of the AFFIRM population reveals a similar negative trend.

Atrial fibriallation ablation, on the other hand, is rarely associated with long-term morbidity, and typically only minor intra-perioperative complications occur [9,19,20]. Table 15.2 shows the most important complications of AF catheter ablation, which in our experience of more than 10,000 cases are very rare (< 1%), with no cases of death. In five recently reported trials, discussed above, that compared ablation strategy to ADT, quality of life was significantly improved in ablated patients with lower morbidity rates in terms of rehospitalizaions and/or thromboembolic events, causing most patients who received ADT to cross over to ablative therapy. These findings are clinically important although older patients and/or those with persistent or permanent AF were excluded from two trials suggesting that these results may not apply to the entire AF population.

Table 15.2 Potential complications of atrial fibrillation ablation.

Arteriovenous fistula
Cardiac perforation/tamponade
Embolic stroke/systemic embolism
Esophageal injury
Femoral pseudoaneurysms
Proarrhythmia
Pulmonary vein stenosis
Sepsis, abscesses, enocarditis
Transient ischemic attack
Valvular injury

Mortality: atrial fibrillation ablation strategy versus antiarrhythmic drug therapy

The impact on mortality of AF by itself is difficult to quantitate as clinical conditions such as severe HF and hypertension are often associated with AF. In addition, mortality in AF may be secondary to stroke rather than hemodynamics. At present, only limited long-term data detailing the impact of catheter ablation of AF on mortality are available. There are no randomized comparative studies on mortality in patients with AF undergoing AF ablation and ADT. One landmark non-randomized study by Pappone et al. [9] reported that AF ablation may reduce mortality as compared to ADT in a large cohort of patients with paroxysmal (69%) or chronic (31%) AF followed up for about 3 years. No cardiovascular disease was found in about one-third of patients and hypertension was the most commonly associated disease. In this study, the survival for ablated patients was longer than among the ADT group, and not different from that expected for healthy persons of the same age and gender. These results are important and indicate for the first time that ablation strategy may indeed result in a mortality benefit, thus achieving one of the most important endpoints. Actually, it is likely that long-term maintenance of sinus rhythm after ablation in the absence of currently available ADT may result in a mortality benefit, which needs to be confirmed in larger, multicenter, randomized trials with a much longer follow-up period. The possibility of performing catheter ablation safely in patients with HF is an important finding. Recently, Hsu et al. [21] reported an improvement in cardiac function among patients who had no AF recurrences after AF ablation. If catheter ablation is safe and results in hemodynamic improvement, it will constitute a novel strategy for the management of patients with both AF and HF in whom morbidity and mortality are highest.

Conclusion

Catheter ablation may provide a true cure rather than only palliative therapy, as ADT does, in patients with AF. The first randomized trials comparing catheter ablation strategy to long-term ADT have demonstrated a striking superiority of ablation with higher efficacy, lower morbidity, and improved quality of life. A mortality benefit for patients with AF, particularly for those with HF, requires larger scale, randomized trials involving several centers worldwide.

References

1 Fuster V, Ryden LE, Cannom DS, et al. ACC/AHA/ESC 2006 guidelines for the management of patients with atrial fibrillation: a report of the American College of Cardiology, American Heart Association Task Force on Practice Guidelines and the European Society of Cardiology Committee for Practice Guidelines (writing committee to revise the 2001 guidelines for the management of patients with atrial fibrillation): developed in collaboration with the European Heart Rhythm Association and the Heart Rhythm Society. *Circulation* 2006;**114**: 257–354.

2 Nattel S, Khairy P, Roy D, et al. New approaches to atrial fibrillation management: a critical review of a rapidly evolving field. *Drugs* 2002;**62**: 2377–97.

3 Carlsson J, Miketic S, Windeler J, et al. STAF Investigators. Randomized trial of rate-control versus rhythm-control in persistent atrial fibrillation: the Strategies of Treatment of Atrial Fibrillation (STAF) study. *J Am Coll Cardiol* 2003;**41**: 1690–6.

4 Corley SD, Epstein AE, DiMarco JP, et al. Relationships between sinus rhythm, treatment, and survival in the Atrial Fibrillation Follow-up Investigation of Rhythm Management (AFFIRM) study. *Circulation* 2004;**109**: 1509–13.

5 Steinberg JS, Sadaniantz A, Kron J, et al. Analysis of cause-specific mortality in the Atrial Fibrillation Follow-up Investigation of Rhythm Management (AFFIRM) study. *Circulation* 2004;**109**:1973–80.

6 Haissaguerre M, Jais P, Shah DC, et al. Spontaneous initiation of atrial fibrillation by ectopic beats originating in the pulmonary veins. *N Engl J Med* 1998;**339**: 659–66.

7 Oral H, Knight BP, Tada H, et al. Pulmonary vein isolation for paroxysmal and persistent atrial fibrillation. *Circulation* 2002;**105**:1077–81.

8 Pappone C, Santinelli V, Manguso F, et al. Pulmonary vein denervation enhances long-term benefit after circumferential ablation for paroxysmal atrial fibrillation. *Circulation* 2004;**109**:327–34.

9 Pappone C, Rosanio S, Augello G, et al. Mortality, morbidity, and quality of life after circumferential pulmonary vein ablation for atrial fibrillation: outcomes from a controlled nonrandomized long-term study. *J Am Coll Cardiol* 2003;**42**:185–97.

10 Wazni OM, Marrouche NF, Martin DO, et al. Radiofrequency ablation vs antiarrhythmic drugs as first-line treatment of symptomatic atrial fibrillation: a randomized trial. *J Am Med Assoc* 2005;**293**:2634–40.

11 Stabile G, Bertaglia E, Senatore G, et al. Catheter ablation treatment in patients with drug refractory atrial fibrillation: a prospective, multi-centre, randomized, controlled study (Catheter Ablation For The Cure Of Atrial Fibrillation Study). *Eur Heart J* 2006;**27**:216.

12 Oral H, Pappone C, Chugh A, et al. Circumferential pulmonary-vein ablation for chronic atrial fibrillation. *N Engl J Med* 2006;**354**:934–94.

13 Pappone C, Augello G, Sala S, et al. A randomized trial of circumferential pulmonary vein ablation versus antiarrhythmic drug therapy in paroxysmal atrial fibrillation. The Ablation for Paroxysmal Atrial Fibrillation (APAF) study. *J Am Coll Cardiol* 2006;**48**:2340–7.

14 Nademanee K, McKenzie J, Kosar E, et al. A new approach for catheter ablation of atrial fibrillation: mapping of the electrophysiologic substrate. J *Am Coll Cardiol* 2004;**43**:2044–53.

15 Oral H, Scharf C, Chugh A, et al. Catheter ablation for paroxysmal atrial fibrillation: segmental pulmonary vein ostial ablation versus left atrial ablation. *Circulation* 2003;**108**:2355–60.

16 Ouyang F, Bansch D, Ernst S, et al. Complete isolation of left atrium surrounding the pulmonary veins: new insights from the double-Lasso technique in paroxysmal atrial fibrillation. *Circulation* 2004;**110**:2090–6.

17 Pappone C, Santinelli V. Atrial fibrillation ablation: a realistic alternative to pharmacologic therapy. *Nat Clin Pract Cardiovasc Med* 2005;**2**:608–9.

18 Flaker GC, Blackshear JL, McBride R, et al. Antiarrhythmic drug therapy and cardiac mortality in atrial fibrillation: the Stroke Prevention in Atrial Fibrillation Investigators. *J Am Coll Cardiol* 1992;**20**:527–32.

19 Pappone C, Santinelli V. How to perform encircling ablation of the left atrium. *Heart Rhythm* 2006;**3**:1105–9.

20 Pappone C, Manguso F, Vicedomini G, et al. Prevention of iatrogenic atrial tachycardia after ablation of atrial fibrillation: a prospective randomized study comparing circumferential pulmonary vein ablation with a modified approach. *Circulation* 2004;**110**:3036–42.

21 Hsu LF, Jais P, Sanders P, et al. Catheter ablation for atrial fibrillation in congestive heart failure. *N Engl J Med* 2004;**351**:2373–83.

CHAPTER 16

Atrial mechanical function after atrial fibrillation ablation

Prashanthan Sanders, Pierre Jaïs, Glenn D. Young, Frédéric Sacher, Martin Rotter, Mélèze Hocini, Li-Fern Hsu, Martin K. Stiles, Bobby John, Dennis H. Lau, Yoshihide Takahashi, Thomas Rostock, Pawel Kuklik, Lorraine Mackenzie, Scott Willoughby, & Michel Haïssaguerre

Atrial fibrillation and stroke risk

Atrial fibrillation (AF) is associated with a variety of adverse clinical consequences, of which the most devastating is thromboembolic stroke. In the absence of rheumatic heart disease the risk of stroke is 5–8-fold greater after adjusting for other stroke risk factors [1], while in patients with rheumatic heart disease there is a 17.5-fold increased risk [2]. The risk of stroke due to AF increases from 1.5% per year between the ages of 50 and 59 years to 24% per year in patients over the age of 80 years [3]. There is also an increased incidence of silent cerebral infarction [4]. Furthermore, evidence suggests that strokes complicating AF result in increased severity of neurological deficit and are twice as likely to be fatal [5].

Anticoagulation in atrial fibrillation

Thromboembolic risk can be effectively reduced with the use of anticoagulation. Several multicenter, prospective, randomized trials have demonstrated significant reductions in the risk of thromboembolic stroke with anticoagulation; warfarin reducing the risk of thromboembolic events by approximately 70% and aspirin conferring a significantly smaller (20% risk reduction) preventative benefit for primary and secondary prevention [6–12]. While effectively reducing the stroke risk, anticoagulation is associated with a significant risk of hemorrhage [13,14]. The significant ongoing morbidity associated with this approach for the treatment of AF has stimulated interest into the potential role of primary catheter ablation of AF in maintaining sinus rhythm and reducing stroke risk.

Tachycardia-mediated atrial cardiomyopathy

Tachycardia-related ventricular cardiomyopathy results from sustained rates in excess of a 100 beats per minute. This is a recognized phenomenon that is defined as an impairment of left ventricular function (with structural, electrical, and metabolic remodeling) secondary to chronic tachycardia, which is partially or completely reversible after normalization of the heart rate or the restoration of sinus rhythm [15,16]. This process demonstrates

Catheter Ablation of Atrial Fibrillation Edited by Etienne Aliot, Michel Haïssaguerre and Warren M. Jackman
 ISBN: 978-1-4501-6349-1.

rate, duration, and species dependency. Several reports about patients with AF have documented improvement in ventricular function with ventricular rate control. The pathophysiological link between increased ventricular rates and cardiomyopathy is not well understood. A similar process of atrial mechanical dysfunction or a tachycardia-mediated atrial cardiomyopathy is increasingly recognized to occur in the atrium and promotes the formation of thrombus and subsequent stroke [17].

Atrial mechanical dysfunction as a result of AF could largely be attributed to the structural abnormalities that are known to result from atrial arrhythmia. However, while these processes take weeks to develop, atrial mechanical dysfunction is observed with even short durations of atrial arrhythmia [18–22], suggesting a role for more functional cellular mechanisms in its development.

It has been postulated that the impairment in atrial mechanical function associated with AF is related to the intracellular calcium overload caused by rapid atrial depolarization [23]. Several animal studies have suggested that atrial arrhythmias result in an increase in cytosolic calcium loading [24,25]. Furthermore, rapid atrial rates impair cellular calcium handling and decrease systolic calcium transients [26]. Schotten et al. have demonstrated that treatment with the calcium channel agonist Bay K8644 results in a significant inotropic effect on muscle fibers from patients in sinus rhythm but has no effect in patients with AF [27]. Several investigators have consistently observed a downregulation of the number or function of L-type calcium receptors [28–30], and an upregulation of the sodium–calcium exchanger in atrial myocardial fibers from patients with AF – perhaps a cellular protective mechanism [31]. However, β-adrenoreceptor density, protein content of the ryanodine-sensitive calcium release channel, sarcoplasmic reticulum calcium adenosine triphosphatase, phosphlamban, and calsequestrin remain unchanged [31].

Interestingly, Schotten et al. have studied the contractile function of isolated atrial myocardial fibers from patients with chronic AF taken at the time of surgery and found a 75% reduction in contractility to a given stimulus compared to muscle fibers isolated from patients in sinus rhythm [27]. Importantly, these authors document that these atrial muscle fibers from patients with AF could result in muscle tension comparable to that from patients in sinus rhythm with the use of increasing concentrations of extracellular calcium or isoproterenol, suggesting that this process may be a functional impairment of the contractile apparatus.

Clinical characterization of atrial mechanical function

Echocardiography is frequently employed to visualize the left atrium and atrial appendage for the exclusion of thrombus prior to cardioversion of atrial arrhythmias or for the exclusion of a cardiac source of embolism [32,33]. Pollick et al. found that left atrial appendage thrombus was associated with both dilation and poor left atrial appendage contraction with the left atrial appendage emptying velocities (LAAEVs) utilized as a marker of left atrial appendage function [34] (Figure 16.1). In addition, left atrial spontaneous echocardiographic contrast (LASEC) is recognized as a risk factor for thromboembolic events [35] (Figure 16.1). It is defined as the appearance of swirling clouds of

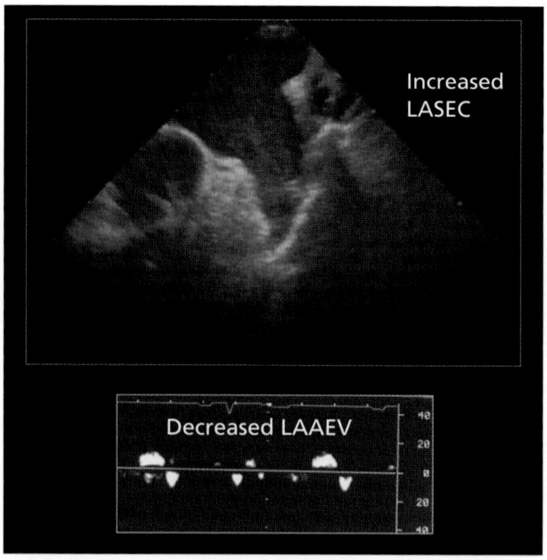

Figure 16.1 Atrial "stunning" after AF ablation. In this patient there is a significantly decreased left atrial appendage emptying velocity (LAAEV) and an increased formation of left atrial spontaneous echocardiographic contrast (LASEC) – factors known to be associated with an increased risk of thromboembolic complications.

echodensity distinct from white noise artifact [36]. Several grading systems have evolved which have been largely dependent on subjective analysis of echocardiographic contrast grade. Fatkin et al. have described the use of an expanded classification of LASEC according to the following criteria [36]: 0 = absence of echogenicity; 1 = minimal echogenicity located in the left atrial appendage or sparsely distributed in the main left atrial cavity; 2 = more dense swirling pattern than grade 1 but with similar distribution; 3 = dense swirling pattern in the left atrial appendage, generally associated with somewhat lesser intensity in the main left atrial cavity; and 4 = intense echodensity and very slow swirling patterns in the left atrial appendage, usually with similar density in the main cavity.

Atrial mechanical dysfunction due to atrial arrhythmias has been best characterized at the time of cardioversion (stunning) as the reduction in both mitral A-wave velocity (MAV) and LAAEV, along with the development of LASEC and thrombus [34,37]. While this phenomenon was initially attributed to the direct current energy utilized for electrical cardioversion, the latter modality has not been observed to cause mechanical dysfunction when used for ventricular tachycardia [38] or in patients in sinus rhythm [39]. Indeed atrial mechanical stunning is also observed following pharmacological cardioversion [40] and in patients with AF who revert spontaneously to sinus rhythm [41].

Atrial mechanical dysfunction after cardioversion

Several studies have examined the recovery of left atrial function following cardioversion of AF to sinus rhythm [42–45]. Omran et al. undertook serial transesophageal echocardiography to demonstrate the return of left atrial and left atrial appendage function 7 days following the endocardial defibrillation of AF [43]. Manning et al., using serial transthoracic echocardiography, identified arrhythmia chronicity as a major determinant of the recovery of atrial function following DC cardioversion of AF [42]. Sanders et al. studied the immediate reversibility of atrial mechanical stunning after cardioversion of AF of short (≤ 6 months) or long (≥ 3 years) duration AF by pacing at faster rates and by administering isoproterenol and calcium [46,47]. These investigators observed that while atrial mechanical function was reversible in patients with short-duration AF, a significantly attenuated response occurred after cardioversion of long-duration AF. Unlike the suggestions in isolated muscle fibers, this study raises the possibility that restoration of sinus rhythm in patients with long durations of AF may not reduce the associated stroke risk.

Potential detrimental effect of ablation on atrial mechanical function

Reports examining left atrial function post maze procedure have suggested that most patients have at least partial left atrial contractile and reservoir function; however, there may be a decline after surgery [48,49]. Thomas et al. studied the recovery of atrial mechanical function in patients undergoing radiofrequency linear ablation during surgery and compared this to the situation in patients undergoing cardioversion [50]. Left atrial function was evaluated by determining the left atrial volume and left atrial ejection fraction. Left atrial function was found to be reduced both after ablation and cardioversion compared to controls. However, the left atrial ejection fraction was lowest in the ablation group (15.8 ± 10%), intermediate in the cardioversion group (26 ± 10%), and highest in the normal controls (33 ± 7%). Although the patients undergoing ablation had a longer duration of AF (51 ± 9 versus 7 ± 2 months; $P = 0.0001$), the investigators raised the concern that the worse atrial mechanical function in the ablation group may be an additional effect of ablation, over and above that caused by chronic AF alone. However, one may expect that a number of factors may have contributed to the impaired atrial function after surgery; trauma from the surgery, including incisions and ischemia, may have independently deleterious effects on the left atrium.

With respect to catheter ablation of AF, several investigators have consistently documented a significant reduction in left atrial size after catheter ablation of AF and the maintenance of sinus rhythm [51–53]. However, the effect of catheter ablation on atrial mechanical function has been limited and varied. Lemola et al. studied patients before and after ablation using contrast-enhanced computed tomography (CT) and determined the left atrial ejection fraction by manually tracing the maximum and minimum sizes [54]. In the 10 patients in whom scanning had been performed in sinus rhythm before and after ablation, the left atrial ejection fraction decreased by approximately 30% (from 30 ± 11% to 19 ± 6%; $P = 0.008$). In addition they confirmed the data observed with surgical ablation that patients with AF, even after restoration of sinus rhythm, had atrial function that was worse than controls. In contrast, Verma et al. utilized both CT and transesophageal echocardiography (TEE) and reported that most indices of left atrial function either remained stable or demonstrated improvement [55]. Unlike the study by Lemola et al., these investigators observed deterioration in left atrial ejection fraction in only a single patient (1%) undergoing catheter ablation of paroxysmal AF.

Determination of left atrial ejection fraction by echocardiography or CT has several limitations that may have contributed to the diverse findings using this parameter; these include the angulations of the image during acquisition and the manual tracing of the left atrial endocardium. In addition, this parameter has not previously been demonstrated to be associated with an increased stroke risk.

Atrial mechanical function after atrial fibrillation ablation

To determine the effect of catheter ablation and the impact of the duration of arrhythmia on the recovery of atrial mechanical function, we performed a serial evaluation of 46 patients undergoing ablation of AF. The LAAEV, LASEC, and presence of thrombus were determined using transesophageal or intracardiac echocardiography. These patients were selected on the basis of the duration of arrhythmia prior to ablation and placed in one of three groups as follows: (1) sinus rhythm: where patients were in sinus rhythm for at least 48 h and no symptoms for 1 week; (2) short-duration AF: where patients were in sustained AF for ≥ 1 month but ≤ 12 months; and (3) long-duration AF: where patients were in sustained AF for ≥ 24 months. The groups were matched for baseline characteristics (Table 16.1). However, they differed in the extent of ablation performed; those with a longer duration of AF underwent more extensive ablation.

The results of LAAEV and LASEC in each group before, immediately after, and ≥ 3 months' post-ablation are shown in Figure 16.2. There was no change in the LAAEV with ablation in sinus rhythm, despite almost half the group undergoing substrate modification. In addition, none of these patients demonstrated LASEC. In contrast, in patients with AF (of short or long duration),

Table 16.1 Characteristics of the three groups.

	Sinus rhythm	*Short-duration AF*	*Long-duration AF*	*P-value*
Number	11	18	17	–
Age (years)	54 ± 14	53 ± 13	58 ± 7	0.4
Male	10	18	15	0.6
Sustained AF (months)	0	5 ± 3	33 ± 13	< 0.0001
SHD	4 (36%)	8 (44%)	4 (24%)	0.4
PVI	11 (100%)	18 (100%)	17 (100%)	ns
CTI	11 (100%)	18 (100%)	17 (100%)	ns
Roofline	5 (45%)	14 (78%)	15 (88%)	0.04
Mitral isthmus	1 (9%)	12 (67%)	12 (71%)	0.003
CFAE	2 (18%)	13 (76%)	10 (59%)	0.07
Follow-up TEE (days)	156 ± 53	138 ± 72	225 ± 165	0.1

AF, atrial fibrillation; CFAE, complex fractionated atrial electrogram; CTI, cavotricuspid isthmus ablation; PVI, pulmonary vein isolation; SHD, structural heart disease; TEE, transesophageal echocardiography.

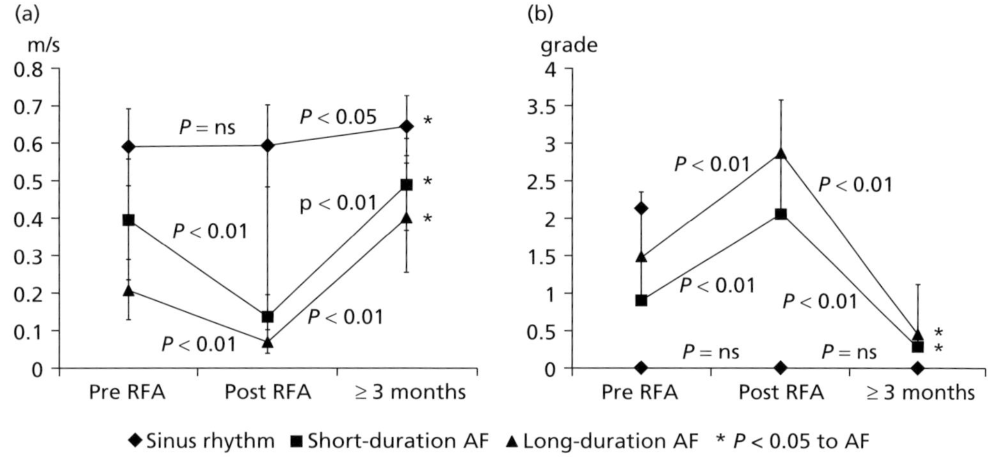

Figure 16.2 The LAAEV (a) and the LASEC (b) before and immediately after ablation and after 3 months or more of maintaining sinus rhythm in patients with sinus rhythm, short-duration atrial fibrillation (AF), and long-duration AF. See text for further details. RFA, radiofrequency ablation.

cardioversion to sinus rhythm was associated with a significant decrease in the LAAEV and was associated with an increase in LASEC with two patients developing left atrial thrombus. With the maintenance of sinus rhythm, atrial mechanical function improved with an increase in the LAAEV and a decrease in LASEC. However, at each time point, patients with longer durations of sustained AF had worse left atrial mechanical function.

These observations suggest: (1) ablation itself has little or no effect on parameters of atrial mechanical function known to be associated with an increased stroke risk; (2) the degree of atrial mechanical dysfunction is determined by the duration of sustained arrhythmia; and (3) atrial mechanical stunning that occurs after ablation to restore sinus rhythm resolves with time, in a time course determined by the duration of sustained arrhythmia.

Risk of stroke post atrial fibrillation ablation

These data on the recovery of atrial mechanical function after ablation to restore sinus rhythm provide the impetus to suggest that such therapy may reduce the risk of stroke associated with this condition. In agreement with this, Oral et al. recently presented observational data in their series of 755 consecutive patients undergoing AF ablation [56]. Of this group, 411 (56%) had at least one risk factor for stroke, with 34 having had a previous stroke. Anticoagulation was ceased in 79% of 256 patients in sinus rhythm with no stroke risk factors and in 68% of 266 patients in sinus rhythm with at least one stroke risk factor. During follow-up, seven of 755 patients (0.9%) had an embolic event within 2 weeks of ablation and a further two (0.3%) had late embolic events (180 and 300 days post-ablation). In the same cohort, two patients (0.3%) had cerebral hemorrhage while anticoagulated.

Conclusion

Impaired atrial mechanical function characterized by a decrease in LAAEV, an increase in LASEC, and the formation of thrombus are established risk factors for thromboembolic stroke associated with AF. Atrial mechanical function is determined by the duration of sustained arrhythmia. Ablation does not significantly affect atrial mechanical function but restoration of sinus rhythm by ablation is associated with an improvement in atrial mechanical function. Recent observational data suggest that this may result in a decrease in the risk of thromboembolic stroke. Further prospective evaluation of high risk individuals is required to determine the effectiveness of catheter ablation of AF in stroke prevention.

Acknowledgments

This project was partly funded by an Affinity Health Research Grant, Affinity Health Foundation, Australia. Dr. Sanders is supported by the National Heart Foundation of Australia. Dr. Rotter is supported by the Swiss National Foundation for Scientific Research, Bern, Switzerland. Dr. Stiles is supported by the National Heart Foundation of New Zealand and the Dawes Scholarship from the Royal Adelaide Hospital. Dr. John is supported by the Biosense-Webster Electrophysiology Scholarship from the University of Adelaide. Dr. Lau is supported by the Earl Bakken Electrophysiology Scholarship from the University of Adelaide. Dr. Mackenzie is supported by a Peter Doherty Fellowship from the National Health and Medical Research Council of Australia.

References

1 Wolf PA, Abbott RD, Kannel WB. Atrial fibrillation as an independent risk factor for stroke: the Framingham Study. *Stroke* 1991;**22**:983–8.

2 Wolf PA, Dawber TR, Thomas HE, Jr., Kannel WB. Epidemiologic assessment of chronic atrial fibrillation and risk of stroke: the Framingham study. *Neurology* 1978;**28**:973–7.

3 Wolf PA, Kannel WB, McGee DL, Meeks SL, Bharucha NE, McNamara PM. Duration of atrial fibrillation and imminence of stroke: the Framingham study. *Stroke* 1983;**14**:664–7.

4 Ezekowitz MD, James KE, Nazarian SM, et al. Silent cerebral infarction in patients with nonrheumatic atrial fibrillation. The Veterans Affairs Stroke Prevention in Nonrheumatic Atrial Fibrillation Investigators. *Circulation* 1995;**92**:2178–82.

5 Lin HJ, Wolf PA, Kelly-Hayes M, Beiser AS, Kase CS, Benjamin EJ, D'Agostino RB. Stroke severity in atrial fibrillation. The Framingham study. *Stroke* 1996;**27**: 1760–4.

6 Stroke Prevention in Atrial Fibrillation Investigators. Stroke Prevention in Atrial Fibrillation Study. Final results. *Circulation* 1991;**84**:527–39.

7 Stroke Prevention in Atrial Fibrillation II Investigators. Warfarin versus aspirin for prevention of thromboembolism in atrial fibrillation: Stroke Prevention in Atrial Fibrillation II Study. *Lancet* 1994;**343**:687–91.

8 Petersen P, Boysen G, Godtfredsen J, Andersen ED, Andersen B. Placebo-controlled, randomised trial of warfarin and aspirin for prevention of thromboembolic complications in chronic atrial fibrillation. The Copenhagen AFASAK study. *Lancet* 1989;**1**:175–9.

9 Connolly SJ, Laupacis A, Gent M, Roberts RS, Cairns JA, Joyner C. Canadian Atrial Fibrillation Anticoagulation (CAFA) study. *J Am Coll Cardiol* 1991;**18**:349–55.

10 Boston Area Anticoagulation Trial for Atrial Fibrillation Investigators. The effect of low-dose warfarin on the risk of stroke in patients with nonrheumatic atrial fibrillation. *N Engl J Med* 1990;**323**:1505–11.

11 Ezekowitz MD, Bridgers SL, James KE, et al. Warfarin in the prevention of stroke associated with nonrheumatic atrial fibrillation. Veterans Affairs Stroke Prevention in Nonrheumatic Atrial Fibrillation Investigators. *N Engl J Med* 1992;**327**:1406–12.

12 EAFT (European Atrial Fibrillation Trial) Study Group. Secondary prevention in non-rheumatic atrial fibrillation after transient ischaemic attack or minor stroke. *Lancet* 1993;**342**:1255–62.

13 Gorter JW. Major bleeding during anticoagulation after cerebral ischemia: patterns and risk factors. Stroke Prevention In Reversible Ischemia Trial (SPIRIT). European Atrial Fibrillation Trial (EAFT) study groups. *Neurology* 1999;**53**:1319–27.

14 Stroke Prevention in Atrial Fibrillation Investigators. Bleeding during antithrombotic therapy in patients with atrial fibrillation. *Arch Intern Med* 1996;**156**:409–16.

15 Packer DL, Bardy GH, Worley SJ, et al. Tachycardia-induced cardiomyopathy: a reversible form of left ventricular dysfunction. *Am J Cardiol* 1986;**57**:563–70.

16 Hsu LF, Jais P, Sanders P, Garrigue S, et al. Catheter ablation of atrial fibrillation in congestive heart failure. *N Engl J Med* 2004;**351**:2373–83.

17 Zipes DP. Atrial fibrillation. A tachycardia-induced atrial cardiomyopathy. *Circulation* 1997;**95**:562–4.

18 Daoud EG, Marcovitz P, Knight BP, et al. Short-term effect of atrial fibrillation on atrial contractile function in humans. *Circulation* 1999;**99**:3024–7.

19 Louie EK, Liu D, Reynertson SI, Loeb HS, McKiernan TL, Scanlon PJ, Hariman RJ. "Stunning" of the left atrium after spontaneous conversion of atrial fibrillation to sinus rhythm: demonstration by transesophageal Doppler techniques in a canine model. *J Am Coll Cardiol* 1998;**32**: 2081–6.

20 Altemose GT, Zipes DP, Weksler J, Miller JM, Olgin JE. Inhibition of the Na(+)/H(+) exchanger delays the development of rapid pacing-induced atrial contractile dysfunction. *Circulation* 2001;**103**:762–8.

21 Sanders P, Morton, JB, Spence SJ, Snelling M, Sparks PB, Edwards GA, Kalman JM. Time course of atrial mechanical remodeling in atrial fibrillation: an intracardiac echo study in a chronic conscious ovine model. *Pacing Clin Electrophysiol* 2003;**26**:951.

22 Schotten U, Duytschaever M, Ausma J, Eijsbouts S, Neuberger HR, Allessie M. Electrical and contractile remodeling during the first days of atrial fibrillation go hand in hand. *Circulation* 2003;**107**:1433–9.

23 Leistad E, Aksnes G, Verburg E, Christensen G. Atrial contractile dysfunction after short-term atrial fibrillation is reduced by verapamil but increased by BAY K8644. *Circulation* 1996;**93**:1747–54.

24 Goette A, Honeycutt C, Langberg JJ. Electrical remodeling in atrial fibrillation. Time course and mechanisms. *Circulation* 1996;**94**:2968–74.

25 Sun H, Chartier D, Leblanc N, Nattel S. Intracellular calcium changes and tachycardia-induced contractile dysfunction in canine atrial myocytes. *Cardiovasc Res* 2001;**49**:751–61.

26 Sun H, Gaspo R, Leblanc N, Nattel S. Cellular mechanisms of atrial contractile dysfunction caused by sustained atrial tachycardia. *Circulation* 1998;**98**:719–27.

27 Schotten U, Ausma J, Stellbrink C, et al. Cellular mechanisms of depressed atrial contractility in patients with chronic atrial fibrillation. *Circulation* 2001;**103**:691–8.

28 Yue L, Feng J, Gaspo R, Li GR, Wang Z, Nattel S. Ionic remodeling underlying action potential changes in a canine model of atrial fibrillation. *Circ Res* 1997;**81**: 512–25.

29 Van Wagoner DR, Pond AL, Lamorgese M, Rossie SS, McCarthy PM, Nerbonne JM. Atrial L-type Ca2+ currents and human atrial fibrillation. *Circ Res* 1999;**85**: 428–36.

30 Bosch RF, Zeng X, Grammer JB, Popovic K, Mewis C, Kuhlkamp V. Ionic mechanisms of electrical remodeling in human atrial fibrillation. *Cardiovasc Res* 1999;**44**: 121–31.

31 Schotten U, Greiser M, Benke D, et al. Atrial fibrillation-induced atrial contractile dysfunction: a tachycardiomyopathy of a different sort. *Cardiovasc Res* 2002;**53**: 192–201.

32 Klein AL, Grimm RA, Black IW, et al. Cardioversion guided by transesophageal echocardiography: the ACUTE Pilot Study. A randomized, controlled trial. Assessment of cardioversion using transesophageal echocardiography. *Ann Intern Med* 1997;**126**:200–9.

33 Grimm RA, Stewart WJ, Black IW, Thomas JD, Klein AL. Should all patients undergo transesophageal echocardiography before electrical cardioversion of atrial fibrillation? *J Am Coll Cardiol* 1994;**23**:533–41.

34 Pollick C, Taylor D. Assessment of left atrial appendage function by transesophageal echocardiography. Implications for the development of thrombus. *Circulation* 1991; **84**:223–31.

35 Fatkin D, Kuchar DL, Thorburn CW, Feneley MP. Transesophageal echocardiography before and during direct current cardioversion of atrial fibrillation: evidence for "atrial stunning" as a mechanism of thromboembolic complications. *J Am Coll Cardiol* 1994;**23**:307–16.

36 Fatkin D, Kelly RP, Feneley MP. Relations between left atrial appendage blood flow velocity, spontaneous echocardiographic contrast and thromboembolic risk in vivo. *J Am Coll Cardiol* 1994;**23**:961–9.

37 Manning WJ, Silverman DI, Katz SE, Douglas PS. Atrial ejection force: a noninvasive assessment of atrial systolic function. *J Am Coll Cardiol* 1993;**22**:221–5.

38 Dodds GA, III, Wilkinson WE, Greenfield RA, Natale A, Kisslo J, Pritchett EL. Evaluation of the effect of transthoracic cardioversion from ventricular tachycardia to sinus rhythm on left atrial mechanical function. *Am J Cardiol* 1996;**78**:1436–9.

39 Sparks PB, Kulkarni R, Vohra JK, et al. Effect of direct current shocks on left atrial mechanical function in patients with structural heart disease. *J Am Coll Cardiol* 1998;**31**:1395–9.

40 Antonielli E, Pizzuti A, Bassignana A, Tanga M, Baralis G, Rovere ME, Di Leo M. Transesophageal echocardiographic evidence of more pronounced left atrial stunning after chemical (propafenone) rather than electrical attempts at cardioversion from atrial fibrillation. *Am J Cardiol* 1999;**84**:1092–10.

41 Grimm RA, Leung DY, Black IW, Stewart WJ, Thomas JD, Klein AL. Left atrial appendage "stunning" after spontaneous conversion of atrial fibrillation demonstrated by transesophageal Doppler echocardiography. *Am Heart J* 1995;**130**:174–6.

42 Manning WJ, Silverman DI, Katz SE, et al. Impaired left atrial mechanical function after cardioversion: relation to the duration of atrial fibrillation. *J Am Coll Cardiol* 1994;**23**:1535–40.

43 Omran H, Jung W, Rabahieh R, et al. Left atrial chamber and appendage function after internal atrial defibrillation: a prospective and serial transesophageal echocardiographic study. *J Am Coll Cardiol* 1997;**29**:131–8.

44 Manning WJ, Silverman DI, Katz SE, Riley MF, Doherty RM, Munson JT, Douglas PS. Temporal dependence of the return of atrial mechanical function on the mode of cardioversion of atrial fibrillation to sinus rhythm. *Am J Cardiol* 1995;**75**:624–6.

45 Manning WJ, Leeman DE, Gotch PJ, Come PC. Pulsed Doppler evaluation of atrial mechanical function after electrical cardioversion of atrial fibrillation. *J Am Coll Cardiol* 1989;**13**:617–23.

46 Sanders P, Morton JB, Morgan JG, et al. Reversal of atrial mechanical stunning after cardioversion of atrial arrhythmias. Implications for the mechanisms of tachycardia mediated atrial cardiomyopathy. *Circulation* 2002;**106**: 1806–13.

47 Sanders P, Morton JB, Kistler PM, Vohra JK, Kalman JM, Sparks PB. Reversal of atrial mechanical dysfunction after

cardioversion of atrial fibrillation: implications for the mechanisms of tachycardia-mediated atrial cardiomyopathy. *Circulation* 2003;**108**:1976–84.

48 Lonnerholm S, Blomstrom P, Nilsson L, Blomstrom-Lundqvist C. Atrial size and transport function after the Maze III procedure for paroxysmal atrial fibrillation. *Ann Thoracic Surg* 2002;**73**:107–111.

49 Albirini A, Scalia GM, Murray RD, et al. Left and right atrial transport function after the Maze procedure for atrial fibrillation: an echocardiographic Doppler follow-up study. *J Am Soc Echocardiogr* 1997;**10**:945.

50 Thomas L, Thomas SP, Hoy M, Boyd A, Schiller NB, Ross DL. Comparison of left atrial volume and function after linear ablation and after cardioversion for chronic atrial fibrillation. *Am J Cardiol* 2004;**93**:165–70.

51 Jayam VK, Dong J, Vasamreddy CR, et al. Atrial volume reduction following catheter ablation of atrial fibrillation and relation to reduction in pulmonary vein size: an evaluation using magnetic resonance angiography. *J Interv Cardiac Electrophysiol* 2005;**13**:107–14.

52 Beukema WP, Elvan A, Sie HT, Misier AR, Wellens HJ. Successful radiofrequency ablation in patients with previous atrial fibrillation results in a significant decrease in left atrial size. *Circulation* 2005;**112**:2089–95.

53 Reant P, Lafitte S, Jais P, et al. Reverse remodeling of the left cardiac chambers after catheter ablation after 1 year in a series of patients with isolated atrial fibrillation. *Circulation* 2005;**112**:2896–903.

54 Lemola K, Desjardins B, Sneider M, et al. Effect of left atrial circumferential ablation for atrial fibrillation on left atrial transport function. *Heart Rhythm* 2005;**2**:923–8.

55 Verma A, Kilicaslan F, Adams JR, et al. Extensive ablation during pulmonary vein antrum isolation has no adverse impact on left atrial function: an echocardiography and cine computed tomography analysis. *J Cardiovasc Electrophysiol* 2006;**17**:741–6.

56 Oral H, Chugh A, Ozaydin M, et al. Risk of thromboembolic events after percutaneous left atrial radiofrequency ablation of atrial fibrillation. *Circulation* 2006;**114**:759–65.

17

CHAPTER 17

Surgery for atrial fibrillation: from scalpel to catheter . . . and back?

Fiorenzo Gaita, Antonio Montefusco, Domenico Caponi, & George J. Klein

Introduction

Atrial fibrillation (AF) is the most common sustained arrhythmia, with an overall prevalence of 4% [1]. This increases with age, ranging from 3% to 5% in people over 65 years of age and reaching 9% in those over 80 [2]. AF is more common with concomitant structural heart disease related to coronary artery disease, heart failure, hypertension, and valvular heart disease. Thirty to 50% of patients undergoing mitral valve surgery have problematic AF [3]. AF is associated with an irregular heart beat, loss of synchronous atrioventricular contraction, and stasis in the left atrium, which increase the risk of stroke and death [4].

The relative role of rhythm control versus rate control in the management of AF has remained controversial. The largest trial to compare these two therapeutic strategies, AFFIRM (Atrial Fibrillation Follow-up of Rhythm Management), failed to show any mortality or other clinical benefit for rhythm control; Nonetheless, this trial was relatively short term and failed to achieve sinus rhythm in a large percentage of the patients randomized to rhythm control. Furthermore, subanalysis suggested improved outcomes in patients in whom sinus rhythm could be maintained, thus supporting the notion that rhythm control would be superior if it could be achieved, especially without antiarrhythmic drugs [5, 6].

Electrophysiology of atrial fibrillation

In order to evaluate the various strategies for AF ablation, it may be useful to consider our understanding of the underlying pathophysiology of AF. Historically, both rapidly firing foci and reentry have been implicated as potential mechanisms [7]. Random reentry with the circuits constantly changing and seeking non-refractory tissue and the concept of the "wavelength of reentry" were subsequently popularized [8,9]. The wavelength is the distance traveled by the electrical impulse in one refractory period. Thus, the wavelength (product of the refractory period and the conduction velocity) is the shortest path length that can sustain reentry. Either reduction of refractoriness or slowing of conduction velocity or both can reduce the wavelength, thus facilitating AF. The number of reentrant circuits in the atria at one time thus depends also on atrial size. Subsequent mapping studies of the atria also showed that the probability of AF perpetuation increased with the number of reentrant wavelets [8].

Atrial mapping during AF in humans showed that certain regions had rapid and fractionated activity (presumably "drivers"), while other regions had slower, regular activity (presumably "passively" activated). Furthermore, permanent AF had more

Catheter Ablation of Atrial Fibrillation Edited by Etienne Aliot, Michel Haïssaguerre and Warren M. Jackman
© 2008 Blackwell Publishing, ISBN: 978-1-4501-6349-1.

regions with a disorganized pattern than paroxysmal AF [10,11].

The importance of local "focal" areas of rapid activity in initiating and maintaining AF has also been recently demonstrated [12–14]. It is currently believed that AF can be mechanistically heterogeneous and that both areas of local rapid activity and abnormal substrate contribute.

Surgical ablation: 20 years' evolution

In 1980, Williams et al. in Cox's laboratory reported a left atrial isolation procedure that confined AF to the left atrium while restoring the rest of the heart to sinus rhythm [15]. Based on the observation that sustained AF requires a critical mass of tissue, Guiraudon et al. introduced the corridor procedure, which was designed to isolate a strip of atrial tissue between the sinus node and the atrioventricular node. The "corridor" presumably had insufficient mass to permit AF. In such a way the sinus impulse travels along the corridor while the remaining atrial tissue remains in AF [16]. It was noted by Guiraudon that after this procedure the left atrial segment frequently remained in AF while the right atrial segments did not, supporting the view that AF, regardless of mechanism, was largely a left atrial disease. This surgery was very successful at restoring sinus rhythm but had theoretical disadvantages of the loss of left atrial kick and continued stroke risk.

Cox et al. [17] subsequently described the maze procedure, which consisted of extensive surgical dissection of both the right and left atria in order to channel the cardiac impulse through a "maze" from the sinus node throughout the atria via a relatively narrow channel incapable of sustaining AF. Clearly, in retrospect, the efficacy of this procedure was related to the isolation of a large part of the left atrium including the pulmonary veins (PVs) and the back of the left atrium and had much less to do with the actual "maze". This procedure was suggested to restore atrial contractility to some degree in spite of the extensive disruption of normal atrial activation sequence. Cox initially reported on 185 patients with a success rate of 93% and a death rate 2.2% [18]. Further experience confirmed a high success rate but a complication rate and perioperative mortality varying from 1.3% to 2.1% [19,20]. Ironically, the maze procedure of Cox and the corridor procedure of Guiraudon were more similar than was apparent since both essentially excluded the arrhythmogenic area of the left atrium. These early successes with operative therapy provided "proof of concept" and paved the way for catheter ablation [21] and less complicated techniques for operative treatment.

Operative therapy after the maze and corridor procedures

A variety of surgical procedures using "lesion sets" and differing ablative tools have since been described (Figure 17.1). All are essentially variants of the earlier procedures, achieving some element of exclusion of the PV region or individual PVs with or without added ablative lines, with the rationale of preventing macroreentrant arrhythmias circulating around the mitral valves and PVs. In general, the operative procedures required for success with persistent AF – especially associated with significant heart disease – are more extensive, incorporating additional lines and also "debulking" atrial tissue.

Sueda et al. [22] essentially excluded the PVs with incision and cryosurgery and added a lesion connecting the encircled pulmonary region to the mitral ring. Importantly, he noted a "higher frequency" of AF in the posterior left atrium suggesting that this "drove" the AF and providing a mechanistic rationale for the success of the procedure. Seventy-eight percent of patients with chronic AF and associated valvular disease remained in sinus rhythm after 18 months of follow-up, with a reduction in the left atrial diameter and some recovery of both right and left atrial contractility. Melo et al. [23] performed bilateral isolation of the PVs using epicardial radiofrequency ablation in patients with permanent AF and associated valvular mitral valve disease. After at least 3 months' follow-up, 10 of 33 patients (30%) remained in sinus rhythm, suggesting that such patients require a more extensive procedure or that the lesions were incomplete. Benussi et al. [24] encircled epicardially the right and left PVs with bipolar radiofrequency probes. Additionally, endocardial lines were performed: one connecting the two

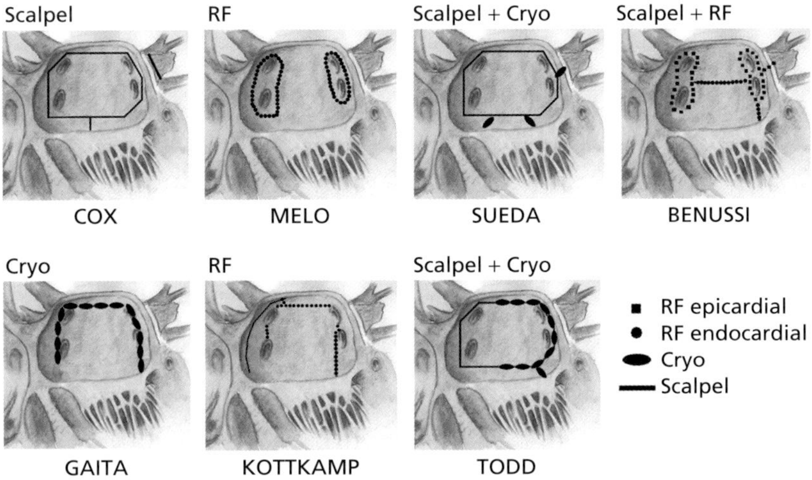

Figure 17.1 Different ablative schemes in surgical ablation of atrial fibrillation. Cryo, cryosurgery; RF, radiofrequency.

encircling lines and the other one connecting the mitral annulus to the left PV encircling line. Furthermore, the left PV encircling line was prolonged to the base of the auricle, when suture of the left atrial appendage was performed. A total of 76.9% of patients were in sinus rhythm at a follow-up of 11 ± 6 months. Gaita et al. [25] reported 32 patients with chronic AF who underwent ablation limited to posterior left atrial cryoablation during valvular heart surgery. A reversed "U" scheme consisting of lesions connecting the four PVs and the mitral annulus was performed. Ninety percent of the patients remained in sinus rhythm after a follow-up of 12 months including one patient requiring additional radiofrequency ablation for atrial tachycardia and five patients taking antiarrhythmic drugs.

With encouraging results in patients with concomitant cardiac disease, interest was kindled in operating on patients with persistent or paroxysmal AF *without* structural heart disease. Kottkamp et al. [26] performed surgical ablation in patients with persistent and paroxysmal AF in the absence of structural heart disease. His group used radiofrequency energy delivered in a unipolar mode and designed a lesion scheme consisting of a line connecting the inferior aspect of the mitral annulus to the left PV and the left lower orifice to the upper PV orifices. This was followed by a line connecting the left and right and the upper and lower right PVs. After 12 months' follow-up, 95% and 97% of patients with paroxysmal and persistent AF, respectively, were free of AF. Unfortunately, a few serious complications were reported, including esophageal perforation and left circumflex coronary artery stenosis. Todd et al. [27] performed isolation of the PVs and posterior left atrium using scalpel incision and cryosurgery. A line connecting the excluded region to the mitral ring was added. The efficacy of the isolation procedure was verified postoperatively. Fourteen patients with drug-refractory lone AF were included. Two patients had early documented recurrent arrhythmia with one showing a gap in the PV area encirclement subsequently completed by catheter ablation. This suggested the importance of complete isolation of the encircled PV area. During long-term follow-up (25.1 months), all patients remained in sinus rhythm. Cox modified the maze procedure twice [28], culminating in the maze III consisting of a surgical incision encircling the PV and a connecting incision to the mitral valve annulus plus atrial appendage excision. This, of course, closely resembled other procedures such as that of Sueda and Todd. Using the maze III procedure, Prasad et al. reported a success rate of 79.6% after a follow-up of 5.4 ± 2.7 years [29].

Although all of these procedures are somewhat variable, the central commonality of the posterior left atrial wall and the PV region is evident. This is probably the most common "culprit" region in AF [14,26,30–32]. It is also reasonably clear that ablation of this region alone is insufficient for persistent and permanent AF. It is evident that almost all the schemes used in surgical ablation for AF involved the PVs. Even when the intended aim was pure modification of the substrate [26,33], it is difficult to claim that the results were totally unrelated to PV isolation. To define the best surgical lesion scheme and to clarify the role of PV isolation, a study was designed to compare three different ablation schemes: (i) a reversed "U" linear cryoablation interconnecting the PV ostia and the right and left lower PVs down to the mitral annulus; (ii) a "7" linear cryoablation interconnecting the PV ostia and the left lower PV only down to the mitral annulus; and (iii) anatomic isolation of the PVs performed just around the PV ostia [34]. At 24 months, sinus rhythm without antiarrhythmic drugs was present in 57% of the first two groups, and in only 20% of the PV isolation group. Carto® mapping after the procedure further showed that the intended lesion was achieved by the surgeon only about 50% of the time. It is noteworthy that when linear lesions connecting the four PVs and the mitral annulus (the "7" scheme) were obtained and confirmed, sinus rhythm without any drugs was achieved long term in 86% of the cases [34], while sinus rhythm was achieved only in 25% of patients with a complete electrical isolation of the PVs (Figure 17.2). In permanent AF with valvular heart disease, PV isolation alone is insufficient. This requirement for lesions in addition to PV isolation is also evident in catheter ablation experience

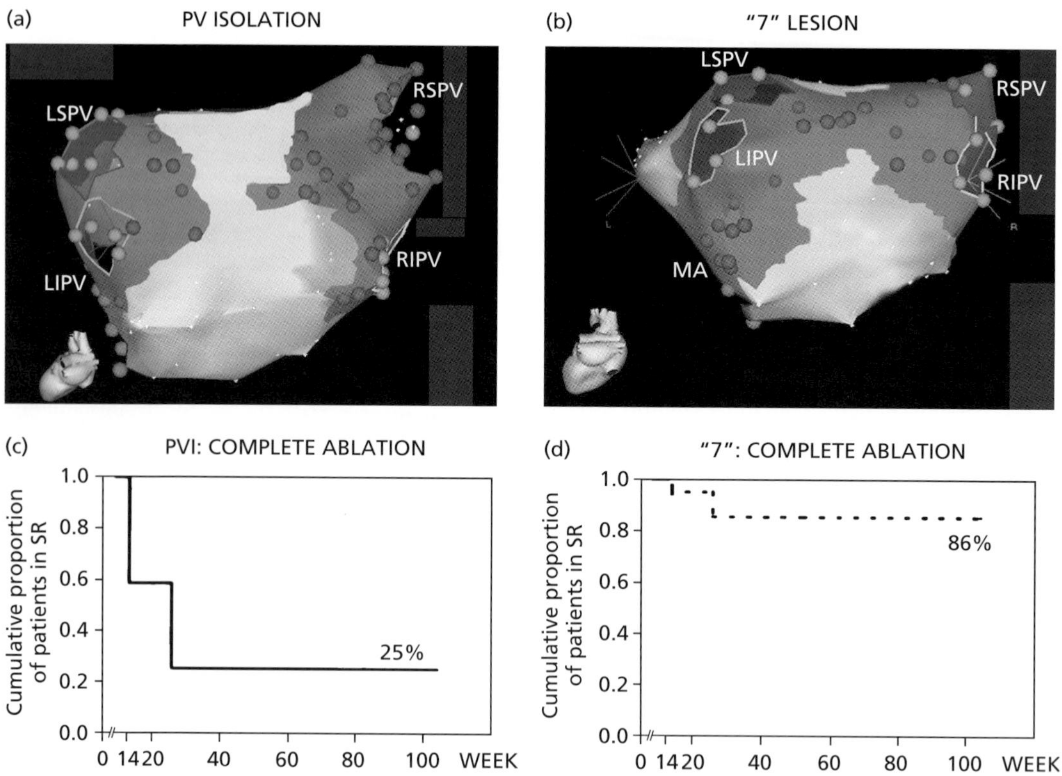

Figure 17.2 (a, b) Ablation lines created during surgical cryoablation. The three-dimensional representations of the left atrium and PVs were obtained with Carto™. (a) Modified posteroanterior view of a gray-coded map in a patient who underwent PV encircling surgical ablation. (b) Modified posteroanterior view of a gray-coded map of a patient who underwent a "7" lesion surgical ablation. (c, d) Long-term follow-up in patients who underwent electroanatomic mapping showing the cumulative proportions of patients in sinus rhythm (SR) without the addition of antiarrhythmic drugs in whom complete PV isolation (c) and "7" lesion (d) were demonstrated. LIPV, left inferior pulmonary vein; LSPV, left superior pulmonary vein; MA: mitral annulus; RIPV, right inferior pulmonary vein; RSPV, right superior pulmonary vein.

in patients with permanent and persistent AF [35–39].

Despite the success of catheter ablation, a simple and safe procedure of ablation to eliminate AF in all patients is not available. This explains the continued interest of surgeons in a minimally invasive procedure [40,41]. Epicardial, minimally invasive, and thoracoscopic procedures offer the advantages of direct visualization of the structures and epicardial ablation eliminates the need for cardiopulmonary bypass. Operative ablation also offers simple left atrial appendage excision, potentially reducing the risk of stroke. PV isolation and excision of the left atrial appendage has been performed using a minimally invasive "keyhole approach" or thoracoscopically without bypass [41,42]. Early results are encouraging with an 80–90% success rate at 6 months' follow-up [41].

Ablative tools

The original operative tool was of course "cut and sew", which has been effective in isolating arrhythmogenic tissue but is considered to be more time-consuming, operator-dependent, and associated with more bleeding. Other tools to ablate atrial tissue have been developed with goals of efficacy, safety, speed, and ease of use. In general, ablation tools can be classified as destroying tissue by heat ("sizzle": radiofrequency, laser, ultrasound, microwave) or by freezing. The former technologies are generally fast and effective but are potentially associated with more collateral damage, while the latter have been slower and more prone to recovery of tissue vitality if not used effectively. While better tools will continue to be developed, they are probably less important than the skill and rationale of the operator.

Radiofrequency

Radiofrequency is the most commonly used technique and employs an alternating electrical current of 100 KHz to 1 MHz to heat and ablate tissue. Several different radiofrequency catheter systems are available, including long flexible probes, rigid probes, pencil-like probes with a cooled tip, and a probe configured as a bipolar clamp. They may be applied endocardially, epicardially, or both simultaneously. The epicardial approach is potentially subject to incomplete endocardial lesion formation due to the cooling effect of blood flow. There is also some concern about collateral damage to surrounding structures such as the esophagus, bronchi, and coronary arteries. Esophageal injury has been reported with unipolar devices, generally following endocardial ablation [26], and it is possible that the risk of this is less with bipolar systems.

Microwaves

Microwaves ablate by heating, causing oscillation of water molecules in tissue and converting electromagnetic energy into heat. The lesion depth is said to be more accurately controlled, improving the probability of transmural lesions. Microwave heating from the endocardium does not cause endocardial surface charring, which may reduce the risk of thromboembolism, but the lesion needs to be accurately "focused" to avoid collateral injury

Cryothermy

Cryothermy ablates by freezing tissue. Cooling is provided by several systems, including expanding nitrous oxide and argon-based systems. Cryoenergy ablates tissue preserving the collagen matrix. Lesions created by cryothermy are dense and homogeneous without charring, potentially reducing the risk of thromboembolism and avoiding damage to surrounding structures (coronary arteries, esophagus, bronchus). The disadvantages potentially include a longer energy application time and reversibility of the lesion if the target temperature is not obtained for complete tissue kill.

High intensity focused ultrasound

High intensity focused ultrasound (HIFU) uses tubular transducers to deliver focused cylindrical zones of ultrasonic waves to produce lesions around PVs. It injures tissue by causing cells to oscillate and generate sufficient heat to destroy tissue. It is apparently capable of ablating atrial myocardium and epicardial fat with equal efficiency, providing a theoretical advantage for epicardial ablation.

Conclusion

Operative ablation of AF is well established and justified in most patients with paroxysmal or persistent AF undergoing cardiac surgery for other reasons. In general, the operative procedure required for AF is centered around some type of PV area exclusion with the addition of other lines and/or atrial debulking for longstanding and well-established AF with significant heart disease. Operative therapy appears especially appropriate in patients with mitral valve disease with tissue valve replacement or valvuloplasty where restoration of sinus rhythm may improve atrial contractility and even obviate the need for anticoagulants in some patients. In patients undergoing non-valvular heart surgery, surgical ablation of AF may well be considered if there is any clinical history of AF, although the benefit of a truly prophylactic concomitant procedure needs to be established.

Good results have been reported with a variety of techniques centered around the PV area and with a variety of ablation tools. It is likely that this type of therapy will continue to evolve with better tools and more widespread use of thoracoscopic techniques. If so, operative therapy may become a serious alternative to catheter ablation, even in patients who do not require a concomitant cardiac procedure [40–42].

References

1 Furberg CD, Psaty BM, Manolio TA, Gardin JM, Smith VE, Rautaharju PM. Prevalence of atrial fibrillation in elderly subjects (the Cardiovascular Health Study). *Am J Cardiol* 1994;**74**(3):236–41.

2 Kannel WB, Wolf PA, Benjamin EJ, Levy D. Prevalence, incidence, prognosis, and predisposing conditions for atrial fibrillation: population-based estimates. *Am J Cardiol* 1998;**82**(8A):2N–9N.

3 Bando K, Kobayashi J, Kosakai Y, et al. Impact of Cox maze procedure on outcome in patients with atrial fibrillation and mitral valve disease. *J Thoracic Cardiovasc Surg* 2002;**124**(3):575–83.

4 Rockson SG, Albers GW. Comparing the guidelines: anticoagulation therapy to optimize stroke prevention in patients with atrial fibrillation. *J Am Coll Cardiol* 2004; **43**(6):929–35.

5 Wyse DG, Waldo AL, Di Marco JP, et al. A comparison of rate control and rhythm control in patients with atrial fibrillation. Investigators. *N Engl J Med* 2002;**347**(23): 1825–33.

6 Corley SD, Epstein AE, DiMarco JP, et al. Relationships between sinus rhythm, treatment, and survival in the Atrial Fibrillation Follow-up Investigation of Rhythm Management (AFFIRM) study. *Circulation* 2004;**109**(12): 1509–13.

7 Moe GK, Rheinboldt WC, Abildskov JA. A computer model of atrial fibrillation. *Am Heart J* 1964;**67**:200–20.

8 Allessie MA, Bonke FI, Schopman FJ. Circus movement in rabbit atrial muscle as a mechanism of tachycardia III. The "leading circle" concept: a new model of circus movement in cardiac tissue without the involvement of an anatomical obstacle. *Circ Res* 1977;**41**:9–18.

9 Allessie MA, Lammers WJEP, Bonke FIM. Experimental evaluation of Moe's multiple wavelet hypothesis of atrial fibrillation. In: Zipes DP, Jalife J., eds. *Cardiac Electrophysiology and Arrhythmias*. Grune & Strutton, New York, 1985:265–75.

10 Gaita F, Calò L, Riccardi R, et al. Different patterns of atrial activation in idiopathic atrial fibrillation. Simultaneous multisite atrial mapping in patients with paroxysmal and chronic atrial fibrillation. *J Am Coll Cardiol* 2001;**37**:534–41.

11 Jais P, Haissaguerre M, Shah DC, et al. Regional disparities of endocardial atrial activation in paroxysmal atrial fibrillation. *Pacing Clin Electrophysiol* 1996;**19**(11 Pt 2): 1998–2003.

12 Mandapati R, Skanes A, Chen J, et al. Stable microreentrant sources as a mechanism of atrial fibrillation in the isolated sheep heart. *Circulation* 2000;**101**;194–9.

13 Nattel S, Li D, Yue L. Basic mechanism of atrial fibrillation – very new insights into very old ideas. *Annu Rev Physiol* 2000;**62**:51–77.

14 Haissaguerre M, Jais P, Shah D, et al. Spontaneous initiation of atrial fibrillation by ectopic beats originating in the pulmonary veins. *N Engl J Med* 1998;**339**:659–66.

15 Williams JM, Ungerleider RM, Lofland GK, Cox JL. Left atrial isolation: new technique for the treatment of supraventricular arrhythmias. *Thoracic Cardiovasc Surg* 1980;**80**(3):373–80.

16 Guiraudon GM, Campbell CS, Jones DL, et al. Combined sino-atrial node atrio-ventricular node isolation: a surgical alternative to His bundle ablation in patients with atrial fibrillation. *Circulation* 1985;**72**(Suppl 3):220 (abstract).

17 Cox JL, Canavan TE, Schuessler RB, et al. The surgical treatment of atrial fibrillation. Intraoperative electrophysiologic mapping and description of the electrophysiologic basis of atrial flutter and atrial fibrillation. *J Thoracic Cardiovasc Surg* 1991;**101**:406–26.

18 Cox JL, Schuiessler RB, Lappas DG, et al. An 8 1/2-year clinical experience with surgery for atrial fibrillation. *Ann Surg* 1996;**224**:267–73.

19 McCarthy PM, Gillinov AM, Castle L, Chung M, Cosgrove D, III. The Cox-maze procedure: the Cleveland Clinic experience. *Semin Thoracic Cardiovasc Surg* 2000;**12**(1):25–9.

20 Schaff HV, Dearani JA, Daly RC, Orszulak TA, Danielson GK. Cox-maze procedure for atrial fibrillation: Mayo Clinic experience. *Semin Thoracic Cardiovasc Surg* 2000; **12**(1):30–7.

21 Schwartz JF, Pellersel G, Silvers J. A catheter based curative approach to atrial fibrillation in humans. *Circulation* 1994;**90**(4 Pt 2):1–335.

22 Sueda T, Nagata H, Orihashi K, Morita S, Okada K, Sueshiro M. Efficacy of a simple left atrial procedure for chronic atrial fibrillation in mitral valve operations. *Ann Thoracic Surg* 1997;**63**:1070–5.

23 Melo J, Andragao P, Neves J, et al. Surgery for atrial fibrillation using radiofrequency catheter ablation: assessment of results at one year. *Eur J Cardiothoracic Surg* 1999; **15**:851–5.

24 Benussi S, Pappone C, Nasimbene S, et al. A simple way to treat chronic atrial fibrillation during mitral valve surgery: the epicardial radiofrequency approach. *Eur J Cardiothoracic Surg* 2000;**17**(5):524–9.

25 Gaita F, Gallotti R, Calò L, et al. Limited posterior left atrial cryoablation in patients with chronic atrial fibrillation undergoing valvular heart surgery. *J Am Coll Cardiol* 2000;**36**:159–66.

26 Kottkamp H, Hindricks G, Autschbach R, et al. Specific linear left atrial lesions in atrial fibrillation intraoperative radiofrequency ablation using minimally invasive surgical techniques. *J Am Coll Cardiol* 2002;**40**(3):475–80.

27 Todd DM, Skanes AC, Guiraudon G, Guiraudon C, Krahn AD, Yee R, Klein GJ. Role of the posterior left atrium and pulmonary veins in human lone atrial fibrillation: electrophysiological and pathological data from patients undergoing atrial fibrillation surgery. *Circulation* 2003;**108**(25):3108–14.

28 Cox JL, Boineau JP, Schuessler RB, Jaquiss RD, Lappas DG. Modification of the maze procedure for atrial flutter and atrial fibrillation. I. Rationale and surgical results. *J Thoracic Cardiovasc Surg* 1995;**110**(2):473–84.

29 Prasad SM, Maniar HS, Camillo CJ, et al. The Cox maze III procedure for atrial fibrillation: long-term efficacy in patients undergoing lone versus concomitant procedures. *J Thoracic Cardiovasc Surg* 2003;**126**(6):1822–8.

30 Jais P, Haissaguerre M, Shah DC, et al. Regional disparities of endocardial atrial activation in paroxysmal atrial fibrillation. *Pacing Clin Electrophysiol* 1996;**19**(11 Pt 2): 1998–2003.

31 Gaita F, Calò L, Riccardi R, et al. Different patterns of atrial activation in idiopathic atrial fibrillation. Simultaneous multisite atrial mapping in patients with paroxysmal and chronic atrial fibrillation. *J Am Coll Cardiol* 2001;**37**:534–41

32 Haissaguerre M, Shah DC, Jais P, et al. Electrophysiological breakthroughs from the left atrium to the pulmonary veins. *Circulation* 2000;**102**(20):2463–5.

33 Gaita F, Riccardi R, Gallotti R. Surgical approaches to atrial fibrillation. *Cardiac Electrophysiol Rev* 2002;**6**: 401–5.

34 Gaita F, Riccardi R, Caponi D, et al. Linear cryoablation of the left atrium versus pulmonary vein cryoisolation in patients with permanent atrial fibrillation and valvular heart disease: correlation of electroanatomic mapping and long-term clinical results. *Circulation* 2005;**111**(2): 136–42.

35 Pappone C, Oreto G, Rosanio S, et al. Atrial electroanatomic remodeling after circumferential radiofrequency pulmonary vein ablation: efficacy of an anatomic approach in a large cohort of patients with atrial fibrillation. *Circulation* 2001;**104**(21):2539–44.

36 Oral H, Knight BP, Ozaydin M, et al. Segmental ostial ablation to isolate the pulmonary veins during atrial fibrillation: feasibility and mechanistic insights. *Circulation* 2002;**106**(10):1256–62.

37 Lim TW, Jassal IS, Ross DL, Thomas SP. Medium-term efficacy of segmental ostial pulmonary vein isolation for the treatment of permanent and persistent atrial fibrillation. *Pacing Clin Electrophysiol* 2006;**29**(4):374–9.

38 Oral H, Pappone C, Chugh A, et al. Circumferential pulmonary-vein ablation for chronic atrial fibrillation. *N Engl J Med* 2006;**354**(9):934–41.

39 Jais P, Hocini M, Hsu LF, et al. Technique and results of linear ablation at the mitral isthmus. *Circulation* 2004; **110**(19):2996–3002.

40 Saltman AE, Rosenthal LS, Francalancia NA, Lahey SJ. A completely endoscopic approach to microwave ablation for atrial fibrillation. *Heart Surg Forum* 2003; **6**(3):E38–41.

41 Pruitt JC, Lazzara RR, Dworkin GH, Badhwar V, Kuma C, Ebra G. Totally endoscopic ablation of lone atrial fibrillation: initial clinical experience. *Roy Ann Thoracic Surg* 2006;**81**(4):1325–30

42 Balkhy HH, Chapman PD, Arnsdorf SE. Minimally invasive atrial fibrillation ablation combined with a new technique for thoracoscopic stapling of the left atrial appendage: case report. *Heart Surg Forum* 2004;**7**(6): 353–5.

18

CHAPTER 18

Electrogram-guided approach to ablation of atrial fibrillation

David J. Wilber, Joseph Akar, Peter Santucci, & Neil Brysiewicz

Introduction

Catheter-based strategies for ablation of atrial fibrillation (AF) have evolved considerably since the initial successful adaptation of the Cox surgical maze procedure to a percutaneous approach by Swartz and colleagues in 1994 [1]. The identification of rapid repetitive discharges from the pulmonary veins (PVs) as initiating and perpetuating triggers for AF by Haïssaguerre and colleagues in 1998 refocused attention on the importance of the musculature of the PVs and periostial atrium in the genesis of AF [2]. Subsequent investigations confirmed the structural and electrophysiological complexities of this region, capable of supporting automaticity, triggered activity, and small reentrant circuits [3–5], and highly sensitive to autonomic modulation [6,7]. Current consensus of experienced investigators involved in AF ablation indicates that electrical isolation of the PVs and a variable portion of the surrounding posterior left atrium (PV antra) should remain a cornerstone for most AF ablation procedures [8].

However, PV/antral isolation alone is associated with subsequent AF recurrence in 20–40% of patients with paroxysmal AF (PAF), and 40–70% of patients with AF of longstanding (> 1 year) duration after a single procedure [8–10]. A substantial portion of recurrences appear to be related to electrical reconnection through previously isolated areas [11–13], with improvement in secondary AF-free survival following repeat PV/antral isolation. Focal sources for initiating and maintaining AF remote from the PVs are also identified [14], and may be more prevalent in patients with persistent or chronic AF [15]. These data have prompted a continued search for adjunctive/alternative strategies to improve outcomes. Linear lesions connecting the PVs to other anatomic barriers (mitral isthmus, left atrial roof, septum, and/or anterior left atrium) have been demonstrated to provide incremental improvements in ablation outcome over PV isolation alone [16,17]. However, conduction block across these lines is often difficult to attain, and regions of incomplete block may be proarrhythmic. For these reasons, recent attention has focused on local electrogram characteristics as a means of identifying atrial sites remote from the PVs responsible for the perpetuation of AF, and hence suitable targets for ablation.

Genesis and significance of fractionated atrial electrograms

Routine conventional isochronal activation mapping of AF is problematic due to the number, small size, and complexity of propagating wavefronts, as well as the requirement for simultaneous dense recordings over large regions of atrial myocardium. Early mapping studies indicated that electrogram

Catheter Ablation of Atrial Fibrillation Edited by Etienne Aliot, Michel Haïssaguerre and Warren M. Jackman

characteristics at individual sites may be linked to specific conduction patterns during AF. In a study of dense right atrial epicardial mapping of human AF during surgery, Konings and colleagues described three types of local atrial electrograms: (1) single deflections, associated with rapid uniform conduction; (2) double potentials, associated with lines of collision or conduction block; and (3) fragmented potentials (multiple deflections with prolonged duration), associated with regions of slow conduction, pivot points, and wave turning [18,19]. During biatrial endocardial catheter mapping of AF, Jais et al. observed that complex atrial electrograms (defined as continuous atrial activity, or electrograms separated by < 100 ms) demonstrated significant spatial and temporal heterogeneity, and were most frequently found in the posterior and septal regions of both atria [20]. Anisotropic conduction in regions of complex changes in local fiber orientation [21–23], enhanced by age-related increases in collagenous septa that diminish side-to-side coupling [24], may also contribute to the appearance of local fractionated extracellular potentials during AF. Such sites could signify the substrate for small reentrant circuits, or, alternatively, regions where wave break and slow conduction occur driven by wavefronts originating elsewhere in the atria.

More recent experimental data obtained during cholinergic AF in isolated perfused sheep hearts demonstrate that AF may be maintained by a single or small number of stable, organized, high frequency drivers or rotors corresponding to rapid vortex-like reentry around a core of 1–2 mm in the posterior left atrium, with subsequent wave break and fibrillatory conduction to the remainder of the atrium [25]. While electrograms recorded from the highest frequency region (rotor) were organized and regular, electrogram disorganization and fractionation was most prominent at the immediate periphery between this region and sites with lower frequencies and lower levels of organization [25,26]. These data suggest that fractionated atrial electrograms are intimately associated with, though not identical to, sites responsible for the genesis and maintenance of AF. Additional data indicate that the frequency and location of fractionation and adjacent drivers are influenced by the pattern and distribution of myocardial fibrosis [27].

Finally, accumulating evidence suggests that fractionated electrograms are strongly influenced by autonomic stimulation and activation of the intrinsic cardiac autonomic nervous system. The latter is composed of regional ganglionated plexi on the epicardial surface of the heart that are highly interconnected and with axonal projections within the atrial subepicardium (28–30). The gangionated plexuses contain both afferent sensory fibers, and sympathetic and parasympathetic efferents. In the left atrium, the ganglia are aggregated in four major regions: (1) anterior to the right PVs and extending into the interatrial septum; (2) inferior and medial to the right PVs; (3) between the left inferior PV and the mitral annulus; and (4) superior and medial to the left PVs (Figure 18.1). Experimental studies demonstrate that activation of this network plays an important role in PV-mediated AF [6,7,31–33].

Locally applied acetylcholine can produce electrogram fractionation during AF, as can injections of acetylcholine or electrical stimulation of the autonomic ganglia [29,32,33]. Destruction of the ganglia alone without myocardial ablation results in organization of electrograms and termination of AF. While fractionation is most common and extensive in the endocardium adjacent to the ganglionated plexuses, it can also be observed at more remote sites [29,32]. Clinical studies indicate that many, though not all, sites with complex fractionated electrograms observed during AF co-localize with sites of ganglionated plexuses [34–36]. High frequency stimulation at endocardial sites can elicit vagal efferent responses, and serve to locate ganglionated plexuses [35,37,38]. Ablation at sites that produce this response is reported to have had a favorable effect on the outcome of ablation for paroxymal AF, particularly as an adjunct to PV isolation [37–40]. These data raise the possibility that at least some forms of electrogram fractionation may be an epiphenomenon, representing activation of the intrinsic cardiac autonomic ganglia, rather than identifying specific anatomic substrates for AF perpetuation. Electrogram fractionation at the posterior left atrium near the PV ostia may represent a marker for the location of the ganglionated plexuses. Such sites may be incorporated into various PV isolation strategies, particularly those that extend some distance from

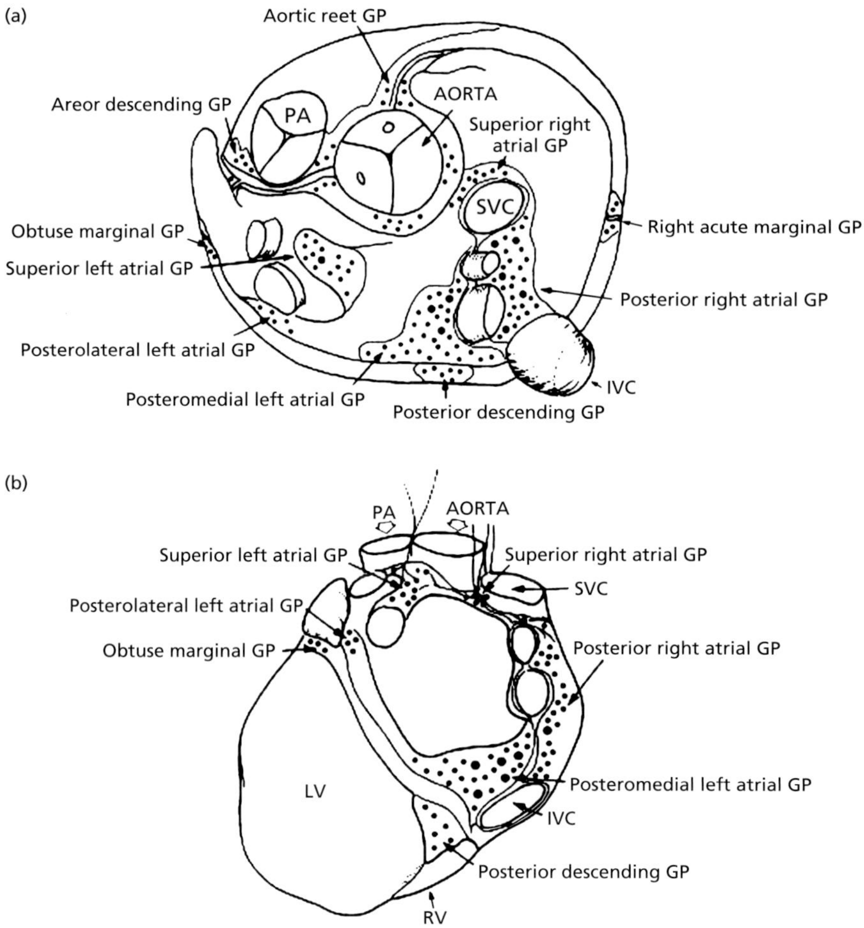

Figure 18.1 Distribution of ganglionated plexuses in the human atria: (a) superior view, and (b) posterior view. GP, ganglionated plexus; IVC, inferior vena cava; LV, left ventricle; PA, pulmonary artery; RV, right ventricle; SVC, superior vena cava. (From [28].)

the PV ostia, and may contribute to the success of PV isolation.

Collectively, these data provide a number of *potential* mechanisms by which complex fractionated atrial electrograms (CFAEs) are generated (Table 18.1). Some of these mechanisms suggest that CFAE sites represent or are closely adjacent to structures critical to the maintenance of AF, while others indicate a more passive role. Multiple mechanisms (and both active and passive) may coexist in the same patient at different sites or times. Rostock and colleagues described dynamic changes in visually identified CFAEs during 60 s recordings of AF at multiple sites during PAF [41]. CFAEs appeared primarily and transiently during periods of local acceleration of the AF rate. Dense local activation mapping around CFAE sites indicated that, in most instances, all local sites accelerated nearly simultaneously with the onset of CFAEs, most compatible with a passive process whereby remote drivers accelerate local myocardium beyond its refractoriness, leading to wave break and fractionation. A minority of sites demonstrated complex local activation patterns occasionally spanning a majority of the local AF cycle length, potentially reflecting a more active local process perpetuating AF (Figure 18.2). These data indicate that all CFAEs may not be the same, and that additional criteria of stability over time, relationship to activity at adjacent sites, and local AF cycle length may all play a role in differentiating sites critical to AF maintenance.

Table 18.1 Potential significance of fractionated electrograms during AF.

Sites of reentrant circuit pivot points, wave turning, and slow conduction
Sites of anisotropic conduction and/or reentry
Sites of wave break at the periphery of high frequency organized rotors
Sites of local autonomic innervation and activation

Targeting complex fractionated atrial electrograms as a primary ablation strategy

Nademanee et al. were the first to propose that targeting sites with fractionated atrial electrograms could be an effective primary strategy for AF ablation [42]. They defined CFAEs as low amplitude, multicomponent potentials (generally 0.05–0.25 mV) that are either continuous or separated by short isoelectric intervals (< 120 ms) averaged over a 10 s recording interval (Figure 18.3). The investigators hypothesized that these sites signified critical anatomic regions that perpetuate reentry. During AF, CFAE sites were most commonly located at the interatrial septum (57%), around the PV ostia (40%), at the proximal coronary sinus (32%), on the roof of the left atrium (32%), and around the mitral annulus (23%). Less common sites were located in the right atrium (crista terminalis, superior vena cava, and appendage). The occurrence of CFAEs at these sites appeared to be stable over the duration of the ablation session. While a proportion of patients had CFAEs in only one or two regions (more common in patients with PAF), a majority had sites in three or more areas. Of note, these investigators used relatively high power (up to 70 W) and extensive ablation of left atrial sites (mean 65 ± 36 radiofrequency applications, range 7–168).

As evidence of an important role in AF maintenance, CFAE ablation resulted in the termination of spontaneous or induced AF (either to sinus, or to an organized atrial tachycardia) in 86% of 57 patients with PAF, and 63% of 64 patients with

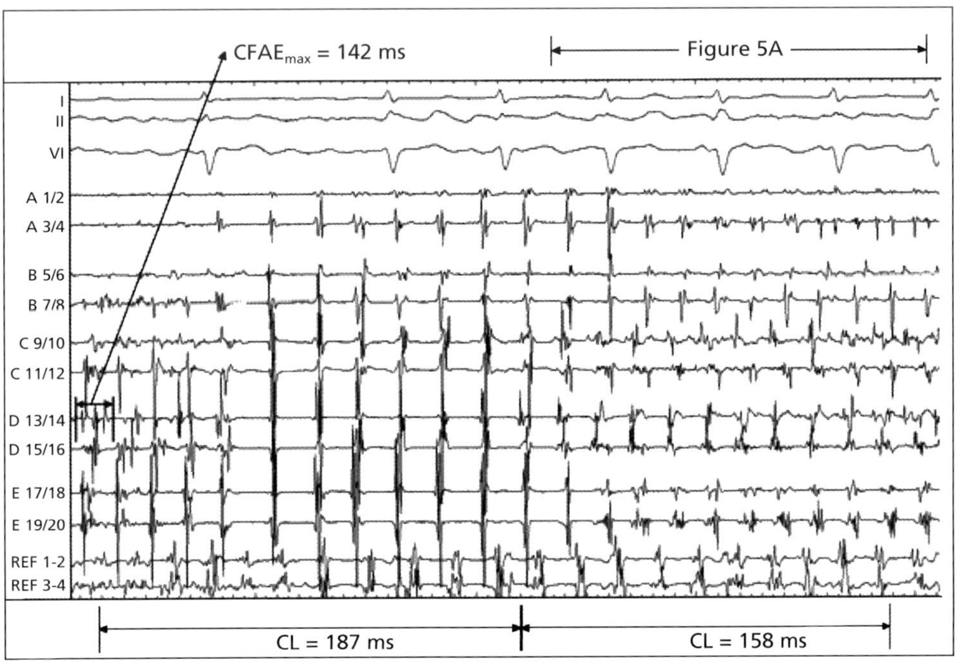

Figure 18.2 Cycle length (CL) dependence of electrogram fractionation. Note the complex, non-simultaneous activation pattern on the right hand side of the panel. See text for additional details. (From [41].)

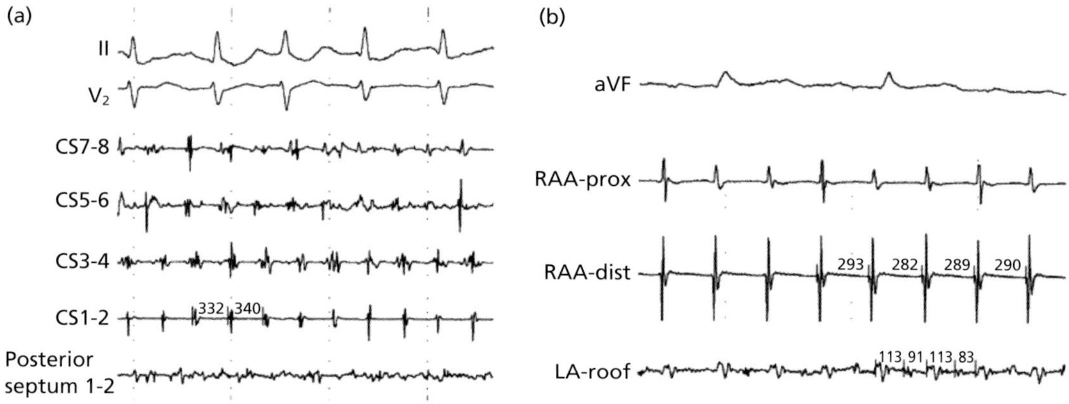

Figure 18.3 Examples of complex fractionated atrial electrograms as defined by Nademanee: (a) continuous fractionated electrical activity, and (b) multicomponent electrograms separated by short (< 120 ms) isoelectric intervals. CS, coronary sinus; LA, left atrium; RAA, right atrial appendage. (From [42].)

persistent/chronic AF [42]. Non-inducibility of AF was used as an additional endpoint for paroxysmal but not persistent AF. During ablation, the endpoint was elimination of fractionated activity, and the authors noted progressive organization of surrounding sites and lengthening of the AF cycle length prior to termination in a majority of patients. When AF converted to an organized atrial arrhythmia (either focal tachycardia or flutter), additional ablation was required before sinus rhythm was achieved. In approximately 15% of patients, additional CFAE sites in the right atrium were ablated. At 1 year of follow-up, 76% of patients were free of symptomatic atrial tachyarrhythmias without antiarrhythmic drugs (AADs), and an additional 15% were AF-free after a second procedure with or without AADs. Of note, more than 70% of recurrences were organized atrial tachycardias rather than AF. These latter tachycardias may have been unmasked in atria that could no longer fibrillate, or represent a proarrhythmic result of residual channels between regions of CFAE ablation.

Nademanee and colleagues recently updated their experience with primary CFAE ablation in an additional 303 patients [43,44]. Of 141 patients with PAF, 83% had acute termination of AF and subsequent non-inducibility; 71% were free of recurrent atrial arrhythmias after a single procedure, and 91% after multiple procedures during long-term follow-up (10% on AADs). Of 161 patients with chronic AF, termination occurred during CFAE ablation in 58%; 57% were free of recurrent atrial arrhythmias after a single procedure, and 85% after multiple procedures (18% on AADs). Similar to their original observations, a majority of recurrences were due to organized atrial arrhythmias rather than AF.

Oral et al. found substantially lower efficacy with CFAE ablation as a primary strategy in 100 consecutive patients with persistent or chronic AF [45]. These investigators employed similar CFAE definitions to the Nademanee study, with an endpoint of voltage reduction to < 0.10 mV. Predominant locations of CFAEs were the anterior atrium in 91%, around the PV ostia (90%), the left septum (75%), the left atrial roof (64%), and the coronary sinus (55%). However, AF terminated during CFAE ablation in only 16% of patients, and only 33% of patients were free of recurrent atrial tachyarrhythmias off AADs during a mean follow-up of 14 ± 7 months. Termination during CFAE ablation did not predict long-term success. Organized atrial tachycardias occurred in 26% of patients during follow-up. Repeat ablation targeting of CFAE sites was performed in 44 patients; these sites were often located near PVs that had no CFAEs at the first ablation. Overall, including repeat procedures, long-term success was achieved in 57% of patients. These investigators concluded that concomitant PV isolation at the time of the initial procedure might have reduced the risk of recurrent arrhythmias, and that CFAE ablation as the sole strategy was not more effective than alternative approaches to chronic AF.

The strikingly dissimilar outcome between the two groups is not easily reconciled. Differences in the extent and duration of radiofrequency applications, mapping density, and pursuit of organized atrial tachycardias at the end of the initial ablation session have all been raised as potential explanations [44]. At this point in time, the role of CFAE ablation as a primary and sole strategy for chronic AF remains controversial.

Targetting complex fractionated atrial electrograms as an adjunct ablation strategy

Several groups have explored the potential role of CFAE ablation as an adjunct to PV isolation strategies in order to improve long-term outcomes and minimize the need for repeat procedures. Oral et al. examined the utility of adding visually identified CFAE ablation to patients with PAF in whom anatomic circumferential PV isolation and linear lesions in the posterior atrium and mitral isthmus failed to eliminate inducible AF [46]. In 60 of 100 consecutive patients, this criterion was met. These patients were randomized to either no further ablation or to additional CFAE ablation in the left atrial roof, septum, and/or anterior wall. AF was rendered non-inducible in 90% of patients undergoing additional CFAE ablation; 86% of patients undergoing CFAE ablation remained free of recurrent atrial arrhythmias without AADs compared to 67% of patients without additional ablation ($P = 0.05$). In a subsequent study of 153 patients with PAF by the same group, a "tailored" strategy was followed, whereby all patients initially underwent ablation of arrhythmogenic PVs (focal, segmental ostial, or circumferential) [47]. In 106 patients (69%) with persistently inducible or spontaneous AF, additional ablation of visually identified CFAE sites in the left atrium, coronary sinus, and/or right atrium was performed, though this resulted in non-inducibility of AF in only 40%. At a mean follow-up of 11 ± 4 months, 77% of patients were free of recurrent arrhythmias without AADs. The extent to which all CFAE sites were systematically sought and identified in these studies is unclear.

Schmitt and colleagues examined the frequency of acute termination during ablation of visually identified CFAEs in 36 patients with PAF and 30 patients with chronic AF [48]. Acute termination was observed in 32 (89%) patients with PAF (19 to sinus rhythm, and 13 to an organized atrial tachycardia), and in 24 (80%) patients with persistent AF (nine to sinus rhythm, and eight to an organized atrial tachycardia). The most common sites of termination in order of frequency were adjacent to the PV ostia, the anterior left atrium adjacent to the appendage, the septum, the posterior mitral annulus, the coronary sinus ostium, and the left atrial roof. Ablation of organized atrial tachycardia was not undertaken, but all patients subsequently underwent circumferential PV isolation at the left atrium–PV junction. During a mean follow-up of 12 ± 3 months, 65% of PAF patients and 54% of chronic AF patients remained in sinus rhythm without AADs.

Two preliminary reports described the impact of CFAE ablation as an adjunct strategy employing computerized on-line automated detection algorithms (discussed in detail below). We found that CFAE ablation alone resulted in acute termination of spontaneous or induced AF in 85% of 34 patients with PAF but in only 10% of patients with persistent/chronic AF [49]. All patients underwent additional ablation following CFAE (wide area PV isolation in PAF patients; wide area PV isolation + mitral and roof linear lesions for persistent AF). At 6 months follow-up, 88% of PAF and 75% of chronic AF patients remained in sinus rhythm without AADs after a single procedure. Verma and colleagues used CFAE ablation as an adjunct to PV antral isolation in patients with PAF ($n = 21$) or persistent/chronic AF ($n = 14$) [50]. Initial CFAE ablation regularized AF in 86% of patients (and resulted in termination of AF or flutter in 57%). After a single procedure, the AAD-free success rate was 83% at a mean follow-up of 10 ± 4 months. A randomized trial of segmental ostial PV isolation alone versus ostial isolation ± CFAE ablation is underway at three German centers [51], but long-term outcome has not yet been reported.

Preliminary findings of randomized studies evaluating adjunctive visually detected CFAE ablation in patients with both paroxysmal and chronic AF have been recently reported. Di Biase et al. found a similar outcome in AF-free survival at 1 year in patients with PAF undergoing PV antral isolation alone, compared to antral isolation combined with CFAE ablation [52]. In contrast, Elayi et al. reported that in patients with persistent/chronic AF, single procedure AF-free survival was 61% in patients undergoing both PV antral isolation and CFAE ablation compared to 42% in patients undergoing antral isolation alone during a mean follow-up of 11 ± 1 months [53]. In the Bordeaux experience with persistent AF, ablation of left atrial sites with CFAEs (particularly along the inferior mitral annulus, within the coronary sinus, and anteromedial to the left atrial appendage) contributed to the progressive slowing of AF cycle length and the termination of AF in 87% of patients during a stepwise approach that also incorporated PV isolation and linear lesions [15,54].

The value of adjunctive CFAE ablation in patients with PAF treated by PV isolation remains unclear, though several studies suggest an additive benefit. The utility of CFAE ablation may be in part related to the extent of the posterior left atrium outside the PVs ablated during ostial, wide area, or antral isolation. Many CFAE sites are within 2–3 cm of the PV ostia [35,42,43], and may be incorporated within the lesions sets of more extensive, particularly antral, approaches to PV isolation. In patients with persistent AF, the success of PV isolation alone is more limited; preliminary data suggest that adjunctive CFAE ablation may play an important emerging role.

Automated detection and classification of complex fractionated atrial electrograms

Most clinical studies to date have relied on subjective and qualitative visual assessment of local electrograms to determine the presence of CFAEs during AF. This approach is highly dependent on operator experience and judgment. None of the published studies have provided measures of inter- or intraobserver variability, and the reproducibility of subjective classification is unknown. An objective quantitative approach would facilitate the comparison of outcomes between investigators, refinement of "high yield" criteria, and a shortened learning curve for new operators.

Computerized algorithms for the automated detection and quantitation of CFAEs have been introduced as integrated modules in three-dimensional mapping systems by both Biosense Webster (Carto®) [49,55,56], and St. Jude Medical (NavX®) [50,57,58]. Both algorithms employ automated identification of low amplitude multi-component complexes, and some measure of local cycle lengths. In the Biosense Webster algorithm, a 2.5 s window is analyzed and CFAE complexes are identified by threshold voltages (programmable, nominally 0.05–1.5 mV) and "isoelectric" intervals (programmable, nominally 60–120 ms) (Figure 18.4). The repetitiveness of CFAE signals (and hence

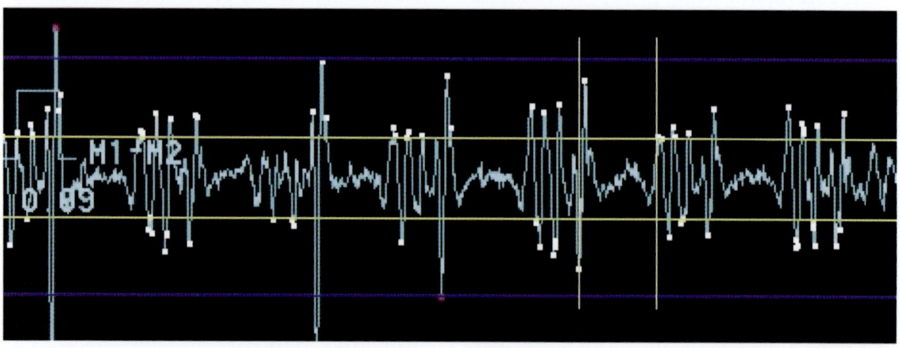

Figure 18.4 Automated algorithm for the detection of complex fractionated atrial electrograms (CFAEs). The middle yellow horizontal lines define the low voltage limit and the outer dark blue lines the upper voltage limit for CFAE detection. Deflections within these boundaries identify the CFAE complex. The interval between the complexes are measured as shown by the vertical yellow lines. In this example, all intervals are less than 120 ms, indicative of highly repetitive CFAEs. See text for details.

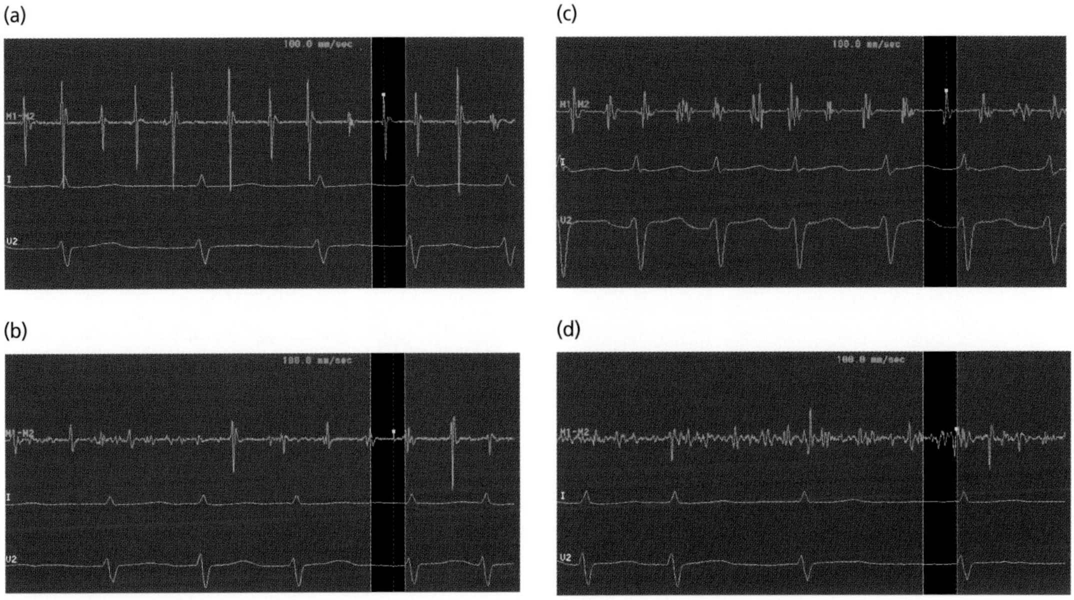

Figure 18.5 Representative 2.5 ms samples at four different sites recorded during automated CFAE mapping. (a) Normal electrograms without CFAEs. (b) Brief period of electrogram fractionation (left side of panel) not meeting criteria for moderate or highly repetitive CFAEs. (c) Low amplitude, discrete, fractionated electrograms with short isoelectric intervals throughout the recording indicative of highly repetitive CFAEs. (d) Near continuous, low amplitude, fractionated electrograms that may not always be detected by nominal automated detection parameters. For automated CFAE detection of this recording, the lower interval boundary must be programmed relatively short, and the voltage criteria modified.

potential suitability as an ablation target) is determined by the number of short coupled intervals (< 120 ms) between CFAE complexes during the 2.5 s recording window (programmable, nominally > 7 for high repetitiveness and 4–7 for moderate repetitiveness) (Figure 18.5). These data are then displayed on a three-dimensional anatomic map, either as focal points, or as gradients of repetitiveness, shortest interval cycle length, or mean interval cycle length (Figure 18.6).

We recently reported our experience in the initial 54 patients undergoing AF ablation utilizing automated CFAE detection (34 with PAF, 20 with chronic AF) [49]. With the nominal criteria outlined above, highly or moderately repetitive CFAEs were identified at a mean of 39 ± 12% of all left atrial or coronary sinus sites, and were significantly more common in patients with chronic AF ($P=0.02$, Figure 18.7). A median of 12 highly repetitive sites (range 1–100) and a median of 36 moderately repetitive sites (range 4–91) were identified per patient. Relying solely on computerized identification of CFAEs, all highly repetitive sites were ablated (3.5 mm open irrigation catheter, maximum power 35 W on the posterior wall and 45 W elsewhere). AF terminated in 29 of 34 (85%) PAF patients (8/29 patients had multiple terminations at different sites) but in only two of 20 (10%) chronic AF patients. Notably, additional ablation (wide area PV isolation ± linear lesions) terminated persistent/chronic AF in nine of the 18 remaining patients. As in previous studies of subjectively identified CFAEs, preferential locations of CFAEs identified by computer algorithm were observed in the left atrial septum, around the PV ostia, in the inferior mitral annulus and proximal coronary sinus, and around the orifice of the left atrial appendage. Representative examples are illustrated in Figures 8.8–18.10. This preliminary experience indicates that ablation guided by automated CFAE detection provides outcomes similar to those previously published for visually identified CFAEs in patients with PAF [42,46,48]. Termination in chronic AF patients was uncommon, similar to

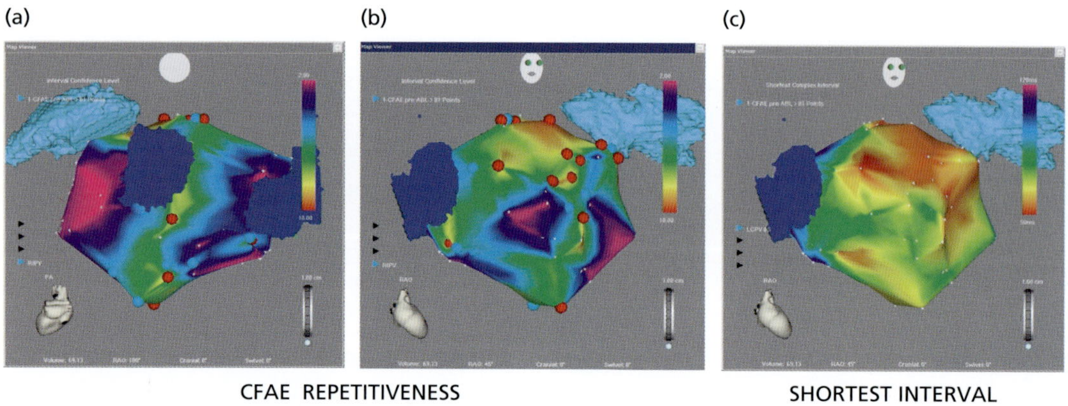

Figure 18.6 Three-dimensional displays of CFAE characteristics on merged Carto/computed tomography images in a patient with PAF acquired prior to ablation. The pulmonary veins are depicted in dark blue, and the left atrial appendage in light blue. (a, b) Posteroanterior and right anterior oblique views displaying CFAE repetitiveness as a continuous variable. The left atrium is color coded, ranging from < 2 short intervals (infrequent CFAE, dark blue) to > 10 short intervals (highly repetitive CFAE, orange). CFAEs can also be depicted as focal points coded for a range of repetitiveness (red dots, highly repetitive; light blue dots, moderate repetitiveness). (c) Right anterior oblique view color coded to depict the shortest isoelectric interval as a continuous variable, ranging from 50 ms (orange) to 120 ms (purple). Taken together these images suggest that the anterior superior left atrium, particularly adjacent to the appendage, has the highest concentration of highly repetitive CFAE sites with the shortest coupling intervals, and should be considered as the initial target for ablation. See text for details.

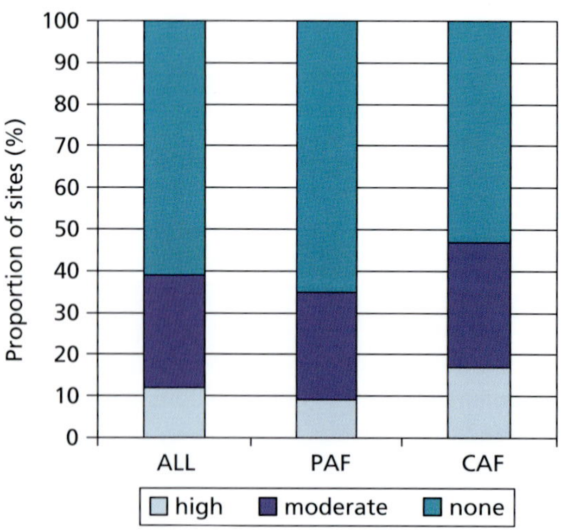

Figure 18.7 Frequency of sites with highly or moderately repetitive CFAEs during mapping of paroxysmal atrial fibrillation (PAF) and chronic atrial fibrillation (CAF). See text for details.

some [45], but not all [42,48], studies guided by subjective CFAE classification. Preliminary data also indicate that CFAEs detected by automated criteria remain relatively stable and reproducible over short (up to 6 s) [57] and longer (30 min) [58] time intervals.

The potential value of objective criteria for CFAE classification was illustrated in a recent study we conducted among five electrophysiologists experienced in CFAE ablation. Recordings from 1030 sites (selected from ~7500 in the above referenced study [49]) were provided, with instructions to evaluate electrograms as indicative of highly repetitive CFAEs with the highest priority for ablation, moderately repetitive CFAEs with an intermediate priority for ablation, or absent or infrequent CFAEs with no target for ablation. The results are shown in Figure 18.11. While there was modest overall interobserver concordance (Kendall W for ordinal response = 0.66, $P < 0.001$), there was substantial variability in the number of sites classified as high priority for ablation between physicians. Of interest, the classification of electrograms by computer algorithm (employing the nominal criteria identified above) fell between the extremes of physician investigators. This variability in subjective CFAE classification may be one cause for divergent outcomes of clinical studies evaluating electrogram-guided ablation strategies.

Automated CFAE detection provides rapid and reproducible identification of potential target sites, and facilitates assessment of the impact of altering threshold criteria on electrogram classification. A

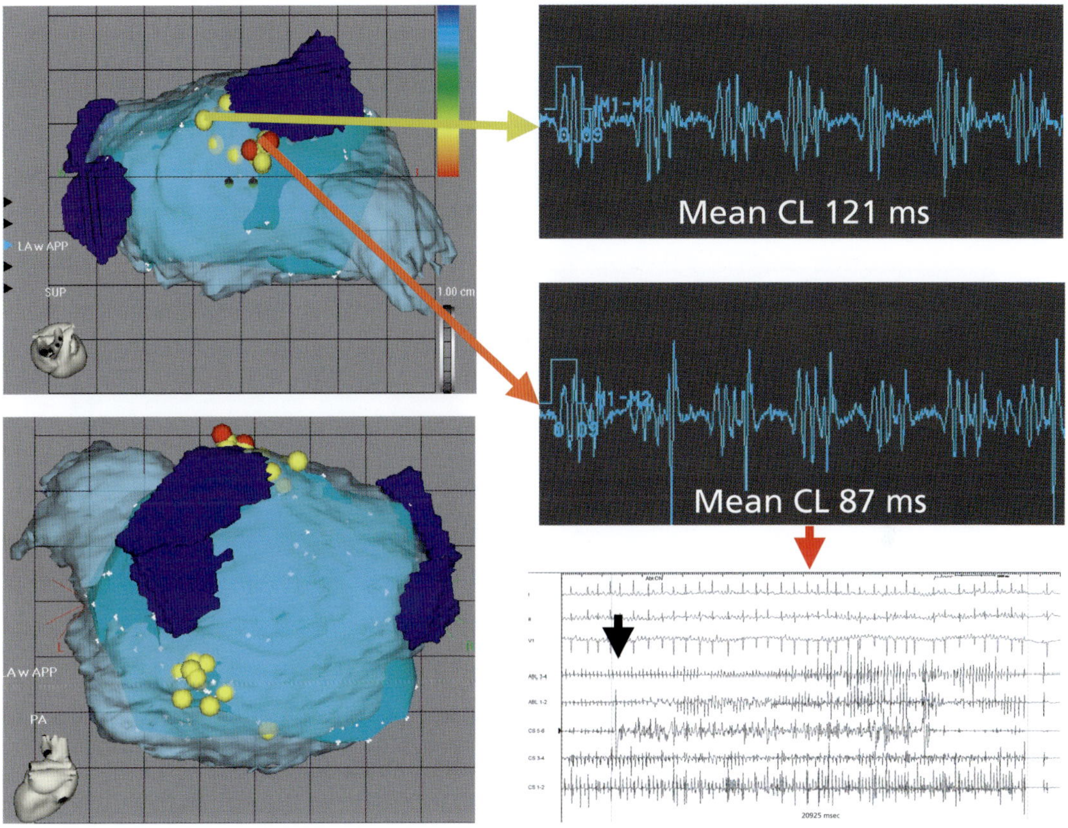

Figure 18.8 Ablation of PAF guided by automated CFAE detection. Fused electroanatomic maps in superior (top left panel) and posteroanterior (bottom left panel) projections demonstrate highly repetitive (red dots) and moderately repetitive (yellow dots) CFAE sites. In this patient these regions were relatively circumscribed. The apparent clustering is due to repetitive sampling at the same and adjacent sites over a 30 min mapping period, indicating a high degree of temporal stability in this patient. On the right, electrograms are shown from moderately repetitive (top right panel) and highly repetitive (middle right panel) CFAE sites, where the latter demonstrates consistently shorter intervals between CFAEs. The bottom right panel shows termination of AF during radiofrequency energy application at the site depicted in the middle right panel. Termination of AF was preceded by slowing of the overall fibrillation cycle length, and required relatively prolonged application (21 s) prior to termination (red arrows, site of termination; black arrow, onset of ablation). Electrograms from the nearby left common ostium were unchanged, and the patient was not inducible following ablation at this site. Note that the distribution of CFAE sites in this patient would have been easily encompassed by circumferential left PV isolation. CL, cycle length.

major challenge for automated CFAE analysis is to improve specificity in identifying target sites critical to the maintenance of AF. In our recent study, ablation of only highly repetitive sites (18%) failed to terminate most persistent/chronic AF [49]. While additional ablation at moderately repetitive sites may have improved the rate of AF termination, it would have resulted in a substantial lesion burden, and ablation at almost 50% of sites. Alternative criteria need to be developed, potentially focusing on stability of electrogram duration and morphology, or specific type of electrogram morphology, rather than primarily on cycle length criteria alone. Longer duration sampling at individual sites may improve assessment of CFAE stability, though preliminary data indicate few differences with sampling times between 2 and 6 s [57]. Current algorithms also have difficulty dealing with near continuous, low amplitude fractionated activity as shown in Figure 18.5d.

A novel approach to electrogram-based ablation of AF was recently proposed by Pachon and

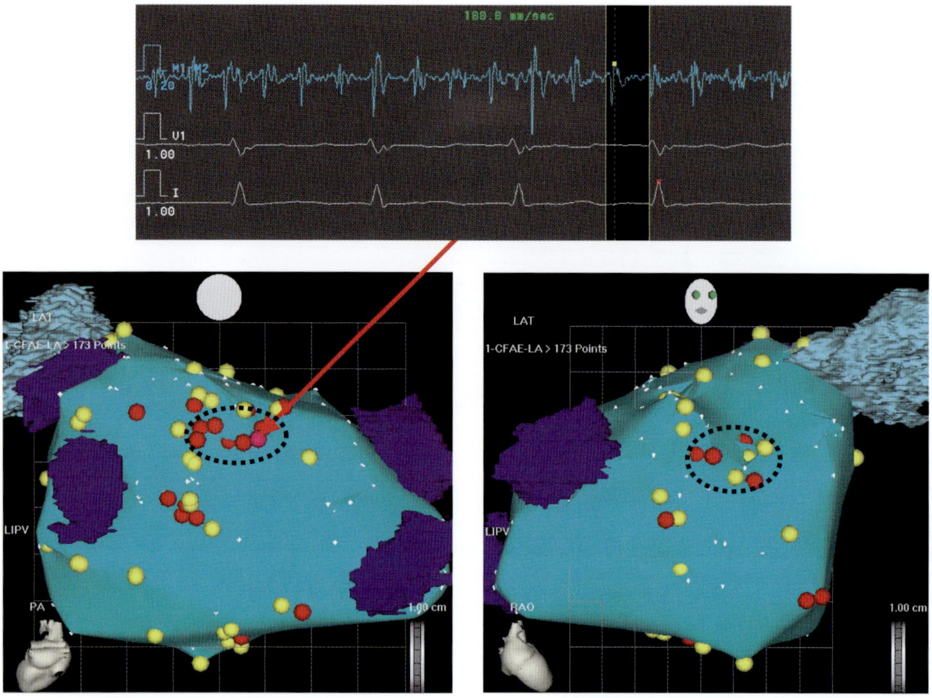

Figure 18.9 Ablation of PAF guided by automated CFAE detection with a format similar to Figure 18.8. In this patient, two primary regions of CFAEs were detected (dashed circles), one in the mid posterior wall, and the other anterior to the right superior PV. Ablation in the posterior wall at sites with highly repetitive CFAEs terminated AF (lower left panel), but it could still be reinduced. Additional ablation directed at highly repetitive sites on the atrial septum (lower right panel), resulted in termination of AF and subsequent non-inducibility. Similar to Figure 18.8, this patient had a high degree of temporal stability during resampling of the same site over the course of the mapping procedure. In contrast, it is unclear that even the widest of antral isolation procedures would have incorporated these sites within the isolated area.

colleagues [59]. These investigators analyzed electrograms during sinus rhythm with fast Fourier transform (FFT). Electrograms were classified into two types based on FFT analysis, one with an in-phase left-shifted FFT, and the other with an out-of-phase right-shifted FFT. The former were hypothesized to arise from normal well-coupled myocardial fibers with normal conduction and relatively long refractoriness, and the latter from "fibrillar" myocardium or "AF nests" with the properties of anisotropic conduction, diminished cellular coupling, and shorter refractoriness. Regions of "fibrillar" myocardium during sinus displayed shorter coupling intervals and more electrogram fractionation during AF compared to surrounding sites. The preferential distribution of these sites was similar to those described for CFAEs. Ablation based solely on the elimination of AF nests and normalization of the FFT in sinus rhythm was reported to eliminate AF recurrence in 94% of 35 patients with PAF during a mean follow-up of 10 ± 5 months. Whether these sites represent regions of fixed structural abnormalities associated with exaggerated anisotropic conduction, or sites with enhanced local autonomic innervation and activation [60] remains to be clarified.

Approach to electrogram-guided ablation

Our current approach is to selectively employ CFAE ablation as an adjunct in patients with PAF who are at high risk for recurrence following PV isolation alone (persistent inducibility following PV isolation, large left atrial size, longstanding history) (Figure 18.12). This strategy is consistent with

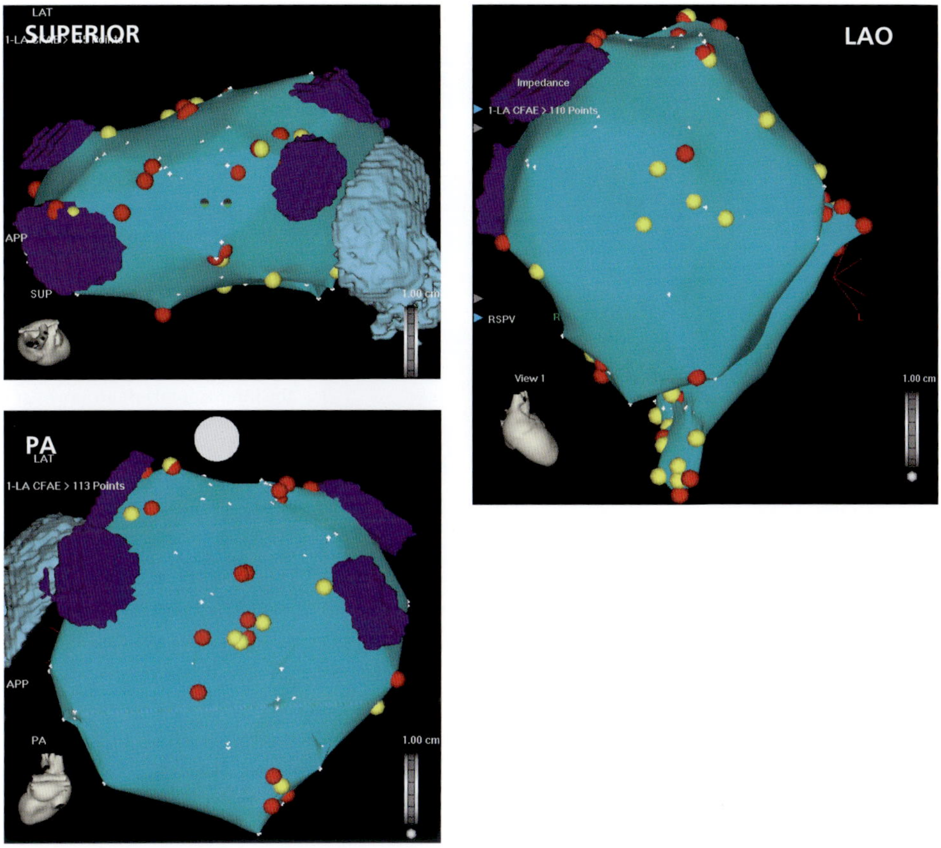

Figure 18.10 CFAE sites detected by automated algorithms in a patient with chronic AF. The format of display is similar to Figure 18.8. There were extensive high and moderately repetitive CFAE sites widely distributed over the left atrium and also prominently in the proximal and distal coronary sinus. Despite extensive ablation of CFAE at all highly repetitive sites, AF did not terminate. LAO, left anterior oblique; PA, posteroanterior.

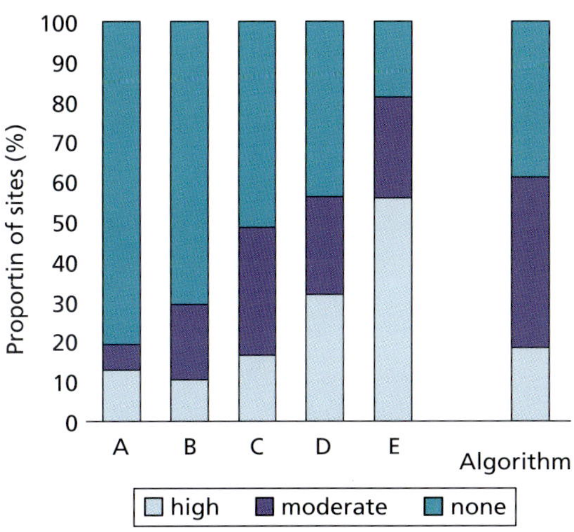

Figure 18.11 (*left*) Individual physician (A–E) ratings of electrograms recorded during AF according to degree of repetitive CFAE activity, and suitability as a target site for ablation. The results were contrasted to classification of CFAEs by automated algorithm. See text for details.

available clinical data, and may reduce the need for repeat ablation in this population. It is recognized that some patients with PAF may benefit from primary CFAE ablation alone [42], particularly those in whom a limited region of CFAE ablation results in non-inducibility and a low lesion burden. The superiority of these strategies relative to PV isolation alone requires additional prospective evaluation.

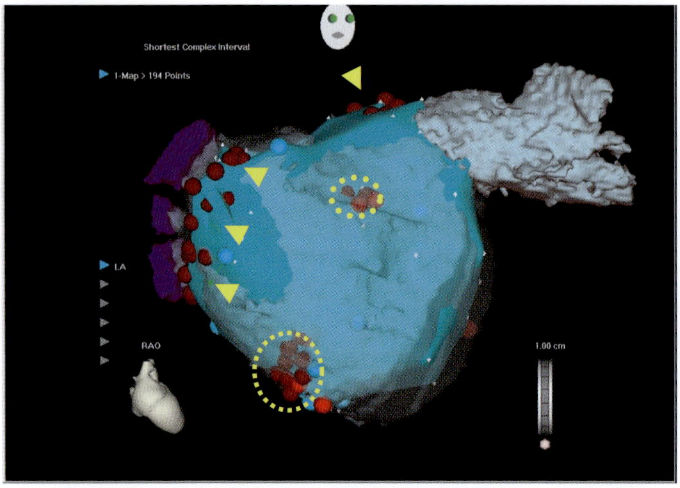

Figure 18.12 Electoanatomic/computed tomography fusion image in the right anterior oblique (RAO) projection of adjunctive CFAE ablation in a patient with a history of PAF. There was continued AF following initial PV isolation despite confirmation of entrance block. The borders of the circumferential isolation are highlighted by yellow arrows. Two regions of CFAEs were identified (dashed circles), one in the high atrial septum and the other at the inferoseptal left atrium near the crux. Ablation of the latter region terminated AF and prevented its reinduction.

CFAE mapping is employed at the onset of ablation procedures in all patients with persistent and chronic forms of AF. CFAE sites are incorporated, where feasible, into the initial wide area PV isolation. Following PV isolation, CFAE regions are ablated, with particular emphasis on sites located in the interatrial septum, anterior to the left atrial appendage, and along the posterior mitral annulus (adjacent to and within the coronary sinus). Linear lesions are reserved for patients in whom AF does not terminate during the initial stages of ablation, or in occasional patients where a series of CFAE ablations may leave a relatively narrow and potentially proarrhythmic isthmus. CFAE ablation alone less frequently terminates AF in this population (10–60%), and no data are yet available regarding the rate of AF termination when CFAE ablation is used as an adjuvant strategy in combination with other techniques.

Several practical issues with CFAE ablation merit additional emphasis. Mapping should be systematic, comprehensive, and of relatively high density (at least one point per cm^2). This allows visualization of CFAEs as regions rather than specific points, further assisted by three-dimensional graphic displays of CFAE properties (see Figures 18.6, 18.8, and 18.9). Catheter stability and adequate contact throughout electrogram recording is critical to avoid spurious observations. Voltage reduction at specific sites may be an insufficient endpoint for ablation, and the persistence of very low amplitude, short coupled electrograms often requires additional ablation at the same or nearby sites, and occasionally requires higher power. The endpoint, where possible, should be complete regional elimination of disorganized electrical activity. We generally renavigate to regions with initially promising CFAE characteristics (see Figures 18.8, 18.9, and 18.12) to confirm the persistence of these characteristics as well as the size and boundaries of the fractionated region. Isolated CFAE points, or regions with poorly reproducible CFAE properties, rarely terminate AF, and are of less interest as targets for ablation.

CFAE ablation has the attractive theoretical advantage of individualizing ablation according the patient's specific arrhythmogenic substrate. Several unresolved issues impede further development. These include: (1) incomplete understanding of the link between electrogram fractionation and critical sites for AF perpetuation; (2) lack of uniform objective and reproducible criteria for CFAE definition (and identification of "high yield" electrogram characteristics); and (3) poorly defined endpoints for the extent and completeness of CFAE ablation. Progress in all of these areas is needed before the ultimate role of electrogram-guided ablation of AF can be ascertained.

Acknowledgments

Supported in part by a grant from the George M. Eisenberg Foundation.

References

1 Swartz JF, Pellersels G, Silvers J, Patten L, Cervantez D. A catheter based curative approach to atrial fibrillation (abstract). *Circulation* 1994;**90**(Suppl I):1–335.

2 Haissaguerre M, Jais P, Shah DC, et al. Spontaneous initiation of atrial fibrillation by ectopic beats originating in the pulmonary veins. *N Engl J Med* 1998;**339**:659–66.

3 Hocini M, Ho SY, Kawara T, et al. Electrical conduction in canine pulmonary veins: electrophysiological and anatomic correlation. *Circulation* 2002;**105**:2442–8.

4 Arora R, Verheule S, Scott L, et al. Arrhythmogenic substrate of the pulmonary veins assessed by high-resolution optical mapping. *Circulation* 2003;**107**:1816–21.

5 Chen YJ, Chen SA. Electrophysiology of pulmonary veins. *J Cardiovasc Electrophysiol* 2006;**17**:220–4.

6 Scherlag BJ, Yamanshi W, Patel U, Lazzara R, Jackman WM. Autonomically induced conversion of pulmonary vein focal firing into atrial fibrillation. *J Am Coll Cardiol* 2005;**7**:1878–86.

7 Patterson E, Po SS, Scherlag BJ, Lazzara R. Triggered firing in pulmonary veins initiated by in vitro autonomic nerve stimulation. *Heart Rhythm* 2005;**2**:624–31.

8 Calkins H, Brugada J, Packer DL, et al. HRS/EHRA/ECAS Expert Consensus Statement on catheter and surgical ablation of atrial fibrillation: recommendations for personnel, policy, procedures and follow-up. *Heart Rhythm* 2007;**4**:816–61.

9 Willems S, Klemm H, Rostock T, et al. Substrate modification combined with pulmonary vein isolation improves outcome of catheter ablation in patients with persistent atrial fibrillation: a prospective randomized comparison. *Eur Heart J* 2006;**27**:2871–8.

10 Bhargava M, Prasad S, Martin DO, et al. Impact of type of atrial fibrillation and repeat catheter ablation on its long term cure rates: results from a prospective multicenter study. *Circulation* 2008, in press.

11 Ouyang F, Antz M, Ernst S, et al. Recovered pulmonary vein conduction as a dominant factor for recurrent atrial tachyarrhythmias after complete circular isolation of the pulmonary veins: lessons from double Lasso technique. *Circulation* 2005;**111**:127–35.

12 Nanthakumar K, Plumb VJ, Epstein AE, Veenhuyzen GD, Link D, Kay GN. Resumption of electrical conduction in previously isolated pulmonary veins: rationale for a different strategy? *Circulation* 2004;**109**:1226–9.

13 Verma A, Kilicaslan F, Pisano E, et al. Response of atrial fibrillation to pulmonary vein antrum isolation is directly related to resumption and delay of pulmonary vein conduction. *Circulation* 2005;**112**:627–35.

14 Callans DJ, Gerstenfeld EP, Dixit S, Zado E, Vanderhoff M, Ren JF, Marchlinski FE. Efficacy of repeat pulmonary vein isolation procedures in patients with recurrent atrial fibrillation. *J Cardiovasc Electrophysiol* 2004;**15**:1050–5.

15 Haïsaguerre M, Hocini M, Sanders P, et al. Localized sources maintaining atrial fibrillation organized by prior ablation. *Circulation* 2006;**113**:616–25.

16 Hocini M, Jais P, Sanders P, et al. Techniques, evaluation, and consequences of linear block at the left atrial roof in paroxysmal atrial fibrillation: a prospective randomized study. *Circulation* 2005;**112**:3688–96.

17 Jais P, Hocini M, Hsu LF, et al. Technique and results of linear ablation at the mitral isthmus. *Circulation* 2004;**110**:2996–3002.

18 Konings KTS, Kirchhof CJHJ, Smeets JRLM, et al. High-density mapping of electrically induced atrial fibrillation in humans. *Circulation* 1994;**89**:1665–80.

19 Konings KTS, Smeets JLRM, Penn OC, et al. Configuration of unipolar atrial electrograms during electrically induced atrial fibrillation in humans. *Circulation* 1997; **95**:1231–41.

20 Jais P, Haissaguerre M, Shah DC, Chouairi S, Clementy J. Regional disparities of endocardial atrial activation in paroxysmal atrial fibrillation. *Pacing Clin Electrophysiol* 1996;**19**:1998–2003.

21 Spach MS, Dolber PC, Heidlage JF. Influence of the passive anisotropic properties on directional differences in propagation following modification of the sodium conductance in human atrial muscle. A model of reentry based on anisotropic discontinuous conduction. *Circ Res* 1988;**62**:811–32.

22 Jacquemet V, Virag N, Ihara Z, et al. Study of unipolar electrogram morphology in a computer model of atrial fibrillation. *J Cardiovasc Electrophysiol* 2003;**14**:S172–S179.

23 Pachon MJ, Pachon ME, Pachon MJ, et al. A new treatment for atrial fibrillation based on spectral analysis to guide the catheter RF-ablation. *Europace* 2004;**6**:590–601.

24 Spach MS, Heidlage JF, Dolber PC, Barr RC. Mechanism of origin of conduction disturbances in aging human atrial bundles: experimental and model study. *Heart Rhythm* 2007;**4**:175–85.

25 Mandapati R, Skanes A, Chen J, Berenfeld O, Jalife J. Stable microreentrant sources as a mechanism of atrial fibrillation in the isolated sheep heart. *Circulation* 2000;**101**:194–9.

26 Kalifa J, Tanaka K, Zaitsev AV, et al. Mechanisms of wave fractionation at boundaries of high-frequency excitation in the posterior left atrium of the isolated sheep heart during atrial fibrillation. *Circulation* 2006; **113**:626–33.

27 Tanaka K, Zlochiver S, Vikstrom KL, et al. Spatial distribution of fibrosis governs fibrillation wave dynamics in the posterior left atrium during heart failure. *Circ Res* 2007;**101**:839–47.

28 Armour JA, Murphy DA, Yuan BX, Macdonald S, Hopkins DA. Gross and microscopic anatomy of the

human intrinsic cardiac nervous system. *Anat Rec* 1997;**247**:289–98.

29 Hou Y, Scherlag BJ, Lin J, et al. The interactive atrial neural network: determining the connections between ganglionated plexi. *Heart Rhythm* 2007;**3**:56–63.

30 Kwaku KF, Verrier RL. The atrial neural network: ablation minefield or strategic target? *Heart Rhythm* 2007;**3**:64–5.

31 Patterson E, Lazzara R, Szabo B, et al. Sodium-calcium exchange initiated by the Ca2+ transient: an arrhythmia trigger within pulmonary veins. *J Am Coll Cardiol* 2006; **47**:1196–206.

32 Lin J, Scherlag BJ, Zhou J, et al. Autonomic mechanism to explain complex fractionated atrial electrograms (CFAE). *J Cardiovasc Electrophysiol* 2007;**18**(11):1197–205.

33 Zhou J, Scherlag BJ, Edwards J, Jackman WM, Lazzara R, Po, SS. Gradients of atrial refractoriness and inducibility of atrial fibrillation due to stimulation of ganglionated plexi. *J Cardiovasc Electrophysiol* 2007;**18**:83–90.

34 Nakagawa H, Jackman WM, Scherlag BJ, et al. Relationship of complex fractionated atrial electrograms during atrial fibrillation to the location of cardiac autonomic ganglionated plexi in patients with atrial fibrillation (abstract). *Circulation* 2005;**112**:SII–746.

35 Lemery R, Birnie D, Tang AS, Green M, Gollob M. Feasibility study of endocardial mapping of ganglionated plexuses during catheter ablation of atrial fibrillation. *Heart Rhythm* 2006;**3**(4):387–96.

36 Lockwood EE, Nademanee K. Determination of key sites of CFAE-targeted AF ablation and correlation with cardiac ganglionic plexi (abstract). *Circulation* 2007;**116**:II–537.

37 Nakagawa H, Scherlag BJ, Wu R, et al. Addition of selective ablation of autonomic ganglia to pulmonary vein antrum isolation for treatment of paroxysmal and persistent atrial fibrillation (abstract). *Circulation* 2004; **110**(Suppl III):III–459.

38 Scanavacca M, Pisani CF, Hachul D, et al. Selective atrial vagal denervation guided by evoked vagal reflex to treat patients with paroxysmal atrial fibrillation. *Circulation* 2006;**114**:876–85.

39 Pappone C, Santinelli V, Manguso F, et al. Pulmonary vein denervation enhances long-term benefit after circumferential ablation for paroxysmal atrial fibrillation. *Circulation* 2004;**109**:327–34.

40 Scherlag BJ, Patterson E, Po SS. The neural basis of atrial fibrillation. *J Electrocardiol* 2006;**39**:S180–S183.

41 Rostock T, Rotter M, Sanders P, et al. High-density activation mapping of fractionated electrograms in the atria of patients with paroxysmal atrial fibrillation. *Heart Rhythm* 2006;**3**:27–34.

42 Nademanee K, McKenzie J, Kosar E. et al. A new approach for catheter ablation of atrial fibrillation: mapping of the electrophysiologic substrate. *J Am Coll Cardiol* 2004;**43**(11):2044–53.

43 Nademanee K, Schwab M, Porath J, et al. Mapping the electrophysiologic substrate to guide AF ablation. In: Wilber DJ, Packer DL, Stevenson WG (eds) Catheter Ablation of Cardiac Arrhythmias: Basic concepts and clinical applications, Third edition, 2008. Blackwell Publishing, Oxford, UK, pp250–60.

44 Nademanee K. Trials and travails of electrogram-guided ablation of chronic atrial fibrillation. *Circulation* 2007; **115**(20):2592–4.

45 Oral H, Chugh A, Good E, et al. Radiofrequency catheter ablation of chronic atrial fibrillation guided by complex electrograms. *Circulation* 2007;**115**(20):2606–12.

46 Oral H, Chugh A, Lemola K, et al. Noninducibility of atrial fibrillation as an end point of left atrial circumferential ablation for paroxysmal atrial fibrillation: a randomized study. *Circulation* 2004;**110**:2797–801.

47 Oral H, Chugh A, Good E, et al. A tailored approach to catheter ablation of paroxysmal atrial fibrillation. *Circulation* 2006;**113**(15):1824–31.

48 Schmitt C, Estner H, Hecher B, et al. Radiofrequency ablation of complex fractionated atrial electrograms (CFAE): preferential sites of acute termination and regularization in paroxysmal and persistent atrial fibrillation. *J Cardiovasc Electrophysiol* 2007;**18**(10):1039–46.

49 Wilber DJ, Brysiewicz NR, Helms RW, Akar JG, Porter M. Prospective study of atrial fibrillation termination during ablation guided by automated detection of complex electrograms (abstract). *Heart Rhythm* 2007;**4**: S14.

50 Verma A, Novak P, Macle L, Whaley B, Beardsal M, Wulffhart Z, Khaykin Y. A multicenter prospective study of ablating complex fractionated electrograms (CFE) during atrial fibrillation using a novel automated mapping algorithm: acute effects on AF and efficacy as an adjuvant strategy (abstract). *Heart Rhythm* 2007;**4**:S345.

51 Deisenhofer I, Schmitt C, Estner HL, et al. Additional ablation of complex fractionated atrial electrograms (CFAE) after pulmonary vein isolation in paroxysmal atrial fibrillation: results of a controlled randomized study (abstract). *Heart Rhythm* 2007;**4**:S115.

52 Di Biase L, Elayi CS, Ching CK, et al. Comparison of atrial fibrillation ablation strategies for paroxysmal patients presenting to the electrophysiology laboratory in atrial fibrillation (abstract). *Circulation* 2007;**116**:II–537.

53 Elayi CS, Verma A, Di Biase L, et al. Results from a randomized study comparing three common ablation strategies for permanent atrial fibrillation (abstract). *Heart Rhythm* 2007;**4**:S15.

54 Haissaguerre M, Sanders P, Hocini M, et al. Catheter ablation of long lasting atrial fibrillation. Critical structures for termination. *J Cardiovasc Electrophysiol* 2005;**15**: 1125–37.

55 Scherr D, Dalal D, Cheema A, et al. Automated detection and characterization of complex fractionated atrial

electrograms in human left atrium during atrial fibrillation. *Heart Rhythm* 2007;**4**(8):1013–20.

56 Scherr D, Dalal D, Cheema A, et al. Temporal stability of complex fractionated atrial electrograms in human left atrium during atrial fibrillation (abstract). *Circulation* 2007;**116**:II–392.

57 Stiles MK, Brooks A, Lau DH, et al. Effect of the duration of electrogram recording on determination of complex fractionated atrial electrograms and dominant frequency (abstract). *Heart Rhythm* 2007;**4**:S348.

58 Roux JF, Gojraty S, Bala R, et al. Complex fractionated electrogram distribution and temporal stability in patients undergoing atrial fibrillation ablation (abstract). *Heart Rhythm* 2007;**4**:S119.

59 Pachon MJC, Pachon MEI, Pachon MJC, et al. A new treatment for atrial fibrillation based on spectral analysis to guide the catheter RF-ablation. *Europace* 2004;**6**(6): 590–601.

60 Lellouche N, Buch E, Celigoj A, et al. Functional characterization of atrial electrograms in sinus rhythm delineates sites of parasympathetic innervation in patients with paroxysmal atrial fibrillation. *J Am Coll Cardiol* 2007;**50**(14):1324–31.

Index

Page numbers in *italics* represent figures, those in **bold** represent tables